HEART TO HEART

Also by Allen B. Weisse

Medicine: The State of the Art
Conversations in Medicine
Medical Odysseys
The Man's Guide to Good Health
The Staff and the Serpent

HEART TO HEART

THE
TWENTIETH-CENTURY BATTLE
AGAINST CARDIAC DISEASE

AN ORAL HISTORY

ALLEN B. WEISSE, M.D.

RUTGERS UNIVERSITY PRESS

New Brunswick, New Jersey, and London

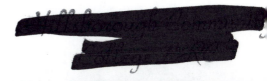

Library of Congress Cataloging-in-Publication Data

Weisse, Allen B.
    Heart to heart : the twentieth-century battle against heart disease : an oral history / Allen B. Weisse.
        p.   cm.
    Includes bibliographical references and index.
    ISBN 0-8135-3157-8 (cloth : alk. paper)
    1. Cardiology—History—20th century.   2. Cardiologists—Interviews.
3. Thoracic surgeons—Interviews.   I. Title.

RC666.5.W456   2002
616.1'2'00904—dc21

2002020161

British Cataloging-in-Publication information is available
from the British Library.

Manufactured in the United States of America

*To the memories of my father, who instilled a love of words,
and of my mother, who brightened so many lives with them*

What has been accomplished does not die,
but too often, alas, the personality of those
who have handed the torch from one generation
to another soon fades into oblivion.

—Harvey Cushing
(as quoted in *Harvey Cushing: A Biography,*
by John F. Fulton, 1947)

CONTENTS

Acknowledgments

The seeds of this book were sown in an earlier oral history, *Conversations in Medicine* (New York University Press, 1984), which covered a fairly wide swath of twentieth-century medical progress. It included a number of interviews with pioneers in the field of heart disease (William Dock, André Cournand, Charles P. Bailey, and Willem J. Kolff), and these interviews formed the core of this new work. The urgent need to complete this medical record dawned on me about the time of my retirement from full-time academic status in 1997. I then realized that many of the medical pioneers still with us had already entered the latter decades of their lives and that their stories had to be told without any further delay.

My profound thanks must be extended to all of the sixteen individuals who gave of their time and trust to be interviewed for this book. Without their full cooperation, the project could never have been started, let alone completed. In some instances, when death intervened before I could review conversations or other important supporting material with those featured in the book, others close to them were kind enough to assist me. In the case of Paul Zoll, his son, Ross, and his engineering associate, Alan Belgard, filled the breach. For C. Walton Lillehei, Dr. Richard DeWall served a similar function, adding depth and further understanding to the John W. Kirklin interview.

My distinguished friend W. Bruce Fye, an expert on the history of cardiology, graciously agreed to review the entire manuscript for errors, as did Dr. John S. Donahoo, director of cardiothoracic surgery at the New Jersey Medical School, for the surgical sections. I am also indebted to my wife, Dr. Laura Weisse, for her keen eye and ear, as well as numerous archivists and librarians who helped along the way. My thanks also to Helen Hsu and Rutgers University Press for their early enthusiasm for this project and for supporting my vision of its design and production. I am also deeply grateful to Victoria Haire for another superb job of editing.

Finally, I owe much to those senior cardiologists who trained me and gave me a sense of medical history, one that I hope I have transmitted in some way to the many medical students, house officers, and fellows who have had to endure my sometimes demanding tutelage throughout my last forty years as an academic internist, cardiologist, and medical historian.

INTRODUCTION

At the beginning of the twentieth century, infectious diseases posed the greatest threat to human health and survival. Tuberculosis alone was the major cause of death in both the United States and western Europe. However, with the introduction of improved sanitary conditions, public health initiatives such as mass immunizations, and finally the introduction of sulfa drugs and then antibiotics, such threats to human life diminished dramatically, at least in the industrialized parts of the world. By midcentury doctors had become much more concerned with cancer as a threat to survival and, even more so, with cardiovascular diseases, which began to account for more deaths than all other causes combined in the United States and elsewhere in the industrialized world. The alarm about cardiovascular disease—coronary disease in particular—had become so great that by the midfifties it was often termed an "epidemic" in medical circles and the mass media as well.

As remarkable as was the sudden appearance of cardiovascular disease as a major health threat, so was the response of medical scientists, who began to address every aspect of the diagnosis, treatment, and, later, the prevention of heart disease. Although cardiovascular disorders have not yet relinquished their position as the number-one killer of our patients, the "epidemic" has abated while progress in this field continues.

The purpose of this book is to present the story of the twentieth-century battle against heart disease through intimate conversations with some of the leading physicians and surgeons who figured so prominently in this effort. The project began in 1979, when the earliest of these interviews were conducted, and concluded in 2000, the beginning of the new millennium. The twentieth century was truly an incredible period of medical research productivity and progress. Methods of diagnosis, treatment, and prevention that at the start of the century were unknown or even scarcely imagined have now been incorporated into daily medical practice. During the thirties and forties "extracardiac" surgery, such as that performed in the "blue baby" operation, progressed to closed-heart operations for some defects, and then, with the introduction of the heart-lung machine, open-heart surgical corrections for congenital and acquired abnormalities became routine.

The implantation of artificial heart valves represented another leap forward, along with the introduction of coronary bypass surgery and even transplantation of the entire heart for otherwise inoperable cardiac disease. A better understanding of cardiac physiology, the ability to catheterize the human heart for more accurate diagnoses, the introduction of electrical methods to resuscitate an arrested heart, pace a dangerously slow one, or terminate potentially fatal arrhythmias complemented the surgical advances of this period. Finally, the recognition of risk factors for certain common types of heart disease and the development of preventive cardiology have enhanced the ability of physicians and their patients to forestall the end results of rheumatic heart disease and, more recently, hypertension and coronary atherosclerosis. The development of various implantable cardiac pumping assist devices as well as an acceptable form of a total artificial heart continue apace for the growing problem of end-stage congestive heart failure. The careers of the contributors to this volume encompass all of these developments, often directly or, at times, indirectly.

One might ask, "Why an oral history?" This approach was used for two main reasons. First, there are already some excellent histories of cardiology available; a number of these works are listed in the "Selected Bibliography" at the end of this book. Second, the conversational approach allowed me, a cardiologist who conducted his professional life during much of this period, to question these individuals in a true give-and-take manner to bring a special kind of freshness and vibrancy to their recollections of the people and events that influenced them, their motivations, their problems, their interactions with their contemporaries, and their hopes and beliefs for the future. These are aspects of medical history that rarely, if ever, are accommodated by conventional historical narratives.

The downside of such an approach is that giving over so much space to such a relatively small number of individuals leads to the exclusion of many others who might merit inclusion. To address this issue, I have included a section at the end of the book that gives short biographies of other prominent physicians and surgeons mentioned in the interviews. As readers come upon their names in the text (identified by the use of small caps), they can turn to the "Biographical Notes" section for more details.

Regarding background sources, it was neither my intent nor within the capacity of this book to provide a listing of the avalanche of honors that has so deservedly descended upon those interviewed. It was also infeasible to include a listing of the thousands of articles and hundreds of books and chapters they have authored or edited. The "Selected Bibliography" provides sources for such material. I have, however, included a "Notes" section, which, although not encyclopedic, is designed to assist readers by indicating some important secondary sources for general information and primary sources when these might be otherwise difficult to find or generally not mentioned by other historians.

Despite such attempts at inclusion, I realize that some slighting of important figures has been inevitable. In the periods preceding both world wars, outstanding individuals on the European scene helped establish cardiology and cardiac surgery as major medical disciplines. These do not appear as contributors to this book, although their importance is documented in the stories of the physicians and surgeons who do. Following World War II, with much of Europe in ruins and the United States still unscathed, the development of the field became primarily an American event even though many medical scientists of European origin, for various reasons, had emigrated to the States; a few of them (e.g., Richard J. Bing, André Cournand, Willem J. Kolff, Eugene Braunwald) are included here, along with a South American, Dr. René G. Favaloro. So, in a sense, although primarily based in the United States during this period, the progress of cardiology can well be considered an international affair.

Also not to be overlooked, although touched on from time to time in the interviews included, are the important contributions made during this period in the field of physical diagnosis of the heart. Especially noteworthy has been the work on acoustic phenomena as exemplified by the careers of W. Proctor Harvey at Georgetown University in the United States and Aubrey Leatham in London. Unfortunately, this aspect of training among more recent cadres of cardiologists is in decline thanks, ironically, to other diagnostic modalities that have revolutionized this aspect of cardiologic practice. Preeminent among these modalities has been echocardiography, as championed by Harvey Feigenbaum at the University of Indiana and his colleagues there and elsewhere. Isotopic imaging of the heart, CT scanning, and magnetic resonance imaging have further expanded our diagnostic capabilities. Finally, we have seen the birth of molecular cardiology in the latter years of the twentieth century. Its full potential will, no doubt, be realized in the first decades of the new century.

A few words about the mechanics of this undertaking might be of interest to readers. After deciding upon a particular contributor and gaining his or her consent, I obtained a copy of the individual's curriculum vitae and bibliography. Reading these documents helped fill in the gaps of my own knowledge of the subject's background. Then time in the library was devoted to reading the subject's published papers. In some instances I also contacted others more familiar with the subject in order to determine the best lines of inquiry. As a result of this intense preparation, the actual interviews could usually be completed within a single sitting of just a few hours. Occasionally a second interview was required in order to compete the task. The rough transcript, prepared from the recorded conversations, served as a basis for reorganizing the material in its final form before submission to the contributor for approval prior to publication. At times, two or three such submissions were required before a completely accurate and acceptable version was obtained. (The one exception to this routine was in the interview of Dr. Paul M. Zoll, conducted a number of years before his death and never submitted to him personally for review. This task was kindly assumed by his son, Ross, and his colleague Alan Belgard, both of whom were involved with his research.) Finally, I wrote an introduction to each interview, providing background on each individual and the medical milieu of the time.

The order of placement of the interviews within the book is roughly chronological—not in terms of when the interviews were conducted, but rather in terms of the order of progress made during the period covered. The two main aspects of this progress were cardiac surgery and medical cardiology, each depending upon the other and therefore interdigitating as chapter entries. For example, in terms of surgery, the story of early, "extracardiac surgery" is related through the interviews of Drs. Mary Allen Engle and Richard Bing. Direct surgery upon the heart then comes in with the mitral commissurotomy of Charles Bailey. Next comes open-heart surgery (John Kirklin) and related advances; valve replacement (Albert Starr), coronary surgery (René Favaloro); then transplantation, the total artificial heart, and ventricular assist devices (Michael DeBakey, Willem Kolff, and Adrian Kantrowitz).

Paralleling the surgical innovations were advances in the medical field. The opening scene is set in the thirties and forties with the William Dock interview. The introduction of cardiac catheterization (André Cournand) allowed for more accurate diagnoses for our surgical colleagues. The Arthur Guyton interview, immediately following that of Kirklin, emphasizes the importance of nonsurgical advances that permitted the successful performance of heart surgery, itself. Electrical means to pace or restore the arrested heart (Paul Zoll) enabled survival of both medical and surgical patients. Since it is now recognized that much of the future progress in the approach to heart disease depends upon preventive measures, the Jeremiah Stamler interview appears toward the end of the book, followed by those of Eugene Braunwald and J. Willis Hurst, two of today's leading cardiologists who reflect the current status of and future expectations in the field.

Please join me now in meeting this group of extraordinary doctors who accomplished such extraordinary medical and surgical feats in a century that, for good and bad, was so extraordinary in itself.

HEART TO HEART

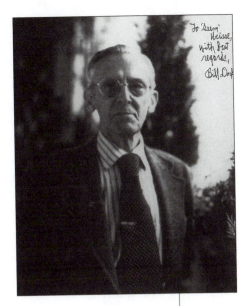

1

William Dock, m.d.
(1898–1990)

On a hot, muggy Saturday morning in July 1960, I boarded the IRT subway in midtown Manhattan, as I had so many times in the past, and headed out to Kings County Hospital in Brooklyn.

Having only one more year to go in my medical residency, I was at a crossroad in my career and greatly needed some solid advice as to where I should go and what I should do next. At the time I was on vacation from my position as a resident in San Francisco and had just finished scouring Boston and New York for possible positions. Time was running out; I was due back on the job in the emergency room of the San Francisco General Hospital the following Monday morning. In desperation I had telephoned the Department of Medicine at the State University of New York Medical Center in Brooklyn the previous afternoon to inquire if any of the senior faculty at my alma mater would be at Kings County Hospital the following morning.

"Dr. Dock is usually in the hospital Saturday mornings" was the reply, and I made an appointment for an interview with him.

Each floor of the main Kings County Hospital was divided into wings containing a large number of beds. At the extreme end of some of these were sun porches that, owing to an overall lack of space for administrative functions, had been converted to offices for the faculty. It was at one of these offices that I found Dr. Dock. He did not remember me, nor should he have. I had not been an exceptional student. Nonetheless, he freely gave of his time and advice. The latter took the form of his own life story, some of it retold here, over a period of several hours, perhaps the most fascinating and rewarding hours I can remember.

No one could be more suitable than William Dock to begin the story about twentieth-century cardiology. Effective medical and surgical treatment for heart disease did not really arrive until the century was well under way, and Dr. Dock, an eminent cardiologist and one of the few great living clinicians, was also well grounded in pathology, which provided the basis upon which such therapy could be devised.

Through his father, a protégé of WILLIAM OSLER, he continued this line of distinguished physicians, and, as will become apparent, he knew just about every great American physician of his time and many of those in Europe as well. His illustrious background was for him neither a crutch nor a heavy burden; it was simply part of the package. His clinical acumen and broad-based knowledge of medicine were legendary. When he appeared at a clinicopathological conference (where a difficult case is presented to the group, discussed by a physician who has been assigned the task of coming up with the correct diagnosis, followed by the disclosure of the pathological findings), unlike most discussants he did not study the protocol beforehand, but entered the conference room "cold," reading aloud the clinical findings, then offering his reasoning and interpretations, and finally, more often than not, coming up with the right answer.

Unlike many others who contributed to this book, he did not occupy a high administrative position, such as department chairman, for many years of his life, nor did he wish to do so. He will be remembered best for his formidably unique mind and for being an inspiring teacher. The following anecdote will give readers a sense of his teaching style.

There was a long-standing controversy in cardiology about the genesis of the first heart sound. It is not a matter of earthshaking consequence; the first heart sound is, after all, just one of countless details concerning human beings about which biologists feel a little happier if they can explain precisely. The details of the dispute are not important here. Suffice it to say that Dock was a major proponent of the view that the sudden tensing of the valves produces the sound and that others disagreed. I vividly recall his small, natty figure pacing animatedly before the blackboard and him suddenly pulling a white handkerchief from his breast pocket. He grasps two opposite sides of the handkerchief, lets it go limp in the center, and suddenly pulls the cloth taut to produce a sound and make his point.

I think the secret of his success with students was related to his enthusiasm and to the fact that he did not talk down to them. If some idea seemed perfectly reasonable to him, he assumed that it should be just as easily grasped by his students. This attitude was very effective, and we worshiped him.

His contemporaries often did not fare as well. He was a superb debater, and although I never saw him in the midst of a public dispute, it was said that his argumentative skill was such that, even when the weight of all the facts was not clearly on his side, he could usually gain the advantage of any adversary. In some quarters this made him feared, and some thought him intolerant and arrogant; perhaps, at times, he was. Perhaps this is why he did not spend many years as a department head, a position where political savvy, rather than scientific acumen, is often the main ingredient of success.

The unsettling aspects of his presence could, however, be turned to advantage; and it was this, undoubtedly, that led Alan Gregg, medical director of the Rockefeller Institute, at one time to suggest that Dock leave the staid and prestigious Cornell Medical College and venture into the medical backwater of Brooklyn to shake things up a bit.

Because Dock worked in a number of locales during the course of his career, the following list may help readers maintain their orientation as they read his interview:

1926–36 Stanford (Medicine)
1936–41 Stanford (Pathology)
1941–44 Cornell (Pathology)
1944–56 Long Island College of Medicine/SUNY Downstate
(Medicine)

1956–57   Palo Alto Clinic (Cardiology)

1957–66   SUNY Downstate (Medicine)

Following his time at Downstate, Dock served at the Brooklyn Veterans' Administration Hospital as chief of the medical service until 1969. Then, for a short period, he worked at the Lutheran Medical Center in Brooklyn before retiring to Paris.

When I visited him in Paris for this interview, I noticed that he had removed the "M.D." after his name in the apartment house directory. But Dock, even in his eighties, could not escape the urgings of his restless and inquiring mind. He was fascinated with the story of the discovery of radioactivity, which he was in the process of putting into book form. He also had read that someone was teaching that the sounds heard in taking the blood pressure were due to a mechanism that he felt was completely wrong. He was in the process of setting up a set of experiments to prove it.

He continued on his own, twice a widower, in his beloved Paris until advancing age finally forced him back to this hemisphere to the home of his son. He died there at the age of ninety-one after surviving his own "cardiac event" by thirty-three years.

Paris, France
June 1979

You came from a medical family: GEORGE DOCK* was your father.

My father was the first full-time professor of medicine in the United States at the University of Michigan in Ann Arbor. When Washington University in St. Louis started with full-time faculty in 1910, he became head of the Department of Medicine there. He was an extremely good department head, and he was an extremely good clinician—and he was a clinician who kept up to date. When ECGs were invented, he didn't say, "What nonsense!" or, like HENRY CHRISTIAN, "Well, SAM [LEVINE], what are the wild waves sayin'?" or "What the hell is your gadget for?" My father was a believer in using polygraphs to record motions of

---

* Names in small caps are listed in the "Biographical Notes" at the back of this book.

arteries and veins and the precordium; he fiddled with this. He was very good with a microscope, and he was a good parasitologist when more people had more parasites. He studied hookworm disease and wrote a good book on it. He also studied pellagra. He was a good hematologist because of his skill with a microscope, but he never made any original observations with it. He had a lot of Negro patients and must have seen dozens of smears of sickle cell anemia, but it was JIMMY HERRICK in Chicago, who hardly saw any Negro patients, who described the disease.

You were a very peripatetic family.

Well, my father liked to travel. I was born and raised in Ann Arbor, Michigan. I spent a year in New Orleans when my father was at Tulane. Then my family was in St. Louis from 1910 to 1922.

There's a well-known story about your father walking around with appendicitis without recognizing it—despite being a great diagnostician. Is this true?

No. It was my brother that walked around with it for three days when we were in New Orleans. His appendix ruptured, and RUDOLPH MATAS, one of the best surgeons in America at that time, heard from my *mother,* who let him know that *he* better see my brother. Matas put him in the hospital and took the appendix out. It was ruptured, so my brother had a drain in for six weeks. The next year, my father was in California, fortunately, and so when I came down with appendicitis at that time, mine came out before it ruptured.

So I had the story right but the characters wrong. It was your father who did not recognize it in your brother!

He didn't even think about it! But, of course, it was the women in our family who were the brightest. My father's sister, Aunt Lavinia, spent a lifetime in nursing and had a tremendous influence on the profession. She graduated from Bellevue and, after being night supervisor there, wrote a materia medica for nurses that became a standard text. She later went down to Hopkins for a few years and wrote a classic multivolume history of nursing with Adelaide Nutting. Although she did most of the work, she preferred to have the authors listed as "Nutting and Dock" because the words seemed to flow better that way. Incidentally, she didn't think much of doctors even though she knew [William] Osler. She hardly ever needed doctors either. Aunt Vinnie lived to ninety-nine and had not seen a doctor for her own care from the age of nine. It was a broken hip she had, but it was not the hip that she died from—it was from indignation!

Was growing up the son of such a famous physician a help or a hindrance to you?

Oh, it was a great help, because in those days doctors were really rich. In 1910 at Washington University in St. Louis a full-time chief was felt to be on miserable pay. He only got ten thousand dollars. But in 1910, before the introduction of the income tax and with the buying power of the dollar then, ten thousand dollars was the equivalent of eighty-five thousand dollars a year after taxes in more recent times. I discussed this in a talk I gave in Atlantic City some years ago. It was entitled, "Hours Rescued from Oblivion."

You went to war before you went into medicine.

Yes. My brother, who was four years older than I, went over in 1915 and finally joined up with a French flying squadron, not the American Lafayette Escadrille. I went over in 1917 as a volunteer ambulance driver for the French army. I had gotten to be pretty good at fixing things, and this came in handy on the job. A few years before that, when I was seventeen, I worked on a ranch that later became Camp Vandenberg in California. The ranches then depended on windmills to keep the cows in water, and I became the best boy on the ranch in repairing windmills. I've been good at gadgets ever since. While I was in France during the war there was a pretty difficult ambulance run from Montzeville to Esnes, and the ambulance drivers always hated getting stuck along the way and perhaps getting hit by a stray shell. I became pretty good at fixing Fords and getting them going again once they got stuck. I offered to be there to help out, go back and forth until the last trip. The other drivers were very appreciative of this. One day when our commanding officer informed us that headquarters intended to pass out a few medals to some of our group on the following day, they selected me to get one. My citation said I was a devoted and conscientious driver et cetera; bravery was not mentioned. I changed tires fast and unclogged carburetors fast.*

What about your early medical training?

I took my first two years of medical school at Washington University in St. Louis. My brother was in France at this time and my mother wasn't feeling very well; so I thought I had better stay home. Then my brother came back safely from the wars, and I realized I couldn't take my clinical years in St. Louis because my father was head of the Department of Medicine. So I shopped around and found that the best place for me was Rush Medical School in Chicago. In this I made no mistake. Rush was a marvelous place; they thought you were an adult, and you could do what you wanted to do in those two years as long as you wrote the examinations at the end of it. I spent almost all my time there doing autopsies with a marvelous pathologist, E. R. LeCount. Although I never took clinical microscopy and was never a clinical clerk, you still could not get better clinical training than they offered there. People like FRANK BILLINGS and James Herrick, who put coronary disease on the map, were active then.

After Chicago I was a house officer at the [Peter Bent Brigham Hospital] between 1922 and 1924. BILL MURPHY was the best internist at the Brigham. He was a resident when I was an intern. HERRMAN BLUMGART was also a fine assistant resident at the time. Murphy, Blumgart, and Samuel B. Grant were the three best residents and internists at the Brigham along with Sam Levine. "Uncle Henry" Christian was a superb executive but was not in the same class as a diagnostician. His rounds were called "shifting dullness."

From Boston I knew I wanted to go into practice in San Francisco and had already made some preliminary arrangements, but first I was

---

* He received the Croix de Guerre.

going to take a *Wanderjahr* on my own. My father, however, insisted that I go work with his old friend K. F. WENCKEBACH, the head of the First Medical Clinic in Vienna. Wenckebach, who was Dutch, was the first man to do clinical electrocardiography. People in Amsterdam wouldn't have anything to do with it when he started. This "silly toy" the physiologists had made! It wasn't movable, you know; you had to bring the patient to it. But "Wencke" persisted. He described atrial fibrillation; he described atrial flutter; he described atrial and ventricular tachycardia. One day one of his patients came in with an attack of atrial fibrillation and told Wenckebach, "Oh, that's nothing. I'll be back tomorrow and it will be all over."

Wenckebach asked, "What do you do for it?"

"I take the quinine I use for my malaria."

Wencke found that quinine was good but quinidine was better. So he introduced the first good antiarrhythmic drug. He was a pioneer in this, and my father was a good friend of his from the time when they were both doing carotid and jugular tracings together—which got them both interested in cardiac arrhythmias.

So my father, as usual, was right in sending me abroad, although at first I was indignant at spending such a long time in Vienna. As it turned out, I had a wonderful time there. I also went there on a honeymoon. I took my wife with me, and she came back highly pregnant.

What was Wenckebach like?

He was a charming person. He was small and thin and quick. He spoke French, German, English, and, of course, Dutch quite fluently. He was a very poor teacher in clinic, however. He would come in and do his cerebration in public; he would think about the patient, and about the disease, and about the history of it. Well, the students didn't take kindly to this rambling. They used to recite:

> In der Klinik Wenckebach
> Nur die erste Bäncke wacht.
>
> [In Wenckebach's clinic
> Only the first row can stay awake.]

But I wouldn't have made a penny when I got back to San Francisco if I hadn't been given the key to some gold nuggets. The mercurial treatment for diuresis was discovered while I was there.[1] And of course it was discovered by the nurses. They used to give mercurials intravenously for the treatment of syphilis, and frequently the syphilitic patients had congestive heart failure resulting from syphilitic aortic insufficiency. They kept jugs at the end of the beds to measure the urine output, and the nurses kept pointing out to the doctors that whenever they gave mercurials to one of these patients in heart failure, he'd have one hell of a diuresis. Eventually, [Paul] Saxl, who really was not one of the brightest men there, thought he better look into this, and they were off to the races and so was I.

When I went into practice I was the only man in San Francisco who could treat pulmonary edema properly. You gave 'em intravenous mercury, and they told all their friends that you were a miracle worker.

How did you switch from private practice to academic medicine?

I originally never intended to go into academic medicine. I thought my father had carried the family as far as they could go in that direction. After being in Boston, I decided that I wanted to do in San Francisco what Sam Levine did: have a connection with a good hospital and a good medical school, but practice in town or a major suburb. I started in San Francisco as the "boy" of Drs. René Bine and Alfred Reed down in Union Square. I did their odds and ends in the afternoons and evenings: lumbar punctures, chest taps, transfusions and whatnot, also seeing some patients. In the mornings I went to the outpatient clinic at Stanford, and some evenings I could also do a little work there, using it as a sort of laboratory.

In the year prior to my arrival, Dr. [ARTHUR] BLOOMFIELD had come out as chief of medicine from Hopkins, and he had anticipated bringing CHESTER KEEFER with him as his first instructor. Chester was at the University of Chicago as a resident. Toward the end of the year Bloomfield asked me to come see him, and when I got there he said, "Bill, I'm in a fix. Chester Keefer has written me and wants to be released from his contract so that he can go to Peking Union Medical

School* as an assistant professor of medicine and stay there for a few years. Of course I released him. Now I've got to have somebody, and you'll have to come back here the first of September."

I had built up quite a practice with my friends in Union Square by that time, so I went home and asked my wife if she could afford to take the cut in income. She said yes, and, with one year's exception, I spent the rest of my professional life in academia.

> **You carried on the peripatetic tradition of your family in more ways than one. You shifted back and forth between the two coasts as well as between internal medicine and pathology. You stayed in medicine at Stanford from 1926 to 1936 and then suddenly shifted to pathology. Why?**

Well, I got into pathology the same way I did academic medicine—by accident. Our dean and professor of pathology at Stanford had been Dr. William Ophüls, the man who discovered coccidiodal granuloma. He was a wonderful dean but, like all good deans, spent far more time teaching in the laboratory than in the dean's office. Well, he died, and they got von Glahn, a Hopkins graduate, to come out from Columbia to look at the job. Dr. von Glahn proceeded to write an insulting but perfectly accurate description of the state of pathology at Stanford as compared to eastern pathology. They got WILLIAM BOYD to come down from Saskatchewan, and he accepted but was snapped up by Toronto as soon as they read the announcement in *Science.*

Finally, President Wilbur of Stanford sent for me and told me, "Dock, you'll have to take over the Department of Pathology the first of September." At the time I was perfectly happy in medicine, but again went home and asked my wife if she would be willing to take another pay cut in going from medicine to pathology. She agreed, and I went into pathology.

Wilbur had promised a great many things to me upon my acceptance of the pathology job, but during the five years I remained there he did not make any change in the income of the department, which

---

* At that time a center for the study of infectious diseases and a highly desirable and exciting place for those in the field to work.

was inadequate for our staff. Each year the promised increase never came. I finally indicated that if this was not straightened out I would resign. I was considering a professorship in pathology at Cornell. Wilbur knew I had been offered some deanships that I had turned down—I was no administrator—and believed that if I had turned down a deanship I would certainly not accept a professorship in pathology. He was wrong. When he did not increase the budget and the only way I could raise the salaries of the other members of the department was to resign, I did.

Why Cornell?

One answer to this might be the one that the "darkie" American who had signed up with the French gave to Mrs. Vanderbilt when she visited him in the hospital in Paris during World War I. He had been a dock-worker in Savannah. Mrs. Vanderbilt asked him, "Mr. Bullard, how did you happen to join the French army?" He said, "Ma'am, it was more through curiosity than intelligence."

But, actually, I had to leave. Wilbur gave me no other choice.

Once I got to Cornell, it was pretty obvious to me that what they needed was a different kind of man. I was interested in the seats and causes of disease, in doing autopsies, in training young surgeons. At Stanford I had always had a prospective surgical resident assigned to me.

At Cornell the surgeons were scared to death of pathologists, and when I gave a talk to the sophomore students on the causes of thrombo-embolic disease and said that everybody should be out of bed as soon as possible after an operation, the surgeons thought I was crazy and couldn't get rid of me soon enough. What they wanted was someone of an entirely different sort: one who would spend all his time studying viruses or enzymes or something like that, rather than bothering the surgeons and obstetricians.

After three years, 1941 to 1944, at Cornell in pathology, you went back to medicine—in Brooklyn, of all places.

Well, I was wasting my time at Cornell, and ALAN GREGG, the head man at the Rockefeller Foundation, got wind of this and sent for me. He said, "Dock, I think you should consider going to the Long Island College of Medicine. There is only one little school in the whole of Long Island. You are worth twenty times as much in Brooklyn as you would be in Boston and ten times as much as you are in Manhattan, and I think you should consider it. You may get thrown out of there in two or three years, but I know you'll land on your feet."

I knew I was in no shape to take over a department of medicine after all those years in pathology, so I arranged through some friends of mine at the University of Southern California to work six months at the Los Angeles County Hospital. I did not bring my family west for this period, and although officially a professor of medicine, I lived the life of a resident again. I was lodged at the Santa Fe Railroad Hospital and started ward rounds there every morning at seven-thirty. I left for the County Hospital at eight-thirty and spent most of the day there, returning about four in the afternoon to complete my work at Santa Fe. I took calls with the residents and gave all those wonderful new drugs that were coming along. I gave sulfadiazine intravenously and, for the first time in my life, saw bacterial meningitis cured. It was the best education in medicine one could get after being away from it for eight years. After the six months were up, I returned east to head the Department of Medicine at the Long Island College Hospital on July 1, 1944. I had good friends there who were sympathetic, and Alan Gregg was right. I was the only one they could have sent there to shake things up a bit; and I had talked to a lot of people there before moving, people like JEAN OLIVER who was probably the world authority on renal anatomy and pathology.

When I arrived in Brooklyn, I recognized that the situation was nowhere near hopeless. But it was clear that this school could not survive as a WASP institution in a community that was predominantly Catholic and Jewish. The faculty were all WASPS, and they needed to recognize the large Jewish community with a lot of doctors—some terrible and some very good—and work with them. George Baehr, an internist at Mount Sinai in New York and a chief adviser to the Federation of Jewish Charities, was helpful, and he had the kind of political clout to help us with Albany. I convinced Jean Oliver and others at the school that this was the way to go, so we affiliated with Maimonides in Brooklyn and finally got the school to become the Downstate Medical Center of the State University of New York.

> I have suggested that you never stayed in one place very long, but actually, except between 1956 and 1957, when you went to Palo Alto, you were continuously at Long Island–Downstate for a period of over twenty years.

After I settled in at Long Island, I resigned the chairmanship of the department in order to get PERRIN LONG to take it over. He was an administrator deluxe. It was political interference from Albany that led to my leaving for a year. They had arranged that in the Open Division at Kings County Hospital they would have the right to appoint their own professors and make their own promotions with no control by the Department of Medicine at the College. Political influence had been brought to bear on the dean, and someone had to do something about it. Once I resigned, I was able to talk freely to the chairman of the board of trustees and then spent my year at the Palo Alto Clinic in private practice. That's what every professor of medicine should do for a sabbatical. He shouldn't go to Oxford to study viruses; he should go to a good private clinic and learn how to take care of sick people.

After a year there, things got straightened out between Albany and the medical school in Brooklyn, and Perrin Long brought me back. And I stayed on there until LUDWIG EICHNA succeeded him. Eichna had a number of good qualities—he was good with medical students, a good committee worker, an executive—but he tried to disaffiliate with the other hospitals, so he antagonized the entire community in Brooklyn. He made it clear to me and BOB AUSTRIAN that we could not get off the faculty too soon to please him. So he got rid of us. But, unlike me, he didn't go away when he was sixty-five.

No one should stick around too long. My father retired at sixty-two; HARVEY CUSHING resigned from Harvard at sixty-two; Osler left Hopkins at fifty-six. Fifty-six was the age that Hippocrates chose as the beginning of senility. Osler was a great Hippocrates and *Religio Medici* man, so that he had firm feelings about what doctors should do and one of them is: "Here's your coat. What's your hurry?"

> Do you really believe, as someone who has worked all his life in biological science, that you can hang a certain age on somebody and say, "All right, now that you are sixty-five or whatever, you're finished"? There are some people who are old when they are fifty, and others who are still young mentally at seventy.

Yes, I'm only too painfully aware of this. The problem is that you are not fit to be the judge of which of these you are. Other people can tell right away whether you're fifty and acting seventy or just the reverse, but you, yourself, have no idea. The only solution is to do what my father and Harvey Cushing did and not stay too long.

Who were the people who influenced you the most?

Dr. E. R. LeCount in Chicago; Dr. Philip Schaefer, biochemist at Washington University; Dr. Opie, who was professor of pathology at Washington University at St. Louis; and FRANK WILSON. Wilson was the greatest man I ever met in medicine.

I guess it was one of the Haldanes who said, "The cosmos is characterized by inexhaustible queerness." And studying the queerness is the fun of being here. Frank Wilson understood that better than all the rest of us. He's the man who introduced the twelve-lead electrocardiogram, but aside from his work in electrocardiography, he was a splendid astronomer and had his own observatory. He was a splendid ornithologist: he knew all the warblers there were in the United States and could recognize their songs, and knew where they wintered and where they summered. He was a splendid botanist. I walked through the Arnold Arboretum in Boston with him, and he could identify every tree at a distance just by its shape. He was a superb mathematician and a very good clinician. You never met such a man. He really had a mind! He spent all of his life in Ann Arbor, except for a few years when he was with my father in St. Louis. I was lucky, because he was in charge of the sophomore students for physical diagnosis and history taking when I was there. It was immediately obvious to me then that, "Boy, this is a man!" and I almost went to Ann Arbor to work with him but got side-tracked in other directions.

What about your own research work?

You have to know what sort of talents you have. I'm not any good at all at biochemistry. I wouldn't be any good at all in bacteriology and virology. My "tricks" are not the ones that are good for you in those areas.

You are good at gadgets. What about the ballistocardiogram?[2]

We have already talked a bit about my way of fixing things. Ballistocardiography is a sad story. Its potential was never realized. It is one of the best methods of studying patients; not just cardiac patients. It's a wonderful cheap toy. I do it in three planes because doing it in one plane is just like taking one lead of the electrocardiogram. I left my three-plane gadget behind me with more regrets than anything else when I retired. No one else had the slightest interest in it.

There is a long-standing dispute between you and ALDO LUISADA about the genesis of the first heart sound.

I refuse to dispute with him. Never argue with a man with an obsession and who won't repeat any experiments that are in the literature. In the 1830s a good Frenchman, Rouanet, pointed out that two leaflets could come together but would not make noise unless you subjected them to tension. I quoted him in my first paper,[3] and this is 140 years old now.

What I like to do is get the answer to things. I've got some new experiments cooking here. I discovered to my horror that people were teaching that when you measure a patient's blood pressure the KOROTKOFF sounds in the artery are due to blood hitting the blood below the cuff. Well, anybody who has ever squirted a hose under the surface of a pool knows that's nonsense. You don't get that kind of noise that way. I'm working on this now.[4]

One particular bit of work, you'll be pleased to know, was performed in 1920 when I was a medical student working with another fellow on our own and not under a professor. We showed that the "bone" that forms in a kidney when you tie a renal artery is not due to calcification of the chalk that precipitates in the kidney but to the cells that lie right under the transitional epithelium in the pelvis of the kidney. Many years later, I think in 1963, CHARLIE HUGGINS in Chicago gave me a flourishing introduction as the man who had made this discovery, and I was quite pleased.

What kind of work makes you the happiest?

Well, I'm happiest with the things that are the least work. There was that talk that caused all sorts of trouble for me at Cornell, "The Abuse of Bed Rest." It all happened quite by accident when I was asked by McKean Cattell, the professor of pharmacology and therapeutics, to give a talk as part of a regularly occurring symposium in 1944.

From my Stanford days as a pathologist I had known that excessive bed rest gave rise to thromboembolic complications, and had lectured on this to students at Stanford since 1936. The death rate from thromboembolism was always much less at the County Hospital than it was at Stanford Hospital. At the County on rounds all you needed to do was ask a patient, supposedly on strict bed rest, "How many times did you get up last night to go to the bathroom?" And he might say, "Well, only *once*, Doc," because there weren't enough orderlies and nurses around the County to bring the urinals to the patients when they wanted them. This wasn't true at the private hospitals. So the patients at the County, when they got up to go to the bathroom, dislodged only tiny clots from their veins and these did not harm them when they got to the lungs and were dissolved, while the wealthier patients, who remained in bed and formed large clots in their legs and pelvises, suffered the major consequences of large pulmonary emboli.

I gave this talk in New York and had no idea it was being written down. It got into the *New York State Medical Journal*[5] and it got into *Time* magazine,[6] and there was my picture, with me looking cuter than ever in 1944 because the picture they used had been taken by my fiancée under a lovely azalea bush twenty years earlier.

Within six months all over the world surgeons were able to get their patients out of bed earlier, and obstetricians were getting their ladies out of bed. The cost of hospitalization went way down. This was during the war, you know, and only at that time, when they couldn't build new hospitals and had a severe shortage of beds, would the surgeons have accepted the idea. After all, they charged the patients for all those daily visits while they were at bed rest.

What I am most proud of is where I saved the most lives. No one ever saved as many lives in twenty minutes as I did with that talk. Incidentally, during the war they were having a rash of thromboembolic complications in a military hospital in young men after surgery, and I was asked to look into it. I found the same thing, but in this instance the medical corpsmen were giving them too much narcotics so that they would not be bothered by them. The patients just lay there for days forming thrombi.

What about the localization of tuberculosis to the right apex?

One morning on rounds at the Long Island College Hospital, one of the students or house staff asked me to explain why it was that pulmonary tuberculosis was so often limited to the apex of the lung rather than the lower lobes. He forced me to think of an explanation. The pulmonary artery pressure had just been measured in man and found to be only one-fifth the systemic pressure, and I looked at the chest X-ray and the location of the main pulmonary artery and the height of the apex above it. I reasoned that the blood supply was less there than the rest of the lung and provided a more favorable culture medium for the tubercle bacillus. Then I was challenged by some of my colleagues on this: "Why the right apex rather than the left apex? They are both the same height above the pulmonary conus." Again I was forced to come up with an answer and reasoned that it was because of the branching of the main pulmonary artery with the branches to the right apex coming off at a much sharper angle and providing less favorable perfusion to the right apex when compared to the left.

The apical localization theory was turned down by a good many TB men at first, but in 1960 Dollery, at Hampstead, England, got a cyclotron in his backyard producing radioactive carbon dioxide. He showed that when you sit up, the blood flow to the right apex is less than that to the left. He wrote, " This exactly confirms Dock's hypothesis in 1946."[7]

That makes you feel better because I never believe any of my own work until other people confirm it with independent methods. Similarly, my work on the localization of coronary disease was confirmed by Minkowsky, who showed that in adults it occurred in the thickest parts, as I had shown in the newborn.[8] So it's nice to have your work confirmed. I get the most satisfaction in knowing I wasn't wrong.

Were you ever wrong?

Yes, at Stanford I was wrong once. Some people in Italy had reported that by giving Congo Red, you could get a remission in pernicious anemia. This was before [George] Minot and [William Parry] Murphy, of course.[9] I tried this on some patients, and their serum bilirubins went down and their reticulocyte counts may have risen. But I never repeated the Congo Red experiments, and it certainly was not the solution to pernicious anemia.

It's funny, sometimes, how discoveries get made.

Like good old Pasteur said, "Chance favors the prepared mind." It helps to recognize something when you stumble over it.

We've talked about Washington University, St. Louis, and Frank Wilson. There was also this fellow there named ALAN CHESNEY. He later went back to Hopkins and ended up as a dean. He was studying something that had to do with rabbits but, along the way, noted that his rabbits got goiters during certain times of the year when they were eating nothing but cabbage for greens. He looked into this and found that it was a thio- compound in the greens that gave them the goiter. And this is where all those antithyroid drugs—thiouricil and so on—come from. He was the one that opened up that field. Chesney was very bright and observant. This was serendipity, but when he stumbled over something he knew that he had "bumped his shins."

Look at the discovery of the Roentgen ray. There were these Crookes tubes all over Europe and America, standard toys in every physics department, a cathode-ray tube. From time to time, one laboratory or another would complain to their photographic supply house that "a lot of the plates you sent us were all fogged." Ilford, the main photographic supplier in England, got the most complaints and always wrote back: "We're sorry, but many other people have lots of the same emulsion and they are having no trouble with it. You better look into the source that is fogging your plates." Not one of these physicists had the sense to put up a plate beside his Crookes tube and leave it there for half an hour and then develop it. [WILHELM] ROENTGEN put a good black cardboard cover over his Crookes tube and went in with a platinocyanide fluorescent screen, and it glowed at three meters. He knew when his shins had been bumped.

Some people have very insensitive shins. Look how long it took them to recognize nonfatal myocardial infarction. My father reported five cases of myocardial infarction diagnosed during life in 1896. He reported this to the Buffalo Medical Society because it was old stuff to him. Pathologists in Germany and France had been studying myocardial infarcts for years but couldn't interest the clinicians. And you know why? Clinicians had believed that coronary occlusion was immediately fatal.* And if a doctor had called one of these attacks a coronary occlusion (or myocardial infarction), he would be making a damn fool out of himself, because in eight out of ten cases the patients would be back to work in a week saying, "That doctor was crazy. He said I had a fatal form of heart disease." It was only after Pardee, in 1920, published "An Electrocardiographic Sign of Coronary Occlusion" that a doctor could make this diagnosis without losing his practice.

Before World War I, Frank Wilson recognized the ECG changes of infarction, as did Sam Levine, FRED SMITH, and Herrick, of course.

Speaking of coronary disease, I've always emphasized to my patients that many have survived for long periods after a myocardial infarction: Dwight Eisenhower, Lyndon Johnson; and Winston Churchill fought a world war after having his fairly early during World War II. You, yourself, must be a record holder of sorts. When did you have yours?

---

* They were probably influenced by the work of experimental pathologist Julius Cohnheim (1839–84), who showed that the coronary arteries of dogs were "end arteries": the animals died almost immediately after the coronaries were ligated.

In 1957. Sam Levine came down from Boston to verify it because I wasn't in a hospital. I would never go to a hospital for a coronary; the death rate is twice as high. TINSLEY HARRISON didn't go to a hospital when he had his infarct.* He's dead now but not from his coronaries. Frank Wilson didn't go into a hospital either, and while we may not all have lived happily ever after, we survived and went back to work.

When they put you in an intensive care unit, the mental stress is far greater than at any time in your life, immobilized and with all those tubes running in and out. That's a terrible thing to do. If a patient has showers of ventricular ectopic beats, I think it's a good idea to monitor him with a defibrillator handy but in a nice quiet single room. The danger period is that time between the time you suddenly realize, "Help, boys, I've had an infarct," and the end of the week. If you live through the week, you've probably got it made.

I am by no means a record holder in terms of survival. Dr. Osler used to treat coronary disease, and, in 1896, he wrote this up. Tinsley Harrison's father was one of his patients and had severe angina at the age of thirty-eight. He went up to Hopkins to visit the great professor, who took a very careful history, including how many children he had, what their ages were, and whether Mrs. Harrison was as plump as he was; and how his weight compared then to what it was during the time he was a high school athlete. After getting all this down and doing a physical examination, Osler said, "Well, I think you'll get over your angina all right when you lose the fifty-five pounds you put on between the time of your marriage and the time this began." He told him to go for walks every Saturday and Sunday and as much as he could during the week, but that he should lose weight steadily by just eating less of all the things he liked to eat. Dr. Harrison did this and lived to the age of ninety-one. JOHN HUNTER lived twenty years after the onset of his angina. So long survival after the onset of angina is not unusual. In my case, I'm a confirmed and practicing coward, so that I

---

* Nor did George Burch (1910–86), another great cardiologist, who might still be with us if, after having diagnosed his own acute myocardial infarction, he had spent a few days in the coronary care unit instead of going home.

promptly went down from 150 to 125 pounds in about six months. I weigh 110 now.

> Your friend WILLIAM BEAN once described your father when he gave the thirty-fourth annual George Dock Lecture a few years ago. In addition to his medical work, he obviously had a rapier wit, and when Bean reported, "He certainly did not suffer fools gladly; he didn't suffer them at all!" I could not help but be struck by the fact that the same might be applied to you. All of your students worshiped you, but you always seemed to have a knack for making your peers very uncomfortable.

Oh, no. People like BILL CASTLE, Art Bloomfield, Jean Oliver, and Perrin Long were not in the least uncomfortable, and they were my peers. Some of these other people were simply not *quite* my peers. I never sought to make people uncomfortable, but I knew I did. I recognized the cause and the result. It was like the father who came home one day and said, "Well now, children, your father has become a professor emeritus," and his young son looked up at him and said, "I know Latin: 'e' means you're out, and 'meritus' means you goddam well deserved it."

> That's perhaps the best definition of "emeritus" I've ever heard. What is nonetheless amazing about your career is that you are so well known despite the fact that, unlike others, such as MAXWELL WINTROBE, you never spent your life at one institution creating your own medical dynasty.

I never had a chance to do this. I was never invited to be a chief of medicine at a new medical school, as my father was at Washington University, St. Louis, or Tinsley Harrison was at Birmingham, or BOB WILLIAMS at the University of Washington in Seattle, or Wintrobe at Utah. I don't know why this was so. Perhaps I was never in the right place at the right time. And perhaps it's just as well. I am not a good administrator; I'm not in a class with people like Wintrobe. You see, when someone is good at organizing a textbook like Williams's *Endocrinology,* or Wintrobe's *Hematology,* or Tinsley Harrison's *Textbook of Medicine,* he is obviously a good organizer. I am completely disorganized and always have been. After heading the Department of

Medicine at Long Island College for a short time, I was more than happy to have Perrin Long take it over.

> We students never thought much of him, you know. We knew he had something to do with the introduction of sulfa drugs during the war, but we thought him something of a buffoon.

But he was an administrator deluxe and the kind of administrator who made ward rounds. And when he made mistakes on rounds and heard about it, he told everyone about it. He didn't pretend to be a brilliant clinician. He once diagnosed an Arthus reaction in a woman who had a swollen arm after receiving an injection. On rounds the next day, Paul Spear, who was chief of medicine at the Brooklyn VA Hospital at the time, stuck in a needle and pulled out a load of pus! Perrin loved to tell that story.

As for sulfa, it was invented in Germany but was very toxic. Then the French made it less toxic. Long brought this to the United States and persuaded three different drug firms to look into analogues. The first one was sulfinpyrazone, which he used at Hopkins to cure pneumonia, but it made the patients awfully sick. Then he got sulfadiazine and hit the jackpot, because this would cure pneumonia *and* meningitis without making you sick. No one made as much of a contribution in saving lives in the United States as Perrin Long did. This was before the war. When World War II broke out, he instantly left Hopkins and served as a medical consultant in North Africa.

> Do you have any regrets about the past?

Regrets? Oh, many of them. I played my cards badly. I don't lose any sleep over it, but I have the ordinary feeling that I could have played that hand better.

> Without meaning any disrespect, may I say something? Your friend Dr. George Pickering spoke very highly of you and very fondly of you, but he did say, "The trouble with Bill Dock was that he never knew when to keep his mouth shut."

Yes, that's perfectly true. I had a disease that is very well described: it is better to keep your mouth shut and be thought a damn fool than to open it and leave no doubt about the question. I had to move around quite a lot in my life, but I didn't mind moving, and I would have missed a great deal in California, New York, and Brooklyn. I learned a lot, and I never worried about moving:

> For to admire and for to see
> And for to behold this world so wide
> It never done no good for me
> But I can't stop it if I tried.*

* Rudyard Kipling.

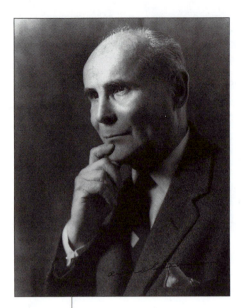

2

ANDRÉ COURNAND, M.D.
(1895–1988)

Dr. Cournand's name and that of his collaborator, DICKINSON W. RICHARDS, will always be associated with the introduction of cardiac catheterization for the study of the circulation and the diagnosis of heart disease. However, the concept of placing tubes or catheters within portions of the cardiovascular system had been an established method of investigation in the animal laboratory for at least a hundred years or more when they began their own work in this field at Bellevue Hospital in the early forties.[1] The major hurdle to the application of such techniques in humans was the question of safety, and it was this impediment to progress that was overcome in 1929.

Werner Forssmann (1904–79) was a twenty-five-year-old surgical house officer in Eberswalde, near Berlin, when he demonstrated that a catheter could be safely passed without danger from an arm vein into the human heart, using himself as the subject. Although opposed by the senior physicians at his clinic, Forssmann managed to deceive a nurse into thinking *she* would be the subject so that he could gain access to the sterile surgical instruments he needed. He persuaded the nurse to allow herself to be tied down on the procedure table but then anesthetized his own antecubital fossa (the inner aspect of the elbow) and passed a ureteral catheter from his arm vein to his heart. He then climbed several flights of stairs to the X-ray department to document his success with a chest film. He repeated the procedure on himself several times to convince others of its safety.

Forssmann's rationale for using heart catheterization was to provide safe and rapid delivery of lifesaving drugs into the heart without risking damage to the heart wall or coronary arteries by sticking needles blindly through the chest wall and into the heart; the use of needles might also result in punctures of the heart wall, through which blood could leak, accumulate, and compress the heart in its own sac (cardiac tamponade). When he came to the Charité Hospital in Berlin, he tried to convince the chief surgeon there, ERNST SAUERBRUCH, of the safety and potential value of the procedure but failed. Sauerbruch is said to have told him, "I'm running a clinic here, not a circus!"

Forssmann, discouraged by the consistent and overwhelming opposition to his ideas, ultimately gave up his attempts to popularize them and was all but forgotten for much of his later life. In 1949, after cardiac catheterization had become a well-accepted procedure, A. J. Benatt, in the British journal *Lancet,* wrote about the early history of cardiac catheterization.[2] He noted that by that time over ten thousand catheterizations had been performed throughout the world and wondered about the fate of that obscure German house officer who had somehow faded from the medical scene. Forssmann was rescued from oblivion in 1956 when he was included in the Nobel Prize for medicine that was awarded to André Cournand and Dickinson W. Richards for their work on catheterization of the human heart.

Cournand and Richards got into the heart by way of the lungs. They were chest physicians; that is, they were primarily interested in lung diseases such as tuberculosis and emphysema. Collaborators since the early thirties, they were attempting to study the relationship of these diseases to cardiac function as well as the results of certain types of treatment for these diseases upon cardiopulmonary function.

One of the things they were determined to measure was the blood flow to the lungs, and after failing to do so by other methods, they decided that the only way to get a true measurement of pulmonary blood flow was by using the direct Fick method. Adolf Fick

(1829–1901) was a German physiologist-physician who, in a one-page communication presented before the Society of Physiology and Medicine in the university town of Würzburg in 1870, stated the principle upon which almost all subsequent methods of measuring cardiac output have been based. Using the Fick principle as applied to pulmonary blood flow, Cournand and Richards would be required to fill in the right side of the following equation:

$$\text{Pulmonary blood flow/minute} \ = \ \frac{\text{oxygen consumption per minute}}{\substack{\text{oxygen content difference} \\ \text{between arterial and venous blood}}}$$

They could measure oxygen consumption by having a patient breathe into a collecting bag and then analyzing the gas contents accordingly. Obtaining arterial blood was not difficult; puncturing an artery in the arm or groin could easily provide a sample. The problem was getting the appropriate sample of venous blood for this calculation. Since each of the body's organs extracts different amounts of oxygen from the arterial blood supply, the veins draining different parts of the body (an arm, a leg, the liver, the kidney, etc.) contain different amounts of oxygen. The sample representing the total body venous sample, the "mixed venous" blood, could only be obtained by drawing blood from the right side of the heart, to which all the venous blood returns and is mixed to give the desired sample. Forssmann's demonstration of the safety of passing a catheter to the heart enabled them to do this.

The development of this technique by Cournand and Richards allowed for the measurement of not only pulmonary blood flow but, in the absence of abnormal shunts within the heart such as septal defects, systemic output as well. These measurements, combined with those of intracardiac pressures and other hemodynamic parameters, provided valuable insights into various aspects of normal and abnormal cardiac physiology. Early on, they conducted important studies of clinical shock and the effects of mechanically assisted ventilation on the cardiovascular system. Cardiac catheterization was also found to be invaluable in the detection of shunts resulting from defects in the walls separating the chambers of the heart (atrial and ventricular septal defects), certain valvular abnormalities, and, with the introduction of left heart catheterization later on, the visualization of the aorta and coronary arteries with the use of radiopaque material injected at appropriate sites. The information gained from such studies provided critical and accurate anatomical road maps to guide the cardiac surgeons as they progressed from the repair of extracardiac abnormalities involving the major vessels connected to the heart (patent ductus arteriosus, coarctation of the aorta, etc.) to intracardiac surgery for repair of congenital and acquired structural diseases of the heart.

Early in my own career, I had a revealing personal encounter with Dr. Cournand. I had just finished a fellowship in cardiovascular diseases at the University of Utah and was looking for a junior position at another institution. Like most beginning investigators, I was not quite sure at this stage of my life which area of research to pursue. I visited Dr. Cournand in his office at Bellevue and approached the great man at his desk. I recall an immense street map of Paris filling the entire wall behind him. He soon asked me about what I wanted to study, and, although I really had nothing definite in mind, I expressed a certain interest in determining the effects of potassium depletion on the heart. Dr. Cournand then proceeded to inquire about all the details of the "proposed investigation," none of which I was equipped to supply at the time. I emerged from his office thinking to myself, "What was that all about?"

During the ensuing years I think I have learned something of what it was all about. During my second interview with Dr. Cournand, the one that follows, I mentioned this episode to him; he naturally had forgotten it among the thousands of others he had no doubt conducted with budding young scientists. He was concerned that I may have been intimidated.

"Was I polite with you?"

"Very polite."

"Good."

"But very rigorous, intellectually rigorous."

Dr. Cournand applied that intellectual rigor to his own work and his interactions with others throughout the course of a brilliant, fruitful, and rewarding career.

New York, New York
December 11, 1979

One tends to think that catheterization of the heart is a rather recent innovation to medicine, but you have pointed out that it has a considerable history.

It is very important to recognize that a lot of work had been done on catheterization of the heart in experimental medicine in the past. The term "heart catheterism" was actually coined by CLAUDE BERNARD in 1847; and in 1876, after over twenty years of animal experiments, he published a book recapitulating a series of twenty-two lectures he had given at the College de France. In the fifth lecture he described the technique of right heart catheterization and left heart catheterization essentially as they are performed today. There is not a word to change. So even before 1900 everything had been done—in animals, of course—but then [ERNEST H.] STARLING came along with his heart-lung preparation, and, for a while, even though it was a great advance, this competed with the use of the catheter in studying the heart in the intact animal.

Once something is well accepted in society or science, it is difficult for people to imagine the amount of resistance that might have met it when it was first introduced. I suppose this was the case with cardiac catheterization.

There was great resistance to this. At the time one did not ordinarily pass tubes into the heart. It was unfortunate for Forssmann to have started something and then see others develop the technique. I first met him in 1952 when I was visiting Heidelberg. He was practicing urology in a small town nearby, and the professor of pharmacology at the university invited him over for me so that we could spend a Sunday afternoon together. Now Forssmann was a very intelligent man and wrote extremely well in German, as is reflected in the English translations of his writings. Like many physicians of his time, he was well prepared in the humanities before he began the study of medicine. But he was obviously not a scientist. What did strike him was the important idea that if heart catheterization could be performed safely in animals, it could also be safely performed in man. He was also the first to have the idea that if you injected a radiopaque substance into the heart, you could get better visualization of X-rays of the cardiac structures and pulmonary vessels.

But he worked alone; he didn't collaborate with a good radiologist in order to get good pictures, and he didn't get reproducible pictures either on himself or animals. You see, he was not prepared to work with other people, and I think that this was his main trouble. When he was working in Berlin and tried to interest Sauerbruch in the possible advantages of heart catheterization in introducing drugs directly into the right atrium, Forssmann probably didn't get support from some key people he needed because of some personal differences between them.

> My former chief, HANS HECHT, at one time carried on an extended corre-spondence with Forssmann and got the impression that, despite his major contribution in demonstrating the feasibility of heart catheteriza-tion in man, he may have overstepped himself later in claiming credit for all the advances it led to.

Professor Eric Berglund once showed me a letter from Forssmann claiming that he had the idea for every development published later on by others in the literature. This is what I call "cryptomnesia," that is, secret memory. It is a term introduced by Robert Merton and refers to the situation in which you read something somewhere and later forget the origin and come to think that the thought was your own. Forss-mann deserves great credit for introducing the catheter into his own right atrium and suggesting the later use of angiography with the injection of radiopaque substances for X-ray pictures. The reason for his use of catheterization, stated in his first paper, was to introduce drugs directly into a heart chamber rather than risk cardiac tampon-ade by inserting a needle into the heart through the chest wall. He vaguely referred to "heart function," but he never mentioned the study of the physiology of the circulation. When he died a few months ago,

I regret to say that, in the article published in the *New York Times* scientific section, the writer attributed to him all the work that was initiated by our group in New York during and after the Second World War.

> Forssmann first catheterized himself in 1929. The following year you arrived in New York from France; in 1932 you had already formed an alliance with Dickinson Richards to study the circulation. How did this come about?

I started my studies in the Faculty of Medicine at the Sorbonne in Paris in 1914. The war had started, and, except for a few of the older professors, most of the faculty had gone off to serve in the army. After about four or five months, I decided to volunteer myself and first went into an infantry regiment. I was then assigned as a medical student to an advanced ambulance service and later made an auxiliary battalion surgeon. We were taught to stabilize fractures and perform a number of other first-aid procedures before shipping the wounded back behind the front lines. There were a tremendous number of casualties among physicians in the army at the front, so that is the reason they put us students there. I was wounded and gassed on the eighth of August 1918, and spent the whole of the winter in Paris before starting in at the beginning to study medicine again in the spring of 1919.

I had a long period of training as a student, intern, and resident. By 1930 I had written my thesis for my M.D., "Acute Disseminated Sclerosis," and was about to start as an assistant in medicine at a hospital in Paris. Before beginning this, I decided that I would like to spend a year in the United States. I had already more or less decided to practice hospital medicine rather than go into private practice in an office setting. The chief of the chest disease service at my hospital in Paris was a friend of Dr. James Alexander Miller at Bellevue Hospital in New York and arranged with him to have me come here. Although I had had thorough training in internal medicine and chest diseases in France, it was decided that I spend my first three months at Trudeau Sanatorium in upper New York State in order to improve my English before moving on to Bellevue.

Did you intend at that time to return to France?

Yes. But while at Bellevue, I published with Oswald Jones a paper on the shrunken middle lobe of the right lung in bronchiectasis. Then Dr. Miller offered me the opportunity to stay on in a full-time research position. "If you succeed," he said, "maybe we'll make something of it. Are you willing to take a chance?" And I agreed. I was thirty-five years of age at the time.

I already had a wife and two children in France and had to arrange to get them settled accordingly.

I started as a fellow in medicine and was supported by a chemical foundation. In 1933 I became chief medical resident of the Columbia Division at Bellevue. At about this time I began my association with Dickinson Richards, who was then an assistant attending physician at the Columbia-Presbyterian Hospital uptown in Washington Heights.

> There are two schools of thought about the conduct of scientific research. The popular one is that scientists plan precisely in advance what they are going to do and then do it. This, at least, is what we all try to imply in our research grant applications, although ALBERT SZENT-GYÖRGY, one of the people I admire most, once admitted, "When I go into the laboratory I'm never quite sure what I am going to do."
>
> To quote you directly: "In 1932, Dickinson Richards, then at the Columbia-Presbyterian Medical Center, and I, chief resident of the Chest Service (Columbia University Division) at Bellevue in New York, agreed on a systematic and comprehensive examination of the cardiopulmonary function in normal and diseased man."[3] You were both thirty-seven then, and it was still fairly early in your careers. Did you really have your whole plan thought out so systematically at that time?

Let me tell you how all this came about. When Dr. J. Alexander Miller, who was head of the Chest Service at Bellevue, asked me to stay, he inquired if I would be interested in doing some work with Dickinson Richards on the following subject: Why is it that some patients undergoing thoracoplasty* die and others do not? What makes the difference in the result?

---

* A therapeutic collapse of the lung, usually performed for tuberculosis at the time.

Richards and I recognized that unless you could study the function of the lung, the chest cage, and the circulation (that is, the heart), the answer would not be forthcoming. You must realize that Richards was superbly prepared to approach such studies. While he was working for his medical degree at Columbia, he also earned a master's degree in physiology. He was greatly influenced by the work of Harvard's Lawrence J. Henderson on the physiology of the blood and respiratory gases. His earliest work, prior to our collaboration, dealt with the effects of anemia on the circulation and the oxyhemoglobin dissociation curve of the blood. He also studied the effects of oxygen therapy in heart failure and pulmonary disease. He spent a year in London with Henry Dale, later Sir Henry Dale, studying the hepatic circulation. So that by the time we got together in 1932, we had a clear idea of what had to be done. We prepared an exhibit for the New York Academy of Medicine in 1933, outlining the problems to be studied, and we constantly referred to it. It was produced years later, in 1938, in the *Journal of Thoracic Surgery*.[4] In it we delineated all the structures involved in circulatory and respiratory function (the chest wall, the muscles, the lung, the heart, the blood, the arteries and veins and tissue, etc.), the function of each of these (ventilation, gas transport, energy exchange, etc.), and the techniques of measurements involved (ventilation, blood gas content, blood pressure, cardiac output, and so on).

These were all the considerations that we had in regard to studying first pulmonary collapse therapy, then prevalent in the treatment of pulmonary tuberculosis, and, later, chronic fibrosis of the lung and emphysema. Still later on, the methods became applicable to a wide variety of lung and heart diseases.

What specifically got you into catheterizing the heart?

A popular method for measuring cardiac output at the time was the "indirect Fick" method, using a rebreathing technique and measuring carbon dioxide in the expired gases. This is an indirect way to find out the concentration of the gas in the blood coming into the right heart from all parts of the body: the mixed venous blood. But in patients with pulmonary disease one could not predict this from the rebreathing method because of the different blood flow and gas distributions through different parts of the lung, normal and abnormal. We realized that we would have to get venous blood samples directly from the right heart in order to get accurate values of gas concentrations to compare with the arterial blood gas concentrations that we could easily get by sticking a brachial or radial artery. Using the difference between the two, we could directly apply the Fick principle.

In 1936 I returned to Paris on a visit with one of my former teachers, Dr. G. Ameuille, who had completed pulmonary angiography in a hundred patients. I spoke with him and reviewed all the cases that had been presented at the Société Médicale des Hôpitaux. His work on this when published, incidentally, had been received very critically by the great cardiologists of the time, who told him it was "monstrous" to do such a thing as introduce a tube into the heart of a patient. But what impressed me was that he had had no complications; the patients had tolerated the procedure very well. So I brought back with me to the United States some ureteral catheters, which at that time were manufactured only in France, and also some large needles with which to introduce them into veins through the skin. Between 1936 and 1940 we studied dogs exclusively, developing the techniques for manipulating the catheters. On one occasion, we also had the opportunity to study a chimpanzee. George Wright, who was a resident on the Chest Service, offered to advance ureteral catheters under fluoroscopic control into the right atrium of human cadavers in order to determine necessary catheter lengths for human studies and establish external reference points for measuring intracardiac pressure.

It was not until 1940 that Dr. Walter Palmer, chairman of the Department of Medicine, gave us permission to attempt a direct Fick determination of cardiac output in a patient, but he insisted that we choose a very ill patient. Unfortunately, the subject, who had cancer, had extensive metastases to the lymph nodes in the axilla, and Dick Richards was unable to get the catheter past them and into the right atrium. Our next opportunity came at Bellevue, where Dr. Herbert Chasis and his associates were interested in measuring cardiac output in hypertensive patients using the ballistocardiograph, the method being promoted by ISAAC STARR. However, they needed a reliable independent method to calibrate the ballistocardiograph before they could make their measurements. They were part of a group directed by HOMER SMITH, the great kidney physiologist; and they were the first ones to have emphasized the importance of blood flow to the kidney in systemic hypertension. I went to the dining room in the Nurses' Home, where all of us at Bellevue ate at the time, and sat down with Homer Smith, who started talking with me about measuring cardiac output. I told him the best way of getting a good Fick cardiac output was by passing a catheter to the right atrium, as had been done by Forssmann and others. Smith said, "If that's the best method, why not do it?" and arranged with the head of the department of medicine to allow us to study some of his hypertensive patients. This led to our first report on the direct Fick method for cardiac output, published in 1941.[5] Between 1941 and 1945 we improved the technique to include the measurement of heart pressures, develop better catheters and needles, provide electrocardiographic monitoring during procedures, and so forth.

We know that Forssmann and Ameuille met with resistance to the procedure of heart catheterization. What was your own experience after you made your initial reports?

Something happened in December 1941, December 7 to be precise, that resulted in the total absence of resistance to the development of cardiac catheterization in this country. This, of course, was the attack on Pearl Harbor and the beginning of World War II for the United States. Immediately after Pearl Harbor there was a meeting of the American Thoracic Surgical Society in New Orleans, and I met there with the surgeon ALFRED BLALOCK. I showed him what we could do with the catheter, because we already had experience measuring cardiac output and pressures, and indicated that there was also the possibility of now measuring blood volume with methods being developed by Gregersen, the professor of physiology at Columbia. Blalock, at that time, was chairman of the "Shock Committee" in Washington, and I told him that we might be able to contribute greatly to the study of shock by the use of these new methods. He said, "You have your grant," because this was precisely what he was interested in, what with the war casualties coming on and all. We were lucky to have a man like Blalock to deal with, a surgeon who was an investigator and had studied shock in dogs, but realized that the situation might be quite different in man.

So we studied all kinds of shock in 125 cases: traumatic shock, hemorrhagic shock, burn shock, ruptured viscus [bowel] leading to shock. We studied all kinds of treatment: plasma, whole blood, saline, gelatin, drugs. In New York City during the first two years of the war there were still a number of automobile vehicles in operation, and we arranged to have all severe traffic injuries studied by us. We had a very good team, with a surgical resident on call twenty-four hours a day. I had my technicians in contact with me by phone, and as soon as a surgical resident had a case, he would call me and I would go to the hospital to see the patient with him. I could then call in my technicians at any time, the middle of the day or night, to study these patients and evaluate their treatment. When traffic decreased with gas rationing, and the number of traumatic cases was reduced, we turned to the study of shock in burns and the other situations I mentioned.

Once the procedure of heart catheterization became well accepted for these cases, and it was realized how well it was tolerated, we were able to turn our attention to the study of a wide variety of pulmonary and heart diseases.

There was another interesting development as a result of the war. In 1944 I was asked by the Air Corps if I would take on with me a captain assigned to study pressure breathing. At that time they were very anxious to find out the best way to assist breathing in personnel who were wounded in the air, and were perhaps in shock or going into shock. Which type of pressure breathing might be the best in terms of effect on the cardiac output?

[Ray] Bennett was the first engineer with whom we worked, and before the final model was constructed, we had a special instrument prepared in which we could control every aspect of pressure breathing: the curve of pressure, the type of release of pressure (sudden or gradual) from peak inspiration to expiration, the volume of each respiration, the rate of respiration, et cetera. We worked on this for almost two years to develop the best system. This resulted in the prototype of all the kinds of ventilation-assisting devices that are now used in hospitals by anesthesiologists and others.

> **You spent virtually your entire career at Bellevue. The popular conception of it used to be that it was just a place they sent mentally deranged people picked up off the streets of the city. What was it really like?**

I have always been a Bellevue-Columbia man. From the time of the early thirties when I began there, Bellevue's reputation constantly improved because Columbia, New York University, and Cornell each had their own divisions there. Now there was a fourth division early on that was later taken over by New York University, and that was the one that might have been called the "political division." The physicians there were not of the same caliber as those on the university divisions. There were always these large wards at Bellevue, each with at least twenty-five beds, and sometimes additional cots were put up in the middle of the ward, so that material conditions were not the best. But the nursing care was excellent, and the attending staff and house staff provided the finest medical care for their patients. I would also emphasize that although there were three university services, this did not affect cooperation among us. Homer Smith, for example, was a New York University man, and I was with Columbia, but that did not prevent our groups from working together. On the shock work all three university services were involved.

> **Medical circles during the years in which you worked were not often very hospitable to women, but one cannot help noting the number of women who have always circulated around you—IRENÉ FERRER, RÉJANE HARVEY . . .**

You're speaking of the women who worked with me? For a moment I thought you wanted to know about "the women in my life"!

> **No, I didn't want to get that personal.**

I don't know if it has anything to do with my being a Frenchman, but at Bellevue, from a very early time onward, I was always in favor of using the best talent I could find regardless of race, religion, or sex.

Throughout my life this has never made any difference to me. I had the first black secretary at Bellevue, and then an Oriental secretary. I worked with Janet Baldwin, because she was a pediatrician interested in congenital heart disease and was interested in applying our method to the diagnosis in that kind of problem. We worked with ELEANOR BALDWIN, who contributed to many other types of studies. Réjane Harvey and Irené Ferrer were interested in acquired heart disease and the influence of pulmonary disease on the circulation and worked with us along those lines.

> **Speaking of your French background, I have always wondered if you ever felt some special affinity for ALEXIS CARREL, who also came from France and was the first "American" to win the Nobel Prize in medicine for his work on experimental vascular surgery and organ transplants. Was he a hero of yours?**

I knew of his work, of course, but I wouldn't say that he was a hero of mine. Incidentally, Carrel's wife seldom came to the United States; she preferred France. And when I was unable to bring my little family with me when I first began working in New York, they remained for a time in the same village in Brittany where the wife of Carrel lived.

Do you have any regrets about your career?

Oh yes. I have missed many things. For instance, I was probably the first one to go into the coronary sinus* from the right atrium. I realized where I was but didn't take advantage of it to study the metabolism of the heart. I should have written a book on clinical shock but never did. You see, I prepared over forty reports for the committee on shock: monthly reports, semiannual reports, annual reports, biannual reports. By 1945, when we prepared our final report, I was so fed up with reports that I never wrote the book, although we did sum up our findings in four or five papers that went into the literature.

Then I began to feel the pressure of other groups of investigators who were going ahead with the study of all kinds of heart disease. We

---

* The main vein draining the heart itself.

realized that we could study cardiac failure, congenital heart disease, rheumatic heart disease, and the pulmonary circulation. But you couldn't do everything. We had to go ahead and prepare papers as the technique was developing, and, in order to "remain liquid" in financing, I had to continuously prepare grant applications et cetera.

Who were the people that influenced you the most?

You asked me if I had a hero in my life. I have written a number of things about Dick Richards. With Robert Debré, a world-renowned pediatrician who was my chief in Paris, Richards was one of the two greatest men I have been in close contact with in my life. He was a humanist; he was a Hellenist; he was a scientist; he was a superb clinician; and he was an outstanding gentleman. I have never met another man as remarkable as he. We had a most unusual collaboration. Initially he taught me many of the techniques we would have to use for our research, and we worked together at Columbia and Bellevue from 1932 to 1973, the year of his death. A collaboration of forty-one years.

Did you ever have arguments?

A lot of arguments, but always "nice" arguments in which we respected one another. Richard Riley, who was Dickinson Richards's brother-in-law, once compared the two of us when he presented the Trudeau Medal to me. We were the same age but totally different people. He was very solid, admirably organized, while I was more prone to go off on a tangent and imagine things. Riley suggested that perhaps I had a bit more imagination than Richards, but that he had a much more solid scientific background than I.

It sounds like a good combination. It certainly worked.

It was a perfect combination.

3

Mary Allen Engle, m.d.
(1922–)

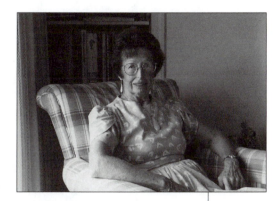

Perhaps there is nothing so heartbreaking as witnessing an infant or small child gasping for breath and dying as a result of heart disease, most often congenital in nature at this time of life. Yet as late as the eighth edition of William Osler's *Principles and Practice of Medicine* (1912), only four and a half of the 1,226 pages were devoted to the subject. Congenital heart diseases, Osler explained, "have only a limited clinical interest, as in a large proportion of the cases the anomaly is not compatible with life and in others nothing can be done to remedy the defect or even to relieve the symptoms."

Given this dismal outlook, there was little incentive to investigate the types and catalog the clinical aspects of these malformations that led to such tragic ends so early in life. Nevertheless, there were some, notably outstanding women, who contributed early on to our understanding and recognition of congenital heart disease even when no surgical relief for these conditions was envisioned. One of them was the Canadian Maude Abbott, an 1894 graduate of the medical school at Bishop's College in Montreal. An admirer of Osler, she was encouraged by him in her passion for collecting, cataloging, and, equally important, divining the physiological effects of various congenital cardiac malformations at the McGill Medical Museum, where she worked first as assistant curator and then as curator. The culmination of this effort, over a period of about forty years, was a 1936 exhibit of her findings in one thousand cases,

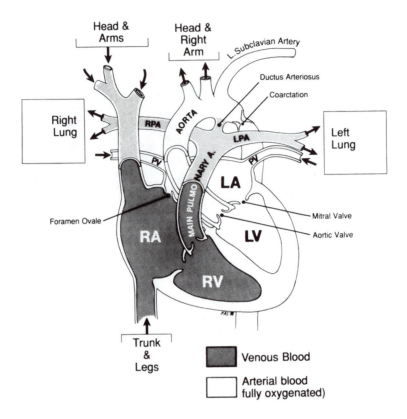

FIGURE 3-1. The heart and its major vessels. A patent ductus arteriosus and co-arctation have been drawn in to illustrate the location of these congenital abnormalities. The foramen ovale between the right and left atria is open in utero and closes after birth. (Abbreviations: RA = right atrium; RV = right ventricle; LA = left atrium; LV = left ventricle; RPA = right pulmonary artery; LPA = left pulmonary artery; PV = pulmonary vein.)

later documented in a publication of the American Heart Association for all future investigators and practitioners.[1]

Not long after this, in 1938, Harvard surgeon ROBERT E. GROSS would usher in a new era by performing the first successful closure of a patent ductus arteriosus* in a seven-and-a-half-year-old child.[2] (Fig. 3-1.) In 1944, six years later, two other momentous surgical feats were achieved. CLARENCE CRAFOORD in Sweden, spurred on by

---

* Persistence of the intrauterine connection between the aorta and pulmonary artery beyond birth.

Gross's work in this area, was the first to repair a coarctation of the aorta (a congenital constriction of the thoracic aorta),[3] and, at Johns Hopkins, the "blue baby" operation for the cyanotic congenital malformation Tetralogy of Fallot* was introduced by surgeon ALFRED BLALOCK and pediatrician HELEN TAUSSIG.[4] This involved creating a connection between the systemic circulation (an aortic branch) and pulmonary artery branch to allow for additional exposure of poorly oxygenated systemic blood to the lungs and relief of the severe cyanosis (hypoxemia or low oxygen content) that characterized this condition.

All three of these surgical procedures, which involved interventions concerning the vessels emerging from the heart (the aorta, pulmonary artery, and their branches), have collectively been called "extracardiac surgery." Direct operation upon the heart, itself, would come later, but these earlier procedures opened the door to such operations for acquired as well as congenital defects of the heart.

Present at that historic first Blalock-Taussig procedure was a senior medical student, originally from Oklahoma but raised in Texas. Mary Allen English, who would later be known as Mary Allen Engle, was one of the earliest of Taussig's fellows and a pioneer in pediatric cardiology.

After earning her B.A. degree at Baylor University in Waco, Texas, she attended Johns Hopkins Medical School, from which she graduated in 1945. Beginning as an intern and then resident in pediatrics, she quickly came under the influence of Dr. Taussig. When she moved to New York Hospital–Cornell with her newly acquired husband, Ralph Engle, in 1948, she began an association with that institution that ran almost without interruption until 1992, the year of her retirement.

In New York she was able to establish a program in pediatric cardiology which developed into a first-rate division, now named for her, within the Department of Pediatrics. The author of many articles on congenital as well as acquired heart disease, she followed in the footsteps of her mentor, Taussig, by training numerous

---

* Basically a ventricular septal defect with narrowing (stenosis) of the pulmonic valve with aortic overriding of the ventricular septum and right ventricular hypertrophy to complete the tetrad.

generations of future specialists in this discipline. Starting at a time when pediatric cardiology was not a recognized specialty, Dr. Engle was instrumental in setting up standards incorporated into what now is the subspecialty Board of Pediatric Cardiology.

Among her many professional accomplishments, perhaps one of the most notable is that she did all this at a time when women were not universally welcome in medicine. Many other women in similar positions attempted to mimic the aggressive behavior of their male counterparts. Through it all, however, Dr. Engle, for all her accomplishments and positions of influence, has never lost the ladylike qualities of grace, consideration, and good cheer.

Easton, Maryland
August 27, 1999

Let's begin this interview with your recollections of HELEN B. TAUSSIG. You were present at the first "blue baby" operation. What was it like?

I was a senior medical student and substitute intern on pediatric surgery at Johns Hopkins Medical School. DENTON COOLEY, who was an intern then, was my immediate superior; Harry Muller was assistant resident; and Bill Longmire the chief surgical resident. It just happened to be the time when Eileen Saxon, a very blue baby, had her operation. She was about a year old and had frequent Tetralogy attacks (hypercyanotic attacks, Dr. Taussig called them), and had to be in an oxygen tent all the time. She had great dyspnea. She was really very sick. It was like a miracle happening that day, with me way out on the perimeter of history being made. It was a tremendously exciting time.

I had known, when I went to medical school, that I wanted to be a pediatrician. I decided then and there that I wanted to be a pediatric cardiologist, and I was lucky that I could be.

ALFRED BLALOCK had sort of been prepared for this operation when he was at Vanderbilt doing shunts with Sanford Levy to produce experimental pulmonary hypertension,[5] working on an operation for coarctation of the aorta and so on.

He did this work with VIVIEN THOMAS, who came with him to Hopkins. There was a lot of talk about Dr. Blalock's work at the time. Dr. Taussig, Dr. Blalock, and Dr. Edwards A. Park, who was chairman of pediatrics then, had discussed the possibilities together. Dr. Park was a very farsighted man, and he saw some promise in this work. So he gave it his approval. Eileen was the properly selected very sick baby who needed help, and they did it successfully. Along with Dr. Taussig, Vivien Thomas was there in the operating room because Blalock depended upon him a lot since they had been partners for such a long time.

> People don't realize it, but I believe Blalock and Thomas worked on a hundred, perhaps two hundred, dogs after arriving at Johns Hopkins before attempting the first of these operations.

He continued working in the experimental surgery laboratory with Vivien.

> How long did it take Dr. Taussig, after being turned down by ROBERT E. GROSS, to get Blalock to perform the operation?

You probably know of Gross's response: "Madam, I close off patent ductuses; I do not create them." And she left. It probably did not take her too long to convince Blalock because he had a prepared mind. He was willing to accept a new concept, and he did it. He was at Hopkins only a few years before he performed the first of these operations.

> One gathers from people who were at Hopkins then that the relationships among the participants might have been strained at times. I have heard that there was a "Blalock camp" and a "Taussig camp." How much of this was real and how much manufactured?

There is some truth to it. But they had great respect for one another. I remember when we rotated through surgery, and Dr. Blalock came upon a patient with congenital heart disease, he would pay great tribute to Dr. Taussig. He would say, "There are few people in the whole world who could make this diagnosis correctly," and she was one of them. And, in turn, she had great respect for his surgical skill. Then you would have to put a third person in this and make it a triangle. Richard

Bing was there running the catheterization laboratory. And while it was a team that accomplished a great deal, there was some friction, and the people that were in the catheterization laboratory supported Bing; the pediatric cardiology fellows supported Taussig; and the surgeons supported Blalock. But we were all smart enough to know that it took a team to make this work, and it did work.

> **If there was friction, Taussig certainly had a number of reasons for it. She had a very tough life: her mother died when she was eight; she was dyslexic; she was denied admission to Harvard Medical School even though her father was a distinguished professor of economics at Harvard; she had growing deafness. One of her former fellows wrote, following her death, "She suffered."[6] What is your take on this?**

I was devoted to her, and as I learned more and more about her, I admired her even more for what she had accomplished. Her mother died from tuberculosis. Her father was so patient with her, teaching her to read so that she could start school. Then she graduated from Stanford Phi Beta Kappa; she graduated from Hopkins AOA (Alpha Omega Alpha, the medical honor society). I guess she was the original women's libber. She was offered the opportunity to audit courses at Harvard, and she said that she would have been seated up in the back so that she wouldn't "contaminate" the male medical students. When she received an honorary degree from Harvard many years later, in her acceptance speech she reminded them of this. She was a survivor, and she prevailed. She continued to learn, and grow and accomplish, and teach. I just admired her tremendously.

Regarding her deafness, I can imagine how devastating it must have been to a budding young cardiologist to realize she was losing her ability to hear. But she coped. Not only did she learn to enhance her senses of sight and touch, but she also obtained an amplifying stethoscope, and a hearing aid about the size of a hand-held television control and twice as thick. She wore it on a cord around her neck, neatly tucked beneath her dress until she pulled it out to hear a conversation better. Later miniaturizations in the 1950s placed hearing aids in temple pieces of eyeglasses. She remarked that it was so nice to have her ears back up where they belonged! The ultimate improvement did not come until shortly before her retirement when she successfully underwent bilateral stapes operations for otosclerosis. She was immensely happy to be able to use the Littman stethoscope.

Regarding her other tools for diagnosis, she had her eyes, hands, the ECG, the blood count, and chest X-ray. But her most important tool was the fluoroscope. When her chairman, Dr. Park, appointed her chief of the cardiac clinic, he gave her a fluoroscope and instructions to learn about congenital heart disease, and not just about rheumatic fever and rheumatic heart disease, of which there were cases aplenty. She developed a most informative technique. As fellows, we donned dark glasses like her for our eyes to accommodate before we crowded behind her into the little fluoroscopy room. There she looked at the child's heart in four views: frontal, lateral, and both right and left anterior oblique views to assess the size of each cardiac chamber. Barium swallows (chocolate-flavored) outlined the esophagus to reveal left atrial enlargement as well as the side of the aortic arch and presence of retroesophageal vessels. She also compared vascularity in each lung field and determined whether it was increased, decreased, or normal. She combined this information with that from the history, physical examination, ECG, blood count, and standard X-rays to reach a usually accurate physiologic and often precise anatomic diagnosis. Unfortunately, in the days before cardiac surgery, there were many opportunities to confirm the diagnosis postmortem, which established her soon renowned reputation for diagnostic skill.

If she had a grudge against men, it was certainly very well founded, and, in fact, I was on the receiving end of that when I asked her to contribute to an oral history of twentieth-century medicine back in the early eighties. She wrote me back that she was only going to do her own work and not other people's work, et cetera. I persisted for a few years, and a couple of weeks after she finally agreed to meet with me regarding another project, she had that tragic fatal auto accident. So I never had the pleasure and privilege of meeting with her personally. Well, so much for Dr. Taussig. Now let's talk about Dr. Engle.

I have always maintained that women were smarter then men, and you provided proof of it, graduating first in your undergraduate class

**from Baylor and first in your medical school class at Hopkins. How many
women were there in your medical school class?**

There were seven in a class of seventy. Seven was all right; there were
some schools then, like Harvard, that had no women; there were others
that might have, among 125 students, only one woman. I would not
have wanted to be that one woman. But seven (10 percent) was acceptable, and I felt comfortable; I never felt that I had to prove myself.

Had did your family feel about your going into medicine back in 1942?

There was some feeling of trepidation because no one in my family had
ever been a physician, and they were a little shocked that I wanted to
become one. "Shocked" may be too strong a word; they were quietly
surprised by my decision but very supportive.

When I decided to apply, I had a chairman of chemistry and a
chairman of physics at Baylor tell me, "You can do it! Johns Hopkins is
the best. Apply there." That was the only medical school I applied to,
and I was fortunate to be accepted.

**Tell me about your experiences as an intern, resident, and fellow, follow-
ing your medical school graduation.**

Well, I felt very lucky about being able to stay in Baltimore. After finishing my internship and assistant residency in 1947, I was asked by Dr.
Taussig to become a fellow in pediatric cardiology. To do so was one of
the best decisions I ever made. One of the most remarkable things was
that she started a program whereby, every two years, former fellows
came back and met the current fellows. It always started with a picnic
on Sunday afternoon out on her front lawn, overlooking Lake Roland;
so everybody became acquainted. Then on Monday, Tuesday, and
Wednesday we had scientific sessions during the day sharing experiences and new knowledge, with socializing and fun during the
evenings. Now that was "continuing education" before that term ever
came into being. It was a wonderful continuing opportunity to learn,
and I appreciated it.

After the war ended in 1945, following his internship, my husband
still had to put two years into the service. When he got out in 1948, he

wanted to go to Cornell Medical College and the New York Hospital for training in medicine. So that's how I became a New Yorker. While my husband was doing a residency in medicine, I completed my pediatric residency requirements there in 1948–49. I then became a fellow in pediatric cardiology and pharmacology under Dr. Harry Gold until 1950. I became director of pediatric electrocardiography in 1949 and gradually worked to establish a cardiology program similar to that at Hopkins. I was appointed to the staff as an attending pediatrician in 1952. For a couple of years I was director for the care of premature infants while doing pediatric cardiology. In 1962 I became director of pediatric cardiology.

Were you involved in cardiac catheterizations?

At Hopkins, we rotated through Richard Bing's laboratory, although most of our training was a clinical fellowship under Dr. Taussig. I was very fond of Richard Bing. He was a charming and a brilliant person, although a little eccentric. But a lot of bright people are a little eccentric. At that time, incidentally, angiocardiography was separate, so we also had time in radiology learning to interpret X-rays and angio-cardiograms with Bob Cooley.

When we got to New York, I intended, at first, to stay only a year, because, as a person who had grown up in Dallas, Texas, I just was not going to like that "great big city" up there. I did take a year off, following the completion of my pediatric residency, because my husband wanted to do a year of hematology research training at Washington University in St. Louis. I was planning to do a pediatric cardiology fellowship in St. Louis, but when we got there in July, the next month my husband became a victim of the last polio epidemic before Dr. Salk's work took effect. So we spent a good bit of time with him in the hospital recovering. Then, in January, our daughter was born prematurely and very small. So I didn't have much time to do pediatric cardiology, although I did write a paper on the Wolff-Parkinson-White syndrome.

After a year in St. Louis, the best opportunities for both of us seemed to be at Cornell–New York Hospital; so we returned to the big city, and I learned to love it. We stayed there on the faculty till retiring, having contributed, as a couple, ninety years of our lives to that medical center.

Regarding your question about a cath lab, initially we did not have our own, but eventually, when pediatric cardiology was elevated to division status, we recruited Aaron Levin from Duke to establish a new state-of-the-art, complete laboratory for cardiac catheterization and selective angiography in infants and children. Before that, our fellows worked in the single cath lab for the hospital under Dan Lukas.

I was very fortunate at Cornell to have a good deal of support. The chairman of pediatrics, Dr. Sam Levine, supported my interest; the chairman of surgery, Dr. Frank Glenn, wanted to develop a program in cardiac surgery; Dr. Barr, the chairman of medicine, was also interested in congenital heart disease and was supportive. At the time of my arrival there was a long-standing rheumatic fever clinic that was being run by Dr. Maye Wilson, and she continued to follow these patients throughout their lives. She continued to take care of the children who had rheumatic fever, and that was fine; my interest was in congenital heart disease, and I pursued this.

We also worked very compatibly with CHARLIE DOTTER and ISRAEL STEINBERG in angiocardiography . . .

> They were both important figures. Steinberg did original work in angiography, and Dotter was probably the father of angioplasty, which he started in the lower limbs. Dotter, supposedly, is a real character.

He was a good friend of mine, and, like many people of genius, he was a character. He was a risk taker—he learned to fly his own plane—but before he took any risk, he thought it through. And he did develop angioplasty! He had early training in internal medicine but later worked full-time in the Department of Radiology with Steinberg.

"Gus" Steinberg was also a very creative person who, in addition to his practice, did a lot of writing and speaking, and shared his pioneering knowledge with the world.

> Who did the congenital heart surgery at Cornell?

Frank Glenn did some, but his skill was mainly directed to the kind of valve surgery that occurred in rheumatic heart disease. The congenital cases were taken on by George Holswade and Frank Redo. I should mention anesthesiology, because this really was a team effort, and Joe Artusio was in charge of anesthesiology, with Ben Marberry and Marge Topkins taking over the congenital heart work.

At one point, early in the development of open-heart surgery for congenital heart disease, Ben Marberry, George Holswade, and I took a trip to Minnesota to visit Lillehei and his team in Minneapolis; and then John Kirklin at Mayo Clinic. That was very early in the fifties, when open-heart surgery was just coming on board, and this was an important learning experience. We also visited Denton Cooley in Houston. I worked in the experimental surgery lab with George Holswade as we were trying to get things going with hypothermia and also the heart-lung machine. We started by using the bubble oxygenator.

Compare Lillehei and Kirklin.

Each, in his own way, contributed enormously to cardiac surgery, and each was my friend. My preference for the intellectual approach to congenital heart surgery was John Kirklin. Lillehei was a little more "unusual" as a person. Some years later he came to Cornell–New York Hospital, and I got to know him more as a colleague on-site. And this was not the happiest time of his career; that time was back in Minnesota, when he was developing all those innovations in congenital heart surgery.

What happened at Cornell?

It just didn't work. It was a little erratic and just didn't work smoothly.

Things changed so much over the years. I recall that, back in the early sixties, when I did my fellowship training at the University of Utah, your friend George Veasy would come in on Friday mornings to do congenitals with us. The rest of the time we either did adults or worked in the dog lab. Then, when I came to Jersey City with the Seton Hall College of Medicine, I suddenly became the consulting cardiologist for the Margaret Hague Maternity Hospital, which, along with Charity in New Orleans, was one of the two biggest in the country. And there I was, without much training in pediatrics, no less pediatric cardiology, responsible for all these infants, but there simply were not many pediatric cardiologists around at the time.

Cardiac catheterization, especially in small, sick infants, was a late development of pediatric cardiology. At first, it was considered a little risky, or possibly dangerous, and so, in the beginning, it was felt that only children over the age of two years could be subjected to these invasive procedures. Then, as techniques developed and improved, we could say with justification that there was no infant too sick or too small to undergo the necessary diagnostic studies.

Putting it all together was also an important advance. It used to be at Hopkins, and initially at Cornell, that the catheterization would be performed on one day, and then angiocardiography would be performed on another day. Finally we were able to combine the two procedures at one sitting.

You helped set up the Board of Pediatric Cardiology in 1960. Who else worked with you on this, and how did you go about it?

It was an outgrowth of my being appointed to the American Academy of Pediatrics Cardiology Committee with JIM DuSHANE as the chairman. By that time, in 1954, there were several places in the country that were starting programs in pediatric cardiology. So our committee requested to establish a Section on Pediatric Cardiology. It was the first section permitted by the academy. In the beginning, if pediatricians could provide evidence of having been involved and proficient in this work, they would be "approved" as section members. But we came to realize that just accepting pediatricians on the basis of their saying "This is what I have done" was not enough. So our Section Committee decided that it would be appropriate to have examinations for board certification in pediatric cardiology. In the Academy of Pediatrics there had not been subspecialty boards prior to this, so it, too, had to go through an approval process. It was approved, and the same committee began giving written and oral examinations in pediatric cardiology. Early board members included "pioneers" such as DAN McNAMARA,

Ed Lambert, Helen Taussig, and FORREST ADAMS.

Dr. Taussig wrote an important book on congenital heart disease.

It was a classic, the bible of pediatric cardiology.[7] The Commonwealth
Fund published it, and I'm sure that when she started writing it and
they decided to publish it, they had no idea that the field would take off
as it did. When it was published in 1947, soon, all over the world, people
were reading her book and learning from it.

**The books by ALEXANDER NADAS and the one by JOHN D. KEITH, RICHARD D.
ROWE, and Peter Vlad were also influential. Did you know them?**

Oh yes. Pediatric cardiologists who started early, like Alexander Nadas
and Jim DuShane, and others I have mentioned all bonded together.
We knew we were all headed in the same direction with the same goals
of helping babies and children become healthy, no matter what they
had been born with. We were all on the same programs; we worked in
different places but in a collegial way.

I told you before about the gatherings at Dr. Taussig's home. Well,
she "adopted" Alex Nadas and John Keith into that community of
"Taussig's knights" even though they hadn't trained with her. Nadas
had a marvelous sense of humor; he was great. Rowe was in New
Zealand before working with John Keith in Toronto, but later came to
work at Hopkins, where he succeeded Dr. Taussig.

**After reviewing your career and your bibliography, I came to the conclu-
sion that you were interested in *everything*: ventricular septal defects,
pulmonic stenosis, the Mustard procedure, the postpericardiotomy syndrome, thalassemia . . .**

And Kawasaki disease; that was the last. And that was a totally
unknown disease before Kawasaki began writing about it. Then it
seemed to advance from Asia to Hawaii, to the West Coast, and finally
we started seeing a number of these patients in New York.* But this was
not until the late eighties. The cause is still unknown; although it seems

---

* Cardiologists were brought in because in about 20 percent of these patients the coronary arteries become involved and, in some cases, this may be fatal.

to act like a virus, this has not yet been proven. We started doing epidemiological studies on it at Cornell, and we also tried to identify a group that could be helped if therapy were to become available. We learned about the course of the disease, and since I was often asked to talk at medical meetings about this new, puzzling, and frightening disease, which could be lethal, patients began to be referred to us. When we became able to do something for it, with a large single dose of intravenous gamma globulin that just stopped the illness in its tracks, we had a substantial number of patients available to us for this therapy. Now the disease is definitely controllable with large doses of gamma globulin. I cannot tell you why it works, but it does.

Have you followed your patients from childhood into adulthood?

Again, I modeled what I did after Dr. Taussig. She continued to see her children as they grew up; she was invited to their graduations, their weddings. If they happened to have someone in the family with congenital heart disease, she also took care of that child. During my time at Cornell, no one was interested in following these patients into adulthood, so I did and learned a lot in the follow-up. My patients still continue to call me. I recently got a letter from someone who wrote, "I am now thirty-one. You met me when I was three with a hole in my heart. I am so grateful for what you did, but in particular, I am so grateful for my scar." And that's something I have to tell you about.

At Cornell, I was lucky to work with surgeons who were aware of how important was the placement of the scar, particularly in girls. These surgeons, Paul Ebert and Bill Gay, were willing, on girls, to make an inframammary incision across the chest instead of straight down the middle of the sternum. Most midsternotomy scars wind up with an obvious keloid from the top of the sternum down. With an inframammary flap, the incision site would become almost invisible and the girls could later wear a bikini or evening gown with no scar showing.

Is there any medical problem where your approach has changed dramatically over the years?

I think we learned the most about ventricular septal defects and their variety over the years. In Dr. Taussig's book, the murmur was well described, but what she was talking about was the very small "maladie de Roger." This is still very common, and fairly well tolerated. However, when I got to Cornell, I started out by looking up the autopsies of anyone that had ever died with that diagnosis, and I was shocked to learn how many babies had died in cardiac failure with an isolated ventricular septal defect. So this was the first realization that there could be large defects, as well. We published this in about 1954.[8] This was the time when we began to succeed in medical management of their cardiac failure and also the time that Lillehei began to close these defects in Minneapolis.

The other remarkable thing we found was that some of these defects actually closed spontaneously. Who would have believed that? So at the same time surgeons were becoming capable of closing them, we learned that, in some patients, you could wait a bit using medical management if they weren't desperately ill, and the hole might get smaller or even close on its own.

When did the pulmonary artery banding operation* come in?

Around the same time, in the midfifties. FRANK DAMMAN, who had been a fellow with Dr. Taussig, overlapping with me during my time there, got together with Dr. Harry Muller, who had concurrently been on the surgical house staff with Dr. Blalock. They worked together when their careers took them to California, and the two of them developed the concept that these babies with large ventricular septal defects would not die if their lungs were not so flooded with blood flow, shunting through the large hole between the two ventricles. So how do you stop this from happening? You put a band on the pulmonary artery and stem the tide (i.e., reduce the amount of left-to-right shunt). So that

---

* In the early days of open-heart surgery, when it was felt to be too dangerous to perform this procedure on very small infants, for these patients with large ventricular septal defects the pulmonary artery was partially occluded to reduce the degree of left-to-right shunting and its attendant complications, with closure of the defect at open-heart surgery anticipated when the infant was larger and at less of a risk for such repair. Today there is essentially no size limit for the performance of open-heart surgery in infants.

operation worked very well until open-heart surgery for tiny babies became a reality and septal defects themselves could be closed.

> Another change that occurred was the ability to diagnose all kinds of heart disease with echocardiography. This was so much easier than had been the case in the past. When I read your first paper with Dr. Taussig, dealing with the diagnosis of Ebstein's disease,[9] what struck me was that premortem you missed the diagnosis in all three cases. The purpose of the paper was to review aspects of the clinical picture that might be helpful in the future. And in the cath lab we went through all sorts of diagnostic contortions with intracardiac ECGs and so on, trying to make the correct diagnosis. Today you put an echo transducer on the chest of the patient, and, within thirty seconds, you can make the diagnosis with ease.

Very true. I didn't talk about the more recent developments in pediatric cardiology when I mentioned combining the other diagnostic entities, but echocardiography, two-dimensional and then with Doppler, has been wonderful. So simple, so painless, and so accurate that many children with congenital heart disease no longer need to be catheterized to confirm the diagnosis.

> There have been so many advances in the treatment of congenital heart disease; what are the problems that we still are unable to deal with?

There are very few that cannot be dealt with. Some patients are cured, while some are palliated by surgery, but not really corrected. Coarctation of the aorta, for instance: if the surgeon can completely remove the obstruction, that's a cure. The same is true for patent ductus arteriosus: ligation provides a complete cure. Closing atrial or ventricular septal defects provides real cures. But other defects continue to pose problems in later life. Take Tetralogy of Fallot, a very common malformation that, even after complete surgical correction, can present problems with arrhythmias or right ventricular dysfunction, and even death later in life in some patients. Then there is the hypoplastic left heart syndrome: it's hard to build a left heart when the mitral valve is atretic [without an opening] and the left ventricle is such a tiny chamber and the ascending aorta is only a thin thread. The Mustard and other similar operations for transposition of the great arteries are highly beneficial but only palliative, not corrective. There are built-in problems, waiting to happen.

I suppose cardiac transplantation is the answer for some of these conditions.

And that works better in little children, remarkably, than in adults. Their immune system seems better able to tolerate transplanted hearts. That's something else in cardiac surgery that has developed, and credit should be given to DR. LEONARD BAILEY and Loma Linda Hospital in California for making us all realize that transplants can be effective in children and that the children grow into their transplanted hearts as they became older.

On the personal side, you seem to have balanced your life very well. You married while in medical school . . .

At Hopkins, classes were arranged in alphabetical order: I was Mary Allen English, and my lab partner for the first two years was Ralph Landis Engle. That turned out to be a good partnership, and, on graduation day, we got our degrees in the morning and had our marriage ceremony in the afternoon. And you met him this morning, about fifty-four years later. It worked.

We had two children. Our son, unfortunately, died, but our daughter and our two grandchildren live in Alexandria, Virginia. That's only an hour and a half away from where we are in Easton; so it's convenient to get together quite often. She thought about medicine but became interested in marine biology; so that has been her career choice.

Well, that's close. My son is a veterinarian and loves it.

While we're on the subject of younger people, I want to give credit to some of our fellows who joined our team upon completion of their training. I am proud of all of them, but especially those who went on to head their own pediatric cardiology divisions, like Charlie Kleinman at Yale and those who continued on as collaborators at New York–Cornell. In our own department Kathryn Ehlers was chief of the noninvasive laboratory; John O'Loughlin and Michael Snyder were in charge of echocardiography; Arthur Klein set up our exercise testing laboratory and outreach programs to other hospitals. To all of them I am grateful and appreciative.

On the surgical side, I worked closely and happily for many years; first with George Holswade and Frank Redo. Then there were PAUL EBERT, and BILL GAY, who succeeded him when Paul went to become chairman of surgery at the University of California in San Francisco. Wayne Isom and Jeff Gold then headed the team.

> When one considers women in medicine, there are some, like Taussig, who, with good reason I might add, were somewhat bitter. Others were like MARIAN ROPES, a rheumatologist at Mass. General I interviewed some years ago, who described herself as having rose-colored glasses throughout her professional life. She was at the other end of the spectrum. Where are you along that spectrum?

I like to think that I am in the middle. Like all medical students, I wanted to be a good doctor and to help people, but I aspired to be as complete a lady doctor as I could be, a lady with a fine husband and a family, and a doctor with a career in academic pediatric cardiology. I was lucky. I was in the right place at the right time, and it worked.

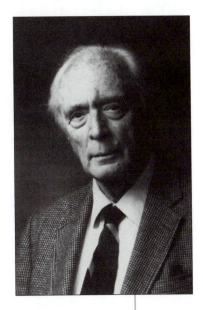

4

RICHARD J. BING, M.D.
(1909–   )

The term "Renaissance man" is one that tends to be applied too casually in attempts to honor public figures. However, in the case of Richard Bing it is impossible to describe him in any other way. Physician, cardiovascular researcher, physiologist, biochemist, teacher, author, composer, humanist; he has been all this and more over a period extending from his formative years in Europe to his present position as director of experimental cardiology and scientific development at the Huntington Medical Research Institutes in Pasadena, California, where he remains active in his tenth decade.

Not only has Dr. Bing excelled in so many different types of endeavor; he seems to have worked with or known an incredible collection of historically prominent people in cardiovascular research and medicine. Who else can one think of who is still living and has rubbed elbows with the likes of ALEXIS CARREL, CHARLES A. LINDBERGH, ALLEN O. WHIPPLE, HOMER W. SMITH, ALFRED BLALOCK, HELEN B. TAUSSIG, and TINSLEY R. HARRISON, among others?

Dr. Bing will be remembered for establishing a diagnostic cardiac catheterization laboratory under Alfred Blalock at Johns Hopkins during the heady early days of cardiac surgery for congenital heart disease. He also produced a distinctive history of cardiology that reflects his personal warmth, humor, and extensive background.[1] However, his inquiring mind and personal odyssey in Europe and then the United States exposed him to a variety of other interests and problems to which he has contributed greatly in our understanding of them.

Throughout this long and very productive career in medical science Dr. Bing has always nurtured his lifelong passion for music, as attested by the more than three hundred classical compositions to his credit.

Because of the many stops along the way during his peripatetic career, it may be helpful for the reader to have an outline of his travels.

1929–34   medical training in Vienna, Munich, Berlin

1935–36   Carlsberg Institute, Copenhagen

1936–37   Rockefeller Institute, New York

1938–39   intern, Columbia-Presbyterian Hospital (New York)

1939–42   New York University (Physiology)

1943–51   Johns Hopkins, Baltimore (U.S. Army, 1943–45)

1951–55   University of Alabama, Birmingham

1956–59   Washington University, St. Louis

1959–69   Wayne State University, Detroit

1969–   University of Southern California and Huntington Research Institutes and Memorial Hospital, Pasadena

Nothing quite prepares one for the delightful experience of spending a day in the company of Dr. Bing, who never tires of discussing his and others' past and present work with incredible recall and large dollops of humor. The only concession to his years was a sturdy cane he employed as he energetically conducted me on a tour of the Huntington laboratories.

In 1999, not long after our meeting, Dr. Bing had the pleasure of seeing the most recent performance of one of his works in Austria. Given the status of the composer, I thought it was very appropriately named: *Magnificat.*

———

Pasadena, California
September 15, 1998

———

As I thought back over your career in cardiology, I tried to think of some kind of analogy, and it occurred to me that if someone went to an aviator and asked him where he had learned to fly and was told, "with the Wright brothers," that would be very close to your own personal history in cardiology. It seems that you have been all over the place and that your career has been personally touched by just about everybody who was anybody in the field during the first half of the twentieth century.

Sometimes when I give a talk or a lecture and am asked if I met this one or that one, I say, "Yes, that is true, but I never met Hippocrates."

Since you have traveled so widely during your career and held so many different positions, it may be wise to approach this interview chronologically. First off, in your education, is it true that you had OTTO FRANK as a professor at one point?

No, he was not one of my professors, but I did hear him lecture. I had already had physiology in Wurzburg, so when I came to Munich this was behind me and I was not subjected to the horror of being examined by Frank. He was extremely tough. To some people he was apparently very comforting and pleasant, but to others he was horrible. WALTER ABELMANN from Boston was helpful to me with my book, and he was a student of Frank.

You have M.D. degrees from both Munich and Bern. How did that come about? Did you have to get out of Germany in the thirties?

Well, I had to get out of Germany for obvious reasons. I took the state board examinations in Munich because I had been a student there. At that time in Germany you moved around, taking different courses in different places in the country, and I finished in Munich. Then Hitler came, and I had to have a diploma. I passed the state board examination in Munich but was not able to get a diploma. So I went to Switzerland to get the diploma and took the examination over again. I knew that if I went to America they would demand to see a diploma indicating I was an M.D.

So you were already planning on going to America?

Oh yes. I left Germany in 1934, and all of my family got out later. Before I went to America, however, I went to the Carlsberg Institute in

Copenhagen, Denmark. I went to work with Albert Fischer to do tissue culture work. It was there that I met ALEXIS CARREL and CHARLES LINDBERGH.

There was an international meeting of biology of some sort to which Fischer, who had been a student of Carrel, invited him and Lindbergh to demonstrate their perfusion system.[2] They had been working on this at the Rockefeller Institute in New York for about a year at the time. I was chosen to help set this up because I spoke Danish and lousy English as well as German.

My role was something between that of a flunky and a young M.D. It was my responsibility to help set up the machine, et cetera. And then, for some reason, both Carrel and Lindbergh sort of took a liking to me and arranged for me to get a grant from Rockefeller to come to New York.

Tell me about Carrel and Lindbergh. What were they like?

Most of the descriptions of Carrel that you read are wrong. Some people make him out to have been a diabolical scientist with a Nazi connection. And some of these reports were related to political considerations at the Rockefeller Institute. But to me, a young kid, he was wonderful. I have many letters of his; nice, supportive, affectionate letters, and I never saw anything of this "diabolical" side to his nature.[3]

He did have a sort of "weirdo" side to his character, though, didn't he? I tried to read his book, *Man, the Unknown,* and I couldn't get through it.

Neither could I. As you say, he was in many ways very weird. He believed in supernatural phenomena and coming back after death. He was a Catholic who interpreted his religion as it suited him, all without guile. To me he was extremely pleasant. You know, a man knows only the side shown to him, and Carrel showed me only interest and affection.

He had already done all that cardiac surgical work and arterial suturing work before this?

It was in 1912 to 1914 that he did most of that work, but no one picked up on it. There was an article written by Julius Comroe called "Alexis Who?" because Carrel had been forgotten and Comroe wanted to revive the memory of what he had done.

How did he work? Was he a loner?

He wasn't a loner, but everyone in his department worked on his ideas. In that sense you might call him a loner, but in my department I say what we are going to work on and we do it, so this isn't unusual for a research laboratory. The boss determines what you will be working on. And Carrel was certainly in no other sense a loner. He loved company. Aside from Lindbergh, he was a great friend of [Albert] Einstein and others. Carrel cultivated famous people as he had that Platonic idea of a superstructure of society.

What about Lindbergh? He had pretty bad press with my generation.

Yes, but to me, again, he was a man who did everything in the world to make things easier for me. He helped get me to the Rockefeller. When I later went to Columbia University, he came over several times to help me with the work. I couldn't think of a more pleasant—actually simple—person, an extremely likable man. I saw only one side of him. Then came this German thing, and I sent him a telegram when he was in Berlin to protest against the inhumanity of the Nazis. After that, our relationship was finished for a while.

During the war I was in the service. He did some military flying, I understood. But after the war we actually became friends, and he had shed some of his misguided political past. The political part of him disappeared, and he became a strong environmentalist.

What happened after your stint at Rockefeller?

Carrel got me a surgical internship at Columbia-Presbyterian with Allen O. Whipple, who became my father-in-law. His daughter and I were married fifty-three years; she died six years ago. Although I was a surgical intern, I did no surgery; it was really a research position. After this, I was an instructor in physiology at Columbia for two years and then went to Bellevue on the NYU service.

At that time Bellevue was a city hospital but had a Columbia Service, an NYU Service, and a Cornell service as well as the regular independent city hospital staff. As an instructor in physiology there, I came under the influence of HOMER SMITH, whose laboratory was across the street from Bellevue on First Avenue—477 First Avenue, to be more precise, and it was the home of an incredible group of researchers at the time.

Homer Smith was a very unusual person.

There you are really on the mark. Homer Smith was extremely unusual. The work "loner" didn't apply to Carrel, but it certainly applied to him. For instance, we spent a summer with him in Maine working on the urinary excretion in the harbor seal, a miserable experience. And Smith woke up my wife and me on a Sunday morning—we had a little baby at the time—and he was very dictatorial and took us up mountain climbing. He never said a word on the trip. Finally, we reached the top of the mountain looking into space and not a word out of him, and we young people had to keep our mouths shut, unable to talk with him. And yet, there was a very romantic side to him. His books on evolution were wonderful.

I'll never forget the passage in *From Fish to Philosopher* where he writes, "With the evolution of the glomerular nephron, there began a battle between the kidney and the reproductive organs that continued for three hundred and fifty million years."

His ideas about why the dinosaurs died out had nothing to do with a big explosion or anything like that. He referred everything to the kidney. He looked at everything through a renal tubule.

There's a story I heard about his death from a nephrologist friend of mine. It seems he had an incapacitating stroke at the end of his life, and because he became so depressed over the limitations this put upon him, he committed suicide. Is this true?

I don't know. I only know that he had a severe problem with alcohol. When I was chairman of medicine at Wayne, I invited him to give a lecture. It was a wonderful lecture, but he appeared drunk when he delivered it. I don't exactly know where it is, but I have a recording of the lecture on tape, and the conclusion was extremely moving. At the end he said, "And now my dear friend, Richard, I bid you farewell," and he died not long thereafter. We had a lot going together, he and I. A strange man, but of all the people I have worked with, he was by far the most brilliant.

> He probably was more eloquent and made more sense drunk than a lot of other people could have who were sober. I gathered from Dr. Cournand that he was a great facilitator in getting research done at Bellevue.

The people who really facilitated the cooperation at Bellevue [between Columbia and NYU] were actually Goldring and Chassis who worked in the department of medicine at NYU and served as a bridge between Smith and the Columbia people, Cournand and Richards.

I was at Bellevue during the time this work was going on, with Richards primarily at "P&S" (Columbia's College of Physicians and Surgeons, with Presbyterian Hospital in Washington Heights) and Cournand at Bellevue. At this time I had no dealings with them at Bellevue, but later on, when I came back from the army and had an appointment at Johns Hopkins, I came back for a visit to Bellevue in preparation for setting up a catheterization laboratory there. I wanted to see how Cournand did cardiac catheterizations, he being the acknowledged master of the technique.

I went there and never saw him perform a cardiac catheterization. This is totally unknown, you know. I don't think he even had a license to practice in New York at the time. Others did a lot of the actual catheterizations, with Cournand directing the proceedings.

There was one episode I watched that I remember with horror. A catheterized man was riding a bicycle, and they wanted to see how the right ventricular and pulmonary artery pressures went up with exercise. All of a sudden the pressure tracings and everything disappeared. They began to fiddle around with the machine until someone had the good sense to look at the patient, who had slumped over and was unconscious!

When you first came to Bellevue-NYU, you did not think of yourself as a cardiologist, did you?

I was primarily a physiologist there, but I always wanted to go back into medicine. When the time came, I had a choice between the departments of medicine at either NYU or Hopkins. In retrospect, I would have loved to have stayed in New York and Smith really wanted me to remain, but the "glory" or whatever of Hopkins was too hard to resist. And it was a good experience. It made the little reputation I have, working with congenital heart disease.

That's getting a little ahead of our story, though. Could you straighten me out on the chronology of your comings and goings in Baltimore?

I know it is a little confusing. From NYU I went to the department of medicine at Johns Hopkins under [WARFIELD T.] LONGCOPE, who was the chief. During that time, for about a year, I acted as an assistant resident, because I needed that to get my license. I had taken the first two parts of my National Board exams in New York, but the third part I took at Hopkins, and once I had the national boards and my license I signed up for the army. I was sent by the army to Edgewood Arsenal, about forty miles outside of Baltimore. I was there when [ALFRED] BLALOCK decided he wanted me back at Hopkins in the department of surgery, and he got me released for this purpose.

There is an interesting story about this, which you may not be aware of: Before you went to work for Blalock, a friend of mine, FRANCIS CHINARD, who was later my chief of medicine, had just been discharged from the U.S. Army Air Corps and had done some work on the effects of altitude and had a really good background in physiology and basic science. He approached Blalock to present his credentials and felt he might contribute to the research program at Hopkins.

Blalock seemed very interested, but when Chinard, who had recently married and, I believe, had a baby on the way, respectfully addressed the question of salary toward the end of the interview, Blalock went off the wall. "Salary? I have no salary to give you. Haven't you got any money? Doesn't your wife have any money?" And that was the end of it.

This story tells us something about the financing for research, or lack of it, before the NIH [National Institutes of Health] really got going in giv-

ing out grants. Chinard has always wondered how you got the job
instead.

I know Chinard; he's a great man. For my part, I was just eating in the
mess hall in Edgewood when I got the call from Blalock asking if I
would like to get out of the army and come to Johns Hopkins. Well, that
was just like offering me Marilyn Monroe on a silver platter. I said, "Of
course," and Blalock took care of the arrangements. I came on as an
assistant professor of surgery, which didn't provide a lot of money, but
I was better off than Chinard in that respect. Now if Chinard had
shown Blalock his pretty wife, he would have been hired because
Blalock had an eye for the ladies.

What Blalock wanted me to do was the physiology of congenital
heart disease, and as long as I did that everything was fine, but then the
catheter slipped into the coronary sinus, and that was something new
altogether.

Up to this time you hadn't done any cardiac catheterizations. Did you go
up to New York to learn the technique?

I visited Cournand's lab three or four times, but, as I said before, I never
saw him do one personally. I was still in uniform at the time and
watched his team perform a few catheterizations before returning to
Hopkins, where I just began doing them myself.

You wrote some of the most important papers on the physiology of congenital heart disease, which many people may not recall. You also
described yourself as a sort of Daniel in the lions' den with Blalock and
Helen Taussig—the big cats.

Well, I did publish about sixteen or eighteen papers on congenital heart
disease while I was there.[4] I was hired by Blalock, not Taussig. Taussig,
like many women in science, never married and never had children,
and her profession was her whole life. She was extremely possessive and
had an ego as big as the Empire State Building. Now Blalock's ego was
of equal magnitude, but he always tried to play it down in a subtle way,
whereas Taussig showed it all the time. So they had tremendous egos
which conflicted, and here I was between the two, and I really never got

any of the credit for what I was doing—it all went to either Taussig or Blalock. So that's what I meant by being Daniel in the lions' den. The lions were around me, and all I could do was let out a squeak once in a while.

> Taussig resented men and had good reason to do so. This was compli-
> cated later on by her increasing deafness, and she also was sort of phys-
> ically clumsy. I tried to get her interview into an earlier book of mine,
> *Conversations in Medicine,* but she put up so many barriers to it that I
> finally had to give up on it. In going over your bibliography, I noted that
> at Hopkins you were doing all this work on congenital heart disease but
> there was only one paper I could find with both yours and Taussig's name
> on it, the one on the Taussig-Bing complex,[5] which you have referred to,
> I believe, as your only tenuous hold on immortality. Incidentally, no one
> seems to know what the Taussig-Bing complex is when you ask them,
> and, as a cardiologist, I don't believe I have ever seen a case of it.

Well, they call it all different sorts of names. I agree with what you said about her problems, but Taussig was extremely jealous of things that we did. At Hopkins there developed two camps, if you will, one pro-Blalock and the other pro-Taussig. W. P. Longmire, [Jr.,] in his book on Blalock, describes it very well.[6] The surgeons loved Blalock; the pediatricians hated him and liked Taussig; and Taussig, in particular, resented anything or anyone that took any little piece of mosaic away from the picture she had constructed. When I started to catheterize the pulmonary artery and made diagnoses of pulmonary hypertension, she resented it and went to Blalock and said she wouldn't send me any more patients.

> Let me make something clear. As I understand it, she didn't think she
> needed cardiac catheterizations to make diagnoses, but I imagine some-
> times mistakes were made and that Blalock wanted a definite diagnosis
> before he "cracked a chest."

Exactly. She stopped sending me patients, and I asked Blalock to give me permission to stop all catheterizations for diagnostic purposes. "That's fine," he said, because of Taussig, but then she came back after two or three weeks and said, "Go ahead."

Why?

Because things didn't go well. You know, once in a while you need a correct diagnosis! She thought she could do everything. It was similar to the case of the British cardiologist PAUL WOOD. He thought he could tell all he had to know from the second heart sound. He worked with me for a while, and after he watched me for a week at Hopkins I said, "Dr. Wood, I hope you enjoyed your time here."

He said, "I didn't learn a damn thing."

I'm sure he did. Now tell me how you got into coronary sinus catheterizations and cardiac metabolism. As I recall it, catheterization of the coronary sinus was originally reported as one of the pitfalls of cardiac catheterization that one had to avoid.

Yes, LEW DEXTER reported that.[7] He missed the opportunity to use this to study cardiac metabolism. I realized this from the work of [C. L.] Evans,[8] who had worked with [ERNEST] STARLING in England and had written a paper on the heart-lung preparation in which he determined the usage of glucose, et cetera, by the heart. I had read that paper and wanted to see what the heart muscle actually uses, and so that was the idea. Of course I also wanted to measure coronary blood flow, and at that time [SEYMOUR] KETY and [C. F.] Schmidt had described the nitrous oxide method of measuring cerebral blood flow at the University of Pennsylvania.[9] I adapted that to the measurement of coronary blood flow in man.[10]

This sort of led to a divorce, more or less, from Blalock, who didn't give a damn about cardiac metabolism so this led to some trouble. And things began to come to a head, especially as I was finishing off the work on congenital heart disease. For example, one problem we had was the spilling of mercury on the floors of the laboratory—we were using the van Slyke method for blood gas measurements—and my staff began to complain about the fumes, which, essentially, Blalock did not want to hear about. He felt I was exaggerating. But the problem really was that he didn't like my going into metabolism. So, you know, when the boss begins to get unhappy, it's time to move on.

So in 1951 you went to Alabama with TINSLEY HARRISON . . .

Tinsley was also a character. He was a little fellow, very mercurial. There was an article published in *Pharos* about Blalock and Harrison, which was quite good. An incident it describes is a dinner given in Atlantic City in honor of Harrison with Blalock giving the main address. I remember that in his talk he said about Harrison, "One thing you can say about him is what the bloomers said to the panties: I have had my ups and downs, but I have never been pushed aside."

By the time I had joined the group, Harrison was only interested in golf and the ballistocardiogram. Tinsley thought he could make a tremendous contribution with the thing, which didn't turn out to be true. I believe he hired me because of my ability at cardiac catheterization, which not many could do at the time. I recall hearing of an old urologist there who was told that I was coming as a catheterization man, and he remarked, "Well, I've been doing that for fifty years!"

While I was in Hopkins I published my papers on coronary sinus catheterization and coronary blood flow. When I got to Birmingham I expanded that work into cardiac metabolism.[11]

You seem to have been happy in Alabama. Why did you leave?

I got an offer to be professor and head of medicine at the Veterans Hospital, Washington University, St. Louis, Missouri. Although I was already a full professor in Alabama, I didn't have much of an opportunity to do any clinical work. And, to me, clinical work was something on the other side of the fence that just had to be greener.

I loved CARL MOORE, the chief of medicine at the university, but the city was awful. For my family Birmingham was a nice place to live; everyone was nice to us at the time. We actually began to set down roots there.

Washington U. was wonderful, but St. Louis was hot and very unpleasant compared to the relative smallness of Birmingham.

Was that what made you leave St. Louis?

What made me leave St. Louis was the opportunity to become chairman of a department at Wayne State in Detroit. That was my big mistake. In Detroit the first five years were pleasant; the dean was a wonderful man, and we got along fine. Then a new dean came in, and no one lasted very long. He got rid of the head of surgery, the head of radiology—they all quit while I hung on with my fingernails a few more years.

I had come with the idea that I would create a department there like that at Johns Hopkins or Washington University at St. Louis with some emphasis on research, but that was a mistake. When things get tough, research is the first thing to go.

And so you finally came to Huntington, where you have remained for about thirty years, a full career span for most people, but only half of yours.

There is always that interplay between two different factors, individual and institution, which can lead to problems. I was initially appointed as chief of cardiology at the Huntington Memorial Hospital as well as chief of medical education. I was all right in the latter role but not really suited for the other. I had done many catheterizations but I hadn't done any coronary arteriography, and they wanted me to set up a clinical operation second to none, and I couldn't do that and I wasn't really interested in doing it. Ten years after I arrived I gave up my position at Huntington Hospital, and I shifted my efforts to the Huntington Medical Research Institutes, where I had had a joint appointment. There they were extremely interested in making things easier for me: I had many grants at the time and money to burn. That made it very attractive to me to shift all my efforts here.

It seems that much of the work you have done is more biochemical than cardiological.

I just picked it up as I went along. I must say I was pretty good in biochemistry all through medical school and later on.

You have done so much work over the last thirty years that it would take another few hours to even touch on this, but what are some of the things you would like to point out that deserve some special attention at this time?

First, let me say something about the Carrel-Lindbergh system. No one has ever used their pump for anything because the original purpose for which it had been devised, the study of the interplay between the environment and different organs, didn't work out. Later on, I thought of other uses of the pump and published articles showing, by use of the pump to perfuse single arteries, that cholesterol uptake by the arterial wall could be influenced by several factors (oxidation products of cholesterol). This never received any attention. But the Lindbergh pump would be ideal to study viruses and their effects on different organs. I regret that I'm eighty-nine because that would be a great lead to follow.

Another thing is something I've worked on for the last six years; before I got into the nitric oxide business, I worked on a new method to replace the conventional use of cell cultures. In my method I implanted cells onto microcarrier beads. For example, I published a paper on how endothelial cells cluster about them. These cells produce tremendous amounts of nitric oxide and all sorts of things! Unfortunately, after two days the cells die, but one day it may have the potential of producing tremendous amounts of these important substances. I published a number of papers on this, but it got as much attention as a flea bite on an elephant's ass.

I was very proud of this work, but no one paid any attention to it. It reminds me of Blalock, who told me many times that he considered his work on shock the most important work in his career but everyone else thought only of "the blue babies."

Right now I'm working on a grant proposal to combine aspirin with nitric oxide. I'm trying to combine aspirin with a nitric oxide donor and see how that works in myocardial infarction.

To shift gears for a moment, clear something up for me. Were you and RUDOLPH BING related?

Not really, as far as I can determine. I met him once and we went over our family backgrounds, and perhaps he was a very distant cousin, but he was from Vienna and my family—the Bings—were actually from Bavaria; some Bings still live in Denmark.

Music has always been important to you.

When I was a young man I thought seriously about a musical career as a performer and had some good training. But I never felt I could sight-read well enough for this, although I could improvise pretty well on the piano. So I gave this up, although later on I began to compose, and I have enjoyed doing this for many years with chamber music and so on.

Music has meant much to me, as much as my research, sometimes even more. My works have been performed in Europe and America. The "Mass" was performed in Vienna; it was written for orchestra, chorus, and solo voices. I think music and medicine complement each other, given the different parts of the soul or persona. Composition of music has been my consolation and joy.

Would you have done anything different in medicine if you had it to do over again?

I think I would have done more clinical work rather than bench research. The publication of scientific results is certainly gratifying, but I would have liked to have had more contact with patients.

Given what I think your philosophy of life is, that is not surprising to me. GEORGE BURCH wrote an article about what the life of a cardiologist should be, in which he described this spartan existence of getting up at five in the morning and running to the hospital to take care of patients, returning home late at night and doing your research, and repeating the process seven days a week without any time for anything else. You wrote a humorous letter to the editor in reply that presented a very different view of what life should be all about. Do you remember it?

Only vaguely, but, as I recall, I pointed out that it is also important to have some leisure in one's life as well as lots of work. After all, if Isaac Newton hadn't taken an afternoon off and gone to sit under that apple tree, he might never have discovered gravity.

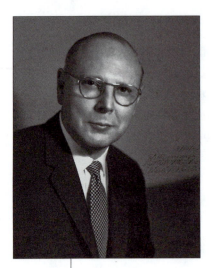

5

CHARLES P. BAILEY, M.D., Sc.D., J.D. (1910–1993)

As exciting and innovative as were the "indirect" surgical procedures for congenital heart disease such as the ligation of the patent ductus and the "blue baby" (Blalock-Taussig) operation, they addressed only a small fraction of the structural problems of the heart that might be surgically corrected in years to come. They did, however, eventually lead to the realization that surgery performed directly upon the heart might be the next major step to be undertaken.

Although as far back as 1896, Ludwig Rehn successfully sutured a wound of the heart, other attempts at heart surgery were rare and often disheartening. One problem that begged for relief was rheumatic heart disease. Rheumatic fever is related to a preceding infection with a common type of bacterium, a streptococcus, following which, in susceptible individuals a type of autoimmune reaction takes place, damaging the heart valves. Until the middle of the twentieth century, rheumatic fever was a serious problem in this country. Since the introduction and free use of antibiotics in the United States, the incidence of rheumatic fever and subsequent rheumatic heart disease has markedly decreased here since the beta-hemolytic streptococcus is very sensitive to antibiotics. However, some cases of rheumatic heart disease continue to occur in the United States, and in the third world, where access to antibiotics is limited, it remains a significant cause of cardiac incapacity and death.

As a result of rheumatic scarring, a valve may become narrowed (stenotic) or fail to close properly (regurgitate). The mitral valve (so-called because anatomists thought its two cusps resembled a bishop's mitre) separates the left atrium and left ventricle, and mitral stenosis is the most common valvular problem in rheumatic heart disease.

Initial surgical attempts at correcting mitral stenosis were made before the introduction of pump-oxygenators and open-heart surgery. The surgeon had to work on the beating heart blindly, by touch. One early attempt was made in 1923 by DR. ELLIOT CARR CUTLER in Boston and cardiologist SAMUEL A. LEVINE.[1] Cutler's approach was from the ventricular side of the valve using an instrument he devised called a cardiovalvulotome. This tube contained a cutting mechanism; it was passed through the ventricular wall and then retrogradely through the mitral valve into the left atrium (see Fig. 3-1). The cutting device was used to remove a piece of the valve and thus reduce the degree of obstruction between the two chambers. The instrument was difficult to use, mortality was high, and with removal of part of the valve substance, a case of severe mitral stenosis could be converted into a problem of severe mitral regurgitation. After several attempts at this procedure, Cutler abandoned it.

Another attempt at surgery for mitral stenosis was made two years later, in 1925, in Great Britain. HENRY S. SOUTTAR at London Hospital operated on a nineteen-year-old girl with a somewhat different method. He approached the mitral valve from above, making a small incision in the left atrium and passing his finger down to the valve, which he then was able to dilate with his finger.[2] This operation, almost forgotten in later years, was actually successful but never repeated because of the prevailing opinion of leading experts that the problem of mitral stenosis was primarily related to the heart muscle and not the deformation of the valve.[3] Although the field lay fallow for the next quarter century, following World War II several surgeons—perhaps encouraged by a 1946 article by DWIGHT E. HARKEN, who reported on the great number of shell fragments he removed with impunity from the hearts of wounded servicemen[4]—began to look at the problem again. These included Harken himself, Charles Bailey, and HORACE G. SMITHY in the United

States, and RUSSELL C. BROCK in Great Britain. Although all deserve credit for establishing the surgical role in mitral stenosis, I found the story of Charles Bailey to be particularly illuminating and worthy of documentation here.

If, during the 1940s, Horatio Alger was still writing stories about poor boys who rose from rags to riches, he could well have based one of his tales on the career of Charles P. Bailey. Born in a small town in New Jersey and growing up in poverty with only a widowed mother to care for him, Dr. Bailey nonetheless achieved, if not riches, the peak of fame and appreciation for his contributions to heart surgery. Bailey, like Souttar, used the atrial approach, but utilized a commissurotomy* knife affixed to the palmar side of his index finger to widen the opening of the valve without punching a hole in it such as had been done by Cutler and his associates. Thus there was a lesser chance of regurgitation developing after this technique, although stenosis did tend to recur in later years in some patients, requiring a second operation. Yet even these patients were able to enjoy a number of years of symptom-free existence.

Bailey just barely pulled off his success with mitral commissurotomy. His first two patients, operated on at Hahnemann in Philadelphia in 1945 and 1946, both died. In 1948 he attempted his third operation at Wilmington Hospital in Delaware, but postoperative complications resulted in another death. After this he was denied privileges to perform such surgery at Hahnemann and knew that any further failures might end all his efforts toward this end. With this thought in mind, he scheduled one mitral commissurotomy in the morning at Philadelphia General Hospital and another for the afternoon at Episcopal Hospital. Then, at the ripe old age of thirty-eight, Bailey contracted measles, necessitating a month's delay in his plans. When the day of judgment finally arrived, the first patient, an elderly man with far advanced disease and other medical problems, did not survive surgery. However, the second patient, a woman who was a much better operative risk,

---

* A commissure is a small space between the adjacent cusps of a valve. These cusps become adherent, scarred, and sometimes calcified, reducing the overall opening area of a valve when it is affected by rheumatic and other types of heart disease.

improved significantly, and with further successes soon reported by Drs. Harken and Brock, the adoption of the surgical approach to the treatment of mitral stenosis was assured.

Besides his work on mitral commissurotomy, Dr. Bailey made many other contributions to cardiac surgery. In 1954 he was one of the first to excise a postinfarction left ventricular aneurysm. In 1956 he performed the first retrograde coronary endarterectomy, attempting to remove the obstructive elements within the coronary artery. (This was before the development of coronary bypass surgery, of course.) He also contributed to the development of techniques for treatment of aortic valve disease, closure of atrial septal defects, and solutions to problems related to prosthetic heart valves which still are amenable to improvements.

Dr. Bailey attended Hahnemann Medical College in Philadelphia and in that city, between 1948 and 1958, did the bulk of his creative work. Between 1959 and 1962 he headed the Department of Surgery at New York Medical College, and then, for a period of ten years, he headed the Section of Thoracic Surgery at St. Barnabas Hospital in the Bronx, New York.

Toward the end of his medical career Dr. Bailey did a complete turnabout. He went to Fordham Law School, from which he obtained a degree in 1973. Although he continued to see some of his old patients, he became a member of a law firm specializing in physicians' problems. In 1986 he founded his own not-for-profit insurance firm, Physicians National Risk Retention Group, in Marietta, Georgia. It is amazing how trenchant and on the mark his thoughts about medical malpractice and doctor-patient relations remain today, after over twenty years.

In 1991 he confronted another aortic valve problem—his own. He was operated on for aortic stenosis by Dr. Denton A. Cooley. Although the surgery went well, Dr. Bailey died in 1993.

New York, New York
August 28, 1979

Could you tell me about the development of the closed mitral commissurotomy operation for mitral stenosis?

When you talk about either me, or DWIGHT HARKEN, or RUSSELL BROCK, you really have to talk about the other two as well because, within a three-month period, entirely independently, each of us came out with the same ideas, both as to concept and as to technique of surgery for mitral valve disease. And this technique proved to be sound and satisfactory until the time when direct vision surgery became possible and later when plastic valves became acceptable as prosthetic replacements. I have often said that if any two of us had died, the remaining one would have kept right on and would have brought out exactly the same final product.

It's still a very valuable procedure in undeveloped countries, where open-heart surgery is not yet feasible and where plastic valves may be too expensive. And it does enable you to do a very good job on about half of all cases of mitral stenosis and a fair job on another quarter, so that, in the sense of logistics, it is still a very valuable method. I just happened to be lucky enough to perform the first one on June 10, 1948. That lady is still alive and still pretty healthy after all these years. Dr. Harken did a similar procedure within a week of that date, and Russell Brock did another one within three months. Neither Harken nor I published our work at the time that we did it.

The reasons I was able to make a contribution to mitral surgery were threefold:

1. I had long been an amateur photographer and was used to working in the darkroom guided by a sense of touch. This helped with a closed procedure where you could not actually look at what you were doing.

2. I had made an extensive study of the anatomy of both the normal and the diseased mitral valve from autopsy material and in the animal laboratory.

3. Having sold ladies' underwear to earn my way as an undergraduate student, I had a good knowledge of such things, and was early on impressed by the similarity of the mitral valve structure to the old-fashioned feminine girdle. Perhaps this is what suggested mitral commissurotomy to me.

The history of heart surgery is fascinating. In 1895 THEODOR BILLROTH, who was no mean surgical innovator himself, was supposed to have said that "no surgeon who wished to preserve the respect of his colleagues would ever attempt to suture a wound of the heart."[5] As late as 1945, when you published a textbook of thoracic surgery, you never even referred to intracardiac surgery. Three years later, you and Harken and Brock were doing precisely that! What was the role of HORACE SMITHY in all this?

First off, I would point out that, despite what Billroth wrote or said, [Ludwig] Rehn in 1896 did successfully suture a wound of the heart. As for Smithy, his work was entirely independent of ours. He was from South Carolina, and it was his survivals with the old Cutler operation for mitral stenosis that really stimulated me to finally do that first successful case.

I reviewed your paper, and I was amazed.[6] I know surgeons must have courage to introduce something new, but I wondered while reading it what kind of a man, or woman for that matter, can take five patients, have four of them die, and then say, "This looks very promising."

Obviously, I felt there were irrelevant reasons for the loss of the first four patients and that the principle was entirely sound and could be developed but just needed further effort. These other cardiac surgeons I mentioned had some unsuccessful cases too. All of us had had a considerable background of animal work before this and, of course, had operated on dead human hearts, so that we were not unfamiliar with the pathology. Finally, however, you have to face the "moment of truth," and the poignancy is so great that I can't really express it. You know that almost all the world is against it; you know that you have a great personal stake and might even lose your medical license, or at least your hospital privileges if you persist. In fact, the thought crosses your mind that maybe you really *are* crazy. And yet you feel that it has to be done and it must be right. At the time I did the last of those five operations, the successful one, I was sure that I was, at the least, in danger of losing all my hospital operating privileges.

Was that fifth operation performed at Hahnemann?

No, that was at the Episcopal Hospital; I had already lost my privileges to do this kind of surgery at Hahnemann because two of the four previous patients had died at Hahnemann. The professor of cardiology there, Dr. George Goeckler, who later became my very good friend, was at that time so bitterly opposed to any further such efforts that he formally invited me to come down to his office to discuss the whole thing with him. First he allowed me the privilege of the floor, which took up practically all of the interview. Then, after I had finished telling him what I thought could be done, he pulled out a previously typewritten sheet of paper on which he had methodically explained that, as a physician, it was his Hippocratic duty not to do harm when he could do no good. He ended up telling me that it was his Christian duty to keep me from doing any more of these operations.

Dr. Goeckler was a great, sincere, and dedicated physician, and he felt he was preventing me from committing manslaughter in this fashion. Realizing that "the jury had been out before the court had been called into session," I responded with some heat. I told him that I believed in this operation, that I was sure I was right, that I knew the results of medical treatment for this condition were so poor as to be worthless, and proclaimed that it was *my* Christian duty to continue with this effort and make it successful; and that I was prepared to spend the rest of my life in that effort. We shook hands and parted.

In the past, many cardiologists thought that rheumatic heart disease was mainly a disease of the muscle and that the valves, narrowed or widened in the process, had little to do with the clinical manifestations.

Yes, and that was why Dr. Samuel Levine was chided by some experts in the twenties for letting Dr. Elliot Cutler of Boston attempt this type of operation on his patients. You see how even the brightest people can be wrong.

There is always the question of priority. Was there any feeling of competition among you and Harken and Brock?

Well, of course there was. It was mainly, I think, between Harken and myself. Brock had more of the dispassionate view of the Englishman, and he maintained good relations with both of us. But I should tell you about Horace Smithy.

At the meeting at which I reported these five cases of mitral stenosis with one survival, Smithy had already operated on eight cases, and it is my recollection that five of them survived surgery. He was called upon to discuss my paper. I hesitate to think of what would have happened if Harken had been the discussant and had Smithy's record with which to clobber me, but Smithy was devoid of that competitive feeling, and, although he had a much better "batting average" than I had at the time, he was most gentlemanly and considerate in mentioning his own work. He didn't present it very fully so that he didn't steal the show. He merely said that he had used the method of Cutler but acknowledged that this converted the stenosis essentially into a regurgitation, and then this wonderful man, who could have outshone me and stolen the day, said, "But I think Dr. Bailey's technique (which was essentially converting the small opening into a Halloween pumpkin type of smiling mouth) is a much more physiological method, and that is the one I am going to use from now on."

His generosity was admirable—especially for a surgeon, I must say.

Well, there are some wonderful people in surgery, but there are no more egotistical and more competitive people than surgeons. But Smithy was not only a southern gentleman, he was a true gentleman; otherwise he would have been unable to resist the temptation to capitalize on the position he was in at that time. After the public session at that meeting, I had a good long talk with him in private, and you can imagine how warmly I felt toward him.

I learned that he, himself, was driven to develop cardiac surgery because he hoped to develop a method applicable to his own case, because he was running out of life. He had me listen to his own heart, and I heard the terrible rumble of aortic stenosis [narrowing of the valve leading from the left ventricle to the main blood vessel, the aorta]. I had to admit to him that I hadn't worked on or considered the problem as yet, so I was not able to offer him any hope or much encouragement in fact. Probably because of this, he subsequently went to Dr.

ALFRED BLALOCK, who wasn't at all willing to operate on Dr. Smithy with his knowledge at the time, which, I suppose, was not much better than mine. There was no pump-oxygenator yet, so this was before open-heart surgery had arrived. Any attempt would have to have been made by a closed method, as with the mitral valve work which was being done. Dr. Smithy subsequently found a patient with aortic stenosis and brought him to Baltimore, where he and Dr. Blalock attempted to operate on him for this condition. Unhappily, the patient died on the operating table, and I'm sure this deterred Dr. Blalock from any further efforts in that direction. It also disappointed Dr. Smithy beyond all belief because, with this man's death, his chance, however remote, to persuade Dr. Blalock to attempt something on him had gone to the grave with the patient. Smithy died in the fall of 1948; I had met him the preceding spring. He was only thirty-four.

What was the source of the friction between you and Dr. Harken?

Well, my mother was redheaded; my daughter is redheaded. I never was, but *Harken was*—that is, until he became gray. And there is an old saying in India that you never find two tigers on the same hill. What they really mean is you don't find two *male* tigers on the same hill; one always drives the other off. And at that time Harken and I had no idea that there was a whole mountain range that would be occupied by heart surgeons in the future, so we just tore at each other with the classical vigor of redheaded people.

There may be another connection. I believe Dr. Harken had some of his medical training in New Jersey at the old Pollak Hospital for Chest Diseases in Jersey City. What about your own early days?

I was born and raised within two miles of Fitkin Hospital in Neptune, New Jersey, and my mother had something to do with my going there for an internship after I finished medical school at Hahnemann. My mother wasn't Jewish, but she was what you might call a "Jewish mother type," in that I was destined to be a doctor before I was born. She thought that was the kind of a son one should have. And she brainwashed me so thoroughly that I never thought of being anything but a doctor for the first forty years of my life. She wanted me to intern at the local hospital because I think she had some idea that she might become a member of the board of trustees there and have some influence on the health and medical care of her neighbors. There was another factor: they paid twenty-five dollars a month in wages to interns at Fitkin, whereas at Hahnemann or Philadelphia General or any other place I might have been interested in, they paid nothing.

Your mother sounds like a pretty strong character. What about your father?

Well, I don't think I ever heard him express himself on the subject, but I'm sure he didn't object. My father was a banker, but at a relatively early age he left banking and I guess you'd say he became a stock market manipulator. The trouble is that one day *he* got manipulated and lost all his money. From then on he had a number of different jobs. He died when I was only twelve and when I saw him coughing up blood into a basin as my mother tried to soothe him, I just stared at this awful exhibition of how mitral stenosis could terminate a young man's life. He was only forty-two. I was already scheduled to be a doctor but was going to go into cancer research up to that time. At that very moment I changed my direction, and my mother was never able to persuade me otherwise. Indeed it seemed to me a much simpler job to solve the mechanical problems of valvular heart disease than the chemical and biological problems of neoplastic development.

Are you saying that, as a boy, you were already thinking of what kind of specialty you were going to go into as a physician?

Oh, my mother had made up my mind for me before I was five; maybe before I was three!

Did any of your teachers encourage you along the lines of cardiac surgery?

No, it was the shock of my father's death and the realization that the heart was only a mechanical pump and certainly would be responsive to physical laws that all mechanical pumps would be subject to. The fact that this hadn't been developed or perhaps even expressed very much did not deter me. I just thought that nobody had thought of it yet. When I was a freshman in medical school, I drew a diagram of a proposed heart-lung machine with these principles in mind and presented it to Dr. John Scott, the professor of physiology there. It was not dissimilar in design to the diagrammatic circulation of our current heart-lung machines.

> Let's get back to the progress of your career. After your internship you went into private practice in Lakewood, New Jersey, for about five years, then took training in thoracic surgery at Seaview Hospital in Staten Island.

Yes, but first I went to the Graduate School at the University of Pennsylvania for an academic year. There they encouraged me, based upon the anticipated coming of the certifying boards in the various specialties, to take residency training on top of postgraduate training. My thesis was titled "Extra-periosteal Pneumothorax for Tuberculosis," for which I received my master's degree in science in 1943. I was a lecturer at Hahnemann from 1940 to 1948 and professor and head of the Department of Surgery there from 1948 to 1958.

> Those must have been pretty heady years, what with the mitral surgery and all that rapid professional advancement.

Actually, the academic rank did not disturb my sense of balance. The fact that I could more or less run my own show was, of course, a comfort. But I could see that this new field was an uncharted area and it was up to me to develop it in all respects that I could, and that was really exciting. People from all over the country and all over the world visited me at Hahnemann, and I was a speaker on a great many medical programs. I turned out to be a pretty good medical writer and speaker. I was invited to lecture in Europe, South America, Canada, Mexico—and what I had to present was usually something new and different from anything they had had before.

> What led you to break with Hahnemann? You had been there for over eighteen years.

Well, a few things happened. One was that we obtained a new professor of surgery, and under his new regime all the surgical subspecialties were to be reincorporated under the general Department of Surgery with the exception of gynecology and thoracic surgery (which included the heart).

Despite these arrangements, I soon found that the new professor of surgery had been given the right to all the lectures on thoracic surgery to the students. My teaching would be limited to residents. Furthermore, since the chairman had been certified by the American Board of Thoracic Surgery, he would be allowed to do his own private chest surgery, and his initial results did not bode well for the future.

I was upset by this and complained to the dean, and when he left for Europe in the spring of the year, I turned to the chairman of the board of trustees but received no satisfaction. Lacking any positive response, I decided to resign my academic position at least until the fall, when everyone would be back and perhaps things could be straightened out. In the meantime, I recommended that my next in command be made acting director of thoracic surgery. I continued to operate at the hospital under my junior's direction, so to speak, but would not be part of the faculty, at least temporarily.

I had reason to believe that there might be some discomforting activities in the fall, so I took certain precautions. I went to the medical school where the new professor had been before, and I met the new dean down there. It seems that there had been a real scandalous situation there, ending up with the resignations of two department heads, one of them our newly arrived professor, and the firing of a third.

Well, the dean gave me copies of newspaper after newspaper with crayon-outlined articles about the scandal, and I had an armful of these when we reconvened at Hahnemann in the fall. I also had another newspaper item with me. Franklin Roosevelt had just swept a previously strongly Republican part of southeastern Pennsylvania and had carried in with him a number of people who would otherwise never have been elected. In Bucks County they had an individual named John Brown running for tax collector on the Democratic ticket, but since there were not too many Democrats in Bucks County, they had simply put the name of a donkey, John Brown, on the ballot. After Election Day, in the newspaper was this picture of him with his ears sticking through this straw hat. My defense was: "You fellows have done the dumbest thing in the world by electing this kind of 'tax collector' for chairman of surgery. If only I had been on the selection committee, I would surely have found this out in advance." And I passed around the newspaper.

> It's amazing how often this happens. Some new guy appears on the scene to head a major department or division, and he is heralded as the greatest thing since sliced bread. Within a year you find out that he is a real "yo-yo," and wonder how someone like this could ever have been hired. You then go back to where he was before and learn all sorts of awful things about him from the people he really worked with at his former institution. It's unbelievable, but I suppose Santayana had it right: those who cannot remember the past are condemned to repeat it.

In the autumn of my years I've become a history buff, and I will swear that's the truth.

What finally happened?

I told them I would go into limbo and remain there until they were ready for a new professor of surgery. I told them that it would be about two years before they realized that this "John Brown" couldn't even collect taxes and they would have to replace him. "When you want a new professor of surgery, you know where you can find me." That's telling off the board of trustees, the dean, and the administration!

But it didn't happen that way. The new professor had been in the Korean War and had made friends with a lot of the brass who were now in a position to help him get grants. Hahnemann had always been shy of grant money. I realized that, despite his past, it would be longer than two years before his exodus. I also realized that I was in no way qualified to head a surgical department. I would have to learn.

I had received an invitation from the New York Medical College to be the chairman of its Department of Surgery. They were in pretty poor shape, and I thought that if I went there, I would do my best and would learn on the job. In any event, I expected that were I to leave after a few years, I'd leave it in a lot better condition than when I arrived there.

The dean at Hahnemann tried to dissuade me, but I went to New York and did get wonderful on-the-job experience in running such a department. I believe I improved the place, and I think I was responsible for the development and maturation of some fine doctors there. However, the dean at New York Medical College was a true tyrant, with autocratic powers such as you don't usually see in these modern times. I had noticed that those people who had come before me had gone through a "honeymoon" period and then had gotten into a period of what I called slavery—and it was! I told my wife before the first year was out to get prepared for another move, and by the end of the 1961–62 academic year I had left.

I had made no prior preparations for the future. I had a number of associations offered to me. I contacted a couple of the new medical schools that were developing then. However, I had had a bellyful of the machinations of high-level academic life, and I thought I'd like to be a free practitioner of medicine. What I wanted was a hospital where I could develop my specialty of cardiovascular surgery without being tied to a medical school. This I found at St. Barnabas Hospital in the Bronx, where I remained for more than ten years.

This brings us up to 1973, when you began the legal phase of your career. How did this happen?

When I was in the Philadelphia area, I had been sued three times for malpractice. None were valid, and I managed to get a defense verdict each time. But neither my lawyers nor my doctor colleagues could explain what was going on. This opened my eyes to a new world, and I made up my mind then that someday, when I had more time, I would go to law school, because this was too complicated to be resolved simply by the reading of a book or two.

When I came to New York there was another malpractice case carrying over from my Philadelphia days, but which had to be fought in the New York courts. Again there was no justification for the case, but my lawyer from Philadelphia was terribly hamstrung by the differing rules in New York, and it was necessary for me to bring in a number of extra medical witnesses to finally get a defense verdict.

Well, the time came that I finally did go to Fordham Law School at night, and I graduated in 1973. But I still did not have the answers to my questions. Law school teaches one how to pass the bar examinations. It doesn't answer fundamental questions such as: Why are there so many malpractice cases? Of course, you might also say that medical school only teaches one how to pass the licensure examinations. It, too, doesn't address some of the philosophical questions, which may have caused one to enter medical school.

So I became a dilettante at law.

Then, two years ago (1977), a case that was absolutely phony was brought up against me eleven years after its occurrence. It was tried in Newark, New Jersey, in federal court. This time the plaintiff got a verdict for thirty-five thousand dollars in a two-million-dollar lawsuit.

The truth is that the diagnosis had been absolutely right: she did have a fistula between the right coronary artery and the right atrium. I did operate it properly and up to all standards and had adequate medical testimony to that effect. And she suffered no injury from the operation except a scar. She had been terribly psychoneurotic and, in fact, had been complaining of chest pains from the age of twenty-two even though the fistula was asymptomatic; it often takes to middle age for these to produce heart failure. Her nonspecific chest complaints led to her being sent to me for a coronary arteriogram, which disclosed this abnormal communication. Now after surgery she was still terribly psychoneurotic, but that was mainly because she was married to the wrong man. Now, I didn't feel any responsibility for her having married the wrong man; she married him before she had ever met me, and she never indicated to me that it was the wrong man, so I never gave her any advice about that. She still had the wrong man after surgery.

After some years, she finally went to a doctor in New Jersey, and he got the idea that maybe she had never had this fistula at all before surgery. So he sent for the preoperative diagnostic movie films, the cineangiograms, and the "dumb-dumb" hospital, without saying a word

either to me or the fellow in charge of the heart catheterization laboratory, sent out the only copy of the film in existence. The doctor in New
Jersey, who happened to be a psychiatrist, turned them over to a cardiologist who was supposed to take them up to another hospital and view
them on a suitable projector. On the way there, he claimed, his car was
burglarized and the film stolen

Now I cannot believe that a theft of that kind would occur. Why
would anyone want to steal a medical movie film? Maybe the plaintiff's
lawyer destroyed it, but even if he did, it seems to me that that's the
responsibility of the patient and her agents or her doctors; it certainly
wasn't mine. And yet, without the film our proof of the preoperative
diagnosis was gone. Now I'm convinced that justice does not exist in
the jury system. The jury is an anachronism abandoned by many other
countries. Plaintiffs' lawyers will argue vigorously about this and shout,
"Preserve the jury system," but that is because they are making their
money out of it, not because it is right.

Long ago before this, I had declared that if I was ever found guilty
of malpractice I would never operate again. So I am finished with surgery, having done my last case in April 1979.

**You're sixty-eight now. What happens to aging surgeons who don't
become lawyers?**

Well, if they get tremors or Parkinsonism, of course they have to quit.
If their brains are not functioning sharply, they have to quit. Usually
hospitals and medical schools retire you at sixty-five. You lose your
chiefship, and, once you do, you find it's hard to go back and become
one of the boys again. From then on the residents may help you, but
they don't give you the kind of respect that they give the fellow who is
chief—and from whom they will have to get their certification and recommendations. They may try to convert you to using the new chief's
methods, or often have ideas of their own and begin to argue with you
about them. It's not as much fun doing surgery after you're sixty-five.

There are some other things that are missing too: the joy of living,
joie de vivre. I used to look forward with anticipation and excitement
to doing an operation. Well, these things seem to take longer as you get

older; my kind of surgery often takes eight hours. So you no longer get that old thrill. And you worry more as you grow more conservative. You think, "My God, there's a 25 percent chance he'll die!" You used to think, "There's a 75 percent chance he'll live and get better." However, with the change in medical practice and the increasing threat of suits, where anything is "dangerous," you don't rush ahead as readily as you once did.

> You edit the monograph *Cardiovascular Advances,* and when the first volume came out, I was surprised to see that the legal section, which you wrote, constituted almost 10 percent of the book's four hundred pages. To summarize the reasons you said we live in such a litigious society: Disappointment in the results realized by the patient or a misunderstanding between doctor and patient. A patient's desire to punish a doctor he or she doesn't like. Avarice of the patient. And frequently all this is complicated by a jury deciding to punish a physician or just to compensate a very unfortunate person even if the doctor was blameless because they feel they ought to give the patient something anyway.

You see, that last one is a "sneaker." Every time you read a medical or surgical textbook about a given disease, particularly things that you treat surgically, they'll give you figures: such and such a chance the patient will survive; such and such a chance he will die; such and such a chance that he will be *better.* The last is not the same as the number that will survive. It never is. And there are varying degrees of improvement; not everybody gets entirely better, and the reasons are many. There may have been too much preexisting disease to correct it entirely. It may be that other tissues and organs have deteriorated secondary to the primary disease or in association with it. Or it may be that the patient has a psychoneurotic element in his symptomatology, and this is not going to go away postoperatively. And all that means is that among the survivors perhaps only 1 percent to 25 percent, depending on what their problems are, will have a perfect or good result. Furthermore, in a recent California study of twenty-one thousand hospital admissions Mills, Rubsamen, and Boyden found that nearly 5 percent suffered medically related injuries associated with their hospitalization.[7] Modern medicine is dangerous. In only 17 percent of these injuries was there any provider fault, but the question is raised: Shouldn't all of these innocent victims receive some compensation?

The jury lumps it all together; they feel that these people ought to have some kind of compensation. Now the doctor doesn't live who can always get ideal results; he can only get up to the level that is reasonably possible. Doctors, if they only understood, would realize that they are in a Catch-22 situation. They can't win; they have to lose. In our fault-based compensation system the plaintiff's lawyers must try to cook up a spurious case of fault, and the jury will be disposed to buy it.

Have modern doctors, in any way, themselves contributed to this problem—as compared to the old-timers, for example?

I don't think doctors are all that different today. I look back on the physicians I knew during my youth, and there were some real sons of bitches. There were some guys who would chew their patients out and say, "Never come back and darken my doorway again. I'll never treat you again." There were patients who would say, "That goddam doctor; he set my leg wrong and look at the crook I've got now in that bone." I think we all make a variety of mistakes, but there was an overall feeling that the doctor had some godly touch and he was like a priest, or minister, or rabbi—and you don't sue them. And they didn't sue doctors in those days except in very rare and unusual cases.

Today's doctors are more successful financially than they were in those days. To that extent patients envy us and don't feel sorry for us as they did when every other patient didn't pay us—and they all knew this. I suppose the fact that doctors don't come out at night time or do house calls may bother them a little. I think that specialization in modern medicine, where you get a whole team working on you instead of just one doctor who is in charge, must depersonalize medical attention. And some doctors treat their patients as diagnoses instead of sick people.

The world has changed, and our position with respect to litigation-proneness is infinitely more vulnerable. We could easily strengthen that position, but so far we haven't done anything for ourselves except to complain and act paranoid. There are some individuals who have done what I have done. They won't operate, and some won't even practice medicine. But until doctors are willing to do this in concert, the overall problem will remain.

I've thought long and hard about this, and I can tell you what they could do. First of all, they'd have to be organized into a great, unified group. Call it a union if you like. It would have to be organized technically as a union, or else legally they would not be able to invoke their rights as citizens. But presently doctors are so prejudiced against unions that I don't see them joining into the equivalent of a union in the foreseeable future. But if they suffer a little more, maybe they will. At any rate, they would have to agree to follow their own leadership. Now in any state, or preferably nationally, that leadership could very simply declare a strike. They could set up emergency centers at hospitals and clinics here and there so no patient would suffer from an acute emergency without medical help. But no elective medical services would be provided until the legislature changed its rules.

The legislature, in two weeks or maybe four, would change the rules because the new rules would be fair and reasonable. Let me ask you: who can judge best whether an orthopedic surgeon has done the right thing in a given case?

I would say another well-qualified orthopedic surgeon.

I would prefer three orthopedic surgeons. Oh yes, they have these so-called Medical Malpractice Panels now, but in New York, for instance, it is composed of a judge, a lawyer, and a doctor of the same discipline as the defendant. You and I, even though we're doctors, wouldn't be too good at judging the work of an orthopedic surgeon. How could two laypeople, two lawyers, ever be expected to know what it's all about?

Having a panel consisting solely of doctors judging other doctors may lay them open to the charge of protecting their own. We always hear complaints about lawyers not being able to get doctors to testify against doctors.

There is no one harsher than a doctor in judging another doctor when he thinks the son of a bitch did something wrong! And there would be safeguards against any kind of prejudice either way on the doctor panel. The doctor panels would be organized in such a way that, each year, an expert could sit on a panel for, let us say, two weeks. They would serve in areas distant from their own so that none of the problems of local relationships would interfere. By having a panel of several doctors instead of only one, other personal biases that might sway one would be counterbalanced by the other doctors. In this way I think you'd have justice.

> **It must be terrible to be sued. I've been lucky, I suppose; I've never been sued.**

Well, the law of averages is warping all the time!*

> **Did you have any great disappointments in your life?**

I regret that I didn't have one or two of my sons go into medicine. I have reflected on some of my past decisions. My father always seemed to have difficulty in holding on to jobs because he had a tendency to argue with his bosses and express his own ideas so vigorously that they found it desirable to separate. I have found some trace of that characteristic in my own personality. I'm probably the only doctor you know who has told two different medical deans where they could stick their professorships!

But I sometimes have mixed emotions about Hahnemann and regret that I left when I did. On the other hand, Hahnemann has just been through another convulsion, and sooner or later I probably would have had my head lopped off there if I hadn't left when I did. I never would have gone to law school had I remained in Philadelphia, but would have liked another ten years to work on the mitral problem; there's a great need for improvement on these prosthetic valves.

> **Your career was unique. When our own professor of surgery gives a lecture on the history of surgery to our medical students, he points out that in American surgery almost all the major figures have descended in a**

---

* In 1981, after twenty-three legally trouble-free years, the law of averages stopped "warping" for me when I found myself named in a suit with four other doctors at my institution. Two years after my retirement in 1997, I was again named in a similar suit.

direct line from one of their great forebears: WILLIAM S. HALSTED, HARVEY CUSHING, and so on. You seem to have developed pretty much on your own.

I was aware of the great things in medicine. I had done a lot of reading about these people; but I didn't come from any of the schools that are supposed to produce great people partly because I didn't have enough money to go to these schools. I was a bright boy: I probably could have made Harvard or Johns Hopkins if I had tried, but I would not have been able to pay the tuition. At that time it was quite inexpensive to go to Hahnemann, which at that time was also teaching homeopathy.* So at least I got two degrees: Doctor of Medicine and Doctor of Homeopathic Medicine.

Anyway, I have the old-fashioned idea that in America you can do whatever you want with your life, and it never bothered me to be in a minority position. In fact, it may even have made me work harder.

---

* Homeopathy is a system of therapeutics, founded by Samuel Hahnemann, in which diseases are treated by administration of minute doses of substances that would in healthy persons produce the same symptoms when given in larger doses.

6

JOHN W. KIRKLIN, M.D.
(1917–   )

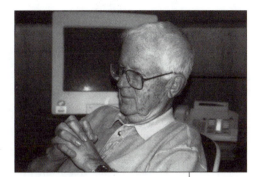

Although surgeons were encouraged by the successes of extra-cardiac operations such as the Blalock-Taussig procedure, and the direct, although blinded, approach of the commissurotomy for mitral stenosis, it became obvious that for the vast majority of surgically approachable cardiac defects—especially those in critically ill infants and young children with congenital heart disease—only full exposure of the internal structure of the heart to the surgeon's eye in a relatively dry operative field would allow such repairs to be performed. This story of open-heart surgery is mainly a tale of two cities. They are not Paris and Vienna; they are not London and Berlin; and they are not New York and Boston. They are Minneapolis and Rochester, Minnesota, smack in the middle of the United States.[1]

At the University of Minnesota Medical School in Minneapolis, DR. OWEN H. WANGENSTEEN presided over the Department of Surgery, where pioneers such as C. WALTON LILLEHEI with key associates began to obtain reliably successful results in the fifties. Because of the uncertainties and limitations in the use of the heart-lung machines and other techniques of that period, between 1954 and 1955 they utilized the technique of cross-circulation, in which an infant or small child with a congenital heart defect would have an adult, usually a parent, serve as the supporting "unit" while the patient's heart was exposed, opened, and repaired.[2] Following the development of a successful bubble oxygenator by RICHARD A. DEWALL at that institution,[3] this was the method used in later open-heart procedures.

Meanwhile, at the Mayo Clinic in Rochester, Minnesota, John W. Kirklin and his team followed their own star in adapting the Gibbon heart-lung apparatus for their operative procedures and called it the Mayo-Gibbon oxygenator.

At both institutions the support of nonsurgical experts was vital to their success. At the University of Minnesota, MAURICE B. VISSCHER, chairman of the Department of Physiology, helped train Lillehei and other surgeons in the basics of hemodynamics. At the Mayo Clinic, physiologist EARL H. WOOD provided similar guidance, and cardiologists such as HOWARD BURCHELL and pathologist JESSE F. EDWARDS also offered their support.

With refinements of surgical technique, instrumentation, and adjuncts such as hypothermia and other means of myocardial preservation, open-heart surgery with complete cardiopulmonary bypass became a routine procedure not only for congenital heart defects but for valvular and coronary disease as well.

Dr. Kirklin's perseverance and brilliant, analytical mind has made him a legendary figure in the field. His intellectual rigor and honesty have been his hallmarks, enabling him and his group to present the first continuous series of open-heart procedures in congenital heart disease[4] at a time when only isolated attempts at open-heart surgery, often unsuccessful, were usually being reported. The Mayo success with the repair of congenital heart defects later led to a leading role for the clinic in the surgical approach to an equally demanding problem, acquired valvular heart disease.

So focused and dedicated has Kirklin been to the goals he set before himself that some people have called him a "human computer." Yet, I learned from an associate, this same man would, at times, go off by himself and become for a time incommunicado following the loss of a patient as he attempted to deal with his disappointment and despair. His earthy responses to my questions convinced me beyond any doubt that it was a flesh-and-blood person and not a computer that was supplying the answers!

After fifteen years at Mayo, Dr. Kirklin moved on to the medical school at the University of Alabama in Birmingham, where, as chief of surgery, he created another citadel of excellence in the field as well as establishing a remarkable clinic that now bears his name. In 1998 Dr. Kirklin became professor emeritus. Although he no longer enters the operating room, his superb textbook, coauthored with DR. BRIAN BARRATT-BOYES of New Zealand, provides an invaluable guide for those who do.[5]

The role of Dr. Lillehei in the field of open-heart surgery and the relationship between him and Dr. Kirklin are topics of great interest to me. I scheduled an interview with Dr. Lillehei, to be included in this book, but he was stricken with a number of debilitating strokes and died before we could have our conversation. To gain more insight into the Minnesota program—and Dr. Lillehei himself—I wrote to Dr. DeWall, who sent back a very helpful letter that expanded upon some of Dr. Kirklin's comments; Dr. Kirklin later received a copy of this letter.[6] References to Dr. DeWall's remarks appear in the endnotes to this interview.

<hr>

Birmingham, Alabama
July 29, 1999

<hr>

Let's begin this interview by going back in time to the early fifties, which was a very exciting period for cardiology. In 1951, CLARENCE DENNIS, who had begun his work on cardiopulmonary bypass in Minnesota and then transferred to the Downstate Medical Center in Brooklyn, attempted the first open-heart repair of a congenital cardiac defect using a pump-oxygenator and failed. In 1952, F. JOHN LEWIS performed the first successful open-heart repair of an atrial septal defect using hypothermia. In 1953, JOHN GIBBON, at Jefferson in Philadelphia, finally had his first successful open-heart repair of an atrial septal defect but was not able to repeat this feat in subsequent patients. In 1954, C. WALTON LILLEHEI began his "cross-circulatory" procedures for the open-heart correction of congenital defects, and in 1955, RICHARD A. DEWALL, with Lillehei's group, introduced the bubble oxygenator for open-heart surgery.

Now at this time you were at the Mayo Clinic, and I would like to know what you were doing then, how were you doing it, and why were you doing it.

Strange as it may seem, we were motivated more by our own experiences, and our own people, than we were by this train of events that you have recounted. Actually, the DeWall oxygenator was introduced *after* we had made our mark in the world, not before.

Whether it was stimulated by our work or vice versa, I am not very interested in arguing.

In about 1952, I operated on a patient who was made the subject of a scientific publication, I think in *Circulation,* a patient with pulmonary stenosis and intact ventricular septum. That patient was an adult in whom, at the time of surgery, I did not feel we had done a very good job. That patient died a day or two later and had an autopsy. EARL WOOD at that time was at the Mayo Clinic and would come to be known to the world as a physiologist. He was known to me as that, also, but he was also a sort of confidant, adviser, fellow conspirator, whatever you want to call it. He called me into his office and said, "John, you're never going to do any better with a heart like this until you get inside of it and can work in there at your leisure."

I said, "Well, that means a heart-lung machine."

"Well," he said, "then we'll have to have one."

As a result of that conversation, it became an integral part of my thinking to develop a heart-lung machine. Since you couldn't buy one, you had no alternative but to develop one. The Mayo Clinic, of course, was visited by lots of people in all walks of "health care," as it's now called, and I very well remember a visit by a group of British people. I don't recall whether they were surgeons or internists, but one of them asked me, "What are you doing?"

I told him that we were working on a heart-lung machine, and he said, "Oh yes, we've heard about those things. We just had a visit to Minneapolis with Dr. Lillehei, and his cross-circulation, and we think that's the exciting world of the future."

We were very aware of Dr. Lillehei's work ninety miles away. I didn't say anything, but I knew very well that that would be a temporary phenomenon. So we made a trip—Earl Wood, myself, David Donald, a guy whom we had been working with in the laboratory for a while, and maybe a few other people. We visited the three places that we knew of in North America that were doing this kind of work. One place we visited was Philadelphia, where Dr. Gibbon was at Jefferson;

the second place we visited was Toronto, where BILL MUSTARD was, and where he was using monkey lungs as the oxygenator; and the third place was Detroit, where DR. [F. DEWEY] DODRILL was located.*

Dewey Dodrill's machine was built for him by General Motors, and it looked like it—it looked like a car engine. Dr. Gibbon's machine had been built by IBM, and it looked like it—it looked like a computer. Be that as it may, we felt that the machine that had the best possibility of becoming a useful tool was Gibbon's. Therefore the Mayo Clinic, where I was quite a junior member at the time, went about the problem of getting all the usual permissions and so on. And then we started to build a Gibbon oxygenator. It wasn't right to call it a "Gibbon" pump-oxygenator, because we made a number of modifications of it. I have never named an instrument after me, and I wasn't about to name a heart-lung machine after me, so it became known as the Mayo-Gibbon oxygenator.

I knew that until we did some patients we were just also rans, so we started in March of 1955 to line up eight patients that we were going to do come hell or high water.

The first one survived, luckily; the second one survived; but they didn't all survive.

I remember very well the night of the first operation, which had been a little hectic, and I got a telephone call at home from DICK VARCO, who was working with Walt Lillehei in Minneapolis. Varco said that there was a distinguished gentleman there who would like to come down to Rochester "if your patient is still alive." I said, "She is," and he said, "Then SIR RUSSELL BROCK would like to come and visit you."

I replied that that would be fine; anybody was welcome.[7] The next day was a Wednesday, as I recall, and Sir Russell arrived and I met him and talked with him. He asked me, "Are you going to do another case while I'm in town?"

I said, "Yes. We're going to do another case tomorrow."

He said, "May I come and watch?"

---

* Another model concept, the rotating-disc oxygenator, was introduced in Sweden by VIKING O. BJÖRK and CLARENCE CRAFOORD, and later modified in the United States by FREDERICK CROSS, who came up with an improved design.

I said, "Sure. Just come at seven, and I'll get you a scrub suit. . . ."

"No, no, no," he said, "I don't want to bother you."

Now Sir Russell Brock was a very famous guy at that time, known to be blustering and difficult. I found him to be none of that. He appeared in the gallery in an inconspicuous spot and sat there quietly all morning while we did the second open-heart operation.

That's about the way it started.

> Gibbon had given up on open-heart surgery at this time, following several failures after his first success. Did he in any formal way pass his mantle to you, asking you to pick up where he had left off on his machine?

Never. I never knew what he thought about us, about me. I remember one day at the American Association of Thoracic Surgery meeting, where Walt Lillehei gave his paper about cross-circulation; I said to Dr. Gibbon, "Dr. Gibbon, the fashion seems to be cross-circulation." He said, "Kirklin, I'm not interested in fashions."

> Another question concerning your early career: reading about the first eight cases that you published in the *Mayo Clinic Proceedings*,[8] I was struck by the 50 percent mortality rate; I thought to myself that, given the current medical climate, anyone who published a series with a 50 percent mortality today might well be run out of town. Would you comment on that?

I don't have any comment on that.

> I suppose that prior to that time, everything having to do with open-heart surgery and the use of the heart-lung machine had been so negative and seemingly hopeless, that even a 50 percent mortality rate was a definite improvement!

Correct. And I think the medical world, if I may use that term, intuitively knew that the cross-circulation technique was not going to be widely accepted and/or used. Against that background there was no other alternative but to go with the heart-lung machine.

> Among the early problems during cardiopulmonary bypass was excessive bleeding into the operative field. Lillehehei emphasized the "azygos fac-

tor," the finding that dogs would survive experiments in which all the venous inflow to the heart except that from the azygos vein was closed off for a time. Lillehei pointed out that this indicated that lower perfusion rates could be used than initially thought, reducing the flooding of the field from excessive perfusion during bypass, and successfully used these lower perfusion rates in his patients.[9] Did that consideration affect your own work?

It did not because we, from the beginning, never believed it.

Isn't that interesting? Many years later, Lillehei recalled that it was one of the major findings that permitted his team to progress successfully without the need to use high perfusion rates.

He couldn't use high perfusion rates. A more accurate statement would be that he didn't because he couldn't; because he could only take so much blood from the donor in his cross-circulation procedures. At Mayo, we never intended to use low flow.

I thought of two other problems that you might have dealt with in 1955. The first was ventricular fibrillation. Were you able to defibrillate your patients at that time? The second was heart block, especially in the repair of ventricular septal defects.

We had defibrillators, so ventricular fibrillation was not really a problem. Heart block *was* a problem. In 1955 or perhaps 1956, I believe, I wrote that the surgery of ventricular septal defects would disappear from the face of the earth if the problem of heart block was not solved or prevented. Now down in Miami there was a guy named MAURICE LEV, and Maurice Lev knew where the bundle of His was, while JESSE EDWARDS, the pathologist at the Mayo Clinic, wasn't sure. Edwards suggested that I go see Dr. Lev. So I got on an airplane and went down to see Dr. Lev, and I found out where the bundle of His was, which enabled us to devise a repair, which avoided damage to the bundle of His [which could result in heart block]. Therefore, the surgery of ventricular septal defects continued.

Did you ever have to resort to inserting pacemakers for those patients?

In the very earliest days pacemakers were the only salvage for a patient, but who is going to subject a beautiful little girl of three months or three years to an operation that is known to require a pacemaker? No question about it; we had to prevent heart block from developing in the first place.[10]

> I knew Dr. Lev from the annual scientific meetings of the American Heart Association. He presented a very gruff exterior; he looked a bit like Edward G. Robinson and even spoke out of the side of his mouth as he did. But Dr. Lev really was a very nice man, and he always brought part of his collection of congenital heart specimens to these meetings and had you put on a pair of rubber gloves so you could explore them with him or one of his assistants. It was quite an educational experience, seeing these defects "in the flesh." He was a wonderful man, I thought.

He was a great man! And you know, he had a younger colleague, SAROJA BHARATI, who has continued his work, I think.

> Another problem you were interested in was "perfusion lung." I know you did a lot of work on that. Could you tell me about your contribution to this subject?

What was my contribution? I believe it remains for others to identify contributions and not the contributor. Who can say? I don't know. Anyway, we developed a lot of knowledge over a period of ten or twenty years, perhaps, about the so-called perfusion lung.[11]

> What is the current status of the heart-lung machine? As an echocardiographer, I go into the operating room to observe the transesophageal echoes of patients and hardly pay attention to the machines whirring away without fanfare. We seem to take it all for granted now.

My opinion is that the current machines suffer terribly from their success, and, as a result, no real improvements have occurred in the last five to ten to fifteen years.

> Something that concerns some of us, even though it is not talked about much, are the effects of bypass on the brain. Not the gross effects like air embolus or thromboembolism, but the subtler effects of open-heart surgery on the central nervous system.

I think it is an enormously complicated subject, and that any pat discussion of it is going to be incomplete and wrong. I think that there are many possible reasons or explanations of brain damage that might occur during cardiopulmonary bypass, but I believe that the facts are that it affects, in an important way, only a minority of patients.

> It's extraordinary that in the whole world, the two places where open-heart surgery got its start were located only ninety miles apart in the heartland of the United States—the University of Minnesota and the Mayo Clinic—rather than in any of the previously recognized academic centers of excellence.

Walt Lillehei tended to refer to those as "the halcyon days."

> I had the pleasure of interviewing DR. OWEN H. WANGENSTEEN many years ago, and apparently he created an atmosphere in Minneapolis with people like Varco, MAURICE VISSCHER, Lillehei, and the rest, that promoted the kind of groundbreaking work they did. Was there a similar situation at the Mayo Clinic when you were a young surgeon there?

Like most questions, the one you put evolves, in part, into a matter of opinion—every word you said. That was one point of view; it was not the only point of view about the University of Minnesota. Other points of view included that they had unbridled financial privileges, and that that led to Walt Lillehei's undoing.

> I don't understand what you mean by "unbridled privileges."

I'm amazed, but perhaps it's because it's so long ago, relatively speaking, that it's forgotten, but Dr. Lillehei made a fortune.[12] Whereas I didn't.

> But I believe you created a different kind of fortune, not personal but in terms of the benefits you brought to the profession and Alabama, especially. But while you were at Mayo you had some very interesting people there: Jesse Edwards, Earl Wood, HOWARD BURCHELL . . .

Yes we did. They were essential. We had, I think for that time, and maybe even for the current time, a small, compact group of highly talented people, the likes of which I don't think existed elsewhere in the world at that time. You've named them: Jesse Edwards, Earl Wood,

Howard Burchell; and I am sure there are a few others—a little later an anesthesiologist named Dick Theye. There were always during my years there this small group that changed a bit over time as people moved—Jesse moved to St. Paul; Howard Burchell went to Minneapolis/St. Paul; I came down here to Birmingham. Why it gradually broke up is an interesting question that I've never thought much about, but I'm sure someone could find a reason. But that group of individuals, during the early to mid fifties and lapping over into the sixties, was a very cohesive, tough group that was integrated in an interesting way. A group to which I owe everything.

I assume that you did get the go-ahead from the upper echelons at Mayo.

Several years ago, a good friend of mine at the Mayo Clinic, Bob Frye, a cardiologist, had a meeting at which, I was told, the question was raised as to how we got the approval of the board of trustees to spend all that money it must have cost to develop that heart-lung machine. We never did! The money came from the Mayo Clinic, of course, but I don't remember ever doing what is such a common everyday practice nowadays, the submission of a grant application and so on. I don't remember ever doing that at the Mayo Clinic. I did [submit a grant application] to the NIH eventually, but the early work was supported by the Mayo Clinic, and your original statement is correct: we got the green light.

You had a very interesting relationship with Lillehei. So many surgeons are competitive with one another, but there was an unusual cooperation between you and Lillehei. . . .

Not really. When you say "cooperation" is when I say "Not really."

How about "appreciation"?

I tend to appreciate the world around me, and a very important part of that world at the time was Walt Lillehei. Walt was a difficult person that, I made up my mind quietly, I needed to know better. I needed to get inside of him somehow and see what really made him tick, not what the newspapers said made him tick. So once I became a little bit established, I invited him to come down to Rochester and give a talk. That was the first time it had ever been done. He couldn't believe it.[13]

Why did I do that? I don't know. It seems to me that the world has enough problems without adding to them by developing interpersonal problems. I had some arguments on airplanes with Dick Varco, more than Walt, who tended to travel in a different milieu than I did. But, yes, I appreciated him, and, eventually, I felt sorry for him because he had been discarded.

> Lillehei had been found guilty on all five counts brought against him by the IRS in 1973 and was treated like some kind of a pariah for several years. Then, when the American Association for Thoracic Surgery, of which you were the president, met in 1979 in Boston, you spotted him in the audience and pointed him out as the "great and pioneering cardiac surgeon" he was, asking him to stand up and acknowledge the great applause that followed.

I resurrected him!

> It had been really a sad train of events when he seemed to go off the deep end in terms of his behavior at a certain point in his life.

Or maybe it just became evident.[14]

> Be that as it may, your action at that meeting, I think, was very much to your credit, if I may say so.

Thank you.

> As we talk about competitiveness among surgeons, I must tell you an anecdote about this, one involving DENTON COOLEY. In the late sixties or early seventies, I was attending an American College of Cardiology course for cardiologists on the latest developments in cardiac surgery. It was held in Philadelphia, and, at one point, all of the approximately twenty-five attendees were sitting in the first two rows of this rather large auditorium as lunchtime approached. Cooley was scheduled to speak around noon on the topic of surgery of the aorta, a field in which he and Michael DeBakey had become the leaders. However, Cooley decided to talk, instead, on coronary bypass surgery, which was the hot topic of the time, and to discuss the first fifty or so surgeries of this type that he had done in Houston.

Meanwhile, DONALD EFFLER of the Cleveland Clinic was scheduled to talk after Cooley, and since the topic of coronary surgery had been assigned to him, he was visibly steaming as Cooley proceeded. After all, at that time it was the Cleveland Clinic that was leading the way in that field. If Cooley had fifty cases to discuss, Effler probably had five hundred.

As Cooley began to talk, people from all over began to drift into the auditorium. I don't know whether it was just lunchtime, or Cooley, or both, but within minutes the auditorium was bursting at the seams, with every seat filled, and people crouching in the aisles and standing in the back. Now, no sooner did Cooley complete his talk as one o'clock approached than, like some old-fashioned movie comedy with the film run rapidly in reverse, the people seemed to empty out in a minute or so, and there again were the two dozen cardiologists in the first couple of rows, with Effler, now, about to begin.

Effler just stood there as the audience fled as if bubonic plague had suddenly broken out, viewing their exit with a wry expression. When the last one left, he glanced over his shoulder at Cooley, who was sitting behind him, and said, "Jesus, Denton, you really drove 'em out of here!"

I thought that was priceless.

Now let's get back to John Kirklin. In the early days of open-heart surgery, almost all of it seemed to be for congenital disease. There certainly was a lot of valvular disease around, but not much was being done. Was that because there were no good artificial valves available?

No. It was because most places, of the few that existed in those early days, had heart-lung machines that couldn't perfuse a big person. That was my opinion—and still is. It is no longer a problem, but the Mayo-Gibbon machine was the first that could perfuse an adult.

That, of course, is very important.

If you're interested in adults.

Let's backtrack for a moment. You were a boy from Muncie, Indiana. How did you get to Minnesota?

My father was a doctor. He was a radiologist, and somehow, at some meeting, DR. WILL MAYO had identified him as an up-and-coming individual in the radiological world. We were living in Muncie at the time, and Dr. Carmen was head of radiology at the Mayo Clinic then, and it was known he was going to die from cancer—this was in the twenties. So Dr. Mayo invited my father to come to Rochester into the radiology department and promised him that when Carmen died, he would become the head. So we ended up in Rochester, Minnesota, in the late twenties.

So you later went to the University of Minnesota for your undergraduate degree and then to Harvard Medical School. Who impressed you there?

Well, it was Harvard even then, so there were tons of them. I spent a lot of time with a man named Logan in the Biochemistry Department. I became, in some interesting way, a little bit of a friend of A. BAIRD HASTINGS, who was the head of biochemistry, and later, I encountered him in a different role when he was at Scripps.

Perhaps it was the war, or perhaps it was you, but you had sort of a peripatetic experience during your years as an intern and resident. Could you take me through that?

It would seem to be peripatetic. I suppose I am, in a way, an "anti" person. At Harvard, if you didn't take a straight internship, you weren't worth anything; so I decided I would take a rotating internship. In Boston they didn't want to talk to you about the best rotating internship, because obviously the best internships were in Boston, and they didn't have any rotating internships. So I went to the University of Pennsylvania Hospital, which was alleged to have the best rotating internship at the time. It was not a fair sample, really, because World War II was on, and a lot of the University of Pennsylvania people were away in the service: in their general hospital in India, and [ISIDORE] RAVDIN [the chief of surgery] was away. It was also the "999 period," which most people today have never even heard of, but the way it worked was that you were approved for nine months at a time to be exempted from the army while you continued your training.

So I stayed in Pennsylvania for the first nine months, and then went to the Mayo Clinic as part of the "999" program, and stayed there a second nine months. I never applied for the third nine months, because the war was on and I figured I needed to be in it. So I became part of the United States Army.

You did neurosurgery in the army. How did that affect you?

I did neurosurgery because, when I went into the army in the spring of 1944, we had the Normandy invasion, and soon there were tons of casualties. So the army plucked some people like me, who had had some general surgery training but weren't sufficiently trained in general surgery to have an army general surgery specialty number. They took us and said, "You guys are going to be neurosurgeons." They sent me back for training to the University of Pennsylvania for six weeks; then to O'Reilly General Hospital in Springfield, Missouri, to the neurosurgical service, where I became a neurosurgeon.

The experience in neurosurgery was very helpful to me. I operated a lot; and I became totally at home in the extremities, where, before that army experience, I had always felt uncomfortable, as did most people. You ordinarily didn't have the opportunity in civilian surgery to wander up and down somebody's hand, arms, axillas, sciatic nerves, and so forth. It helped me a lot, and I think the techniques of cardiac surgery, at least at one time, were the techniques of neurosurgery, because I introduced them.

> I also took a rotating internship, and although it wasn't popular at the time, I felt that, as a later medical resident, I, unlike some of my straight medical confreres, at least knew when I had a surgical problem and knew when to call a surgeon, and would not sit on a case that needed one. I'm sure the patients benefited from this.

I'm sure you're right.

Of course, I neglected to say that, during my residency period, I became acquainted with ROBERT E. GROSS. And if my training was peripatetic, it was because of Robert Gross. I first encountered him as a medical student, of course, and there was one day when suddenly there were 110 future heart surgeons sitting in an amphitheater in the Peter Bent Brigham Hospital . It was the day in our freshman year when there was a lecture being given on a Saturday morning by Robert E. Gross on wound healing. Did you ever see him in person? Well, he walked in, the very image of a surgeon: probably five foot eight or nine, with his hair in perfect order, immaculately dressed in a beautiful blue suit and red tie. He gave a lecture that was not particularly inspiring, but he was clearly Robert Gross, and he was the world's opinion of a surgeon in appearance. And all those medical students were going to be heart surgeons at the conclusion of that lecture because it was only a few weeks before that he had successfully closed a patent ductus.

Years later, after I had returned to Rochester to complete my surgical residency training, I took six months to go to Boston to work with Dr. Gross, before returning to Rochester as an assistant resident in surgery.

> It's interesting how some innovative surgical advances are sometimes planned. When he attempted his first ductus, I believe he had another patient lined up for the next day, just in case the first one failed. It is the tack that you and your associates took at Mayo when you planned your first eight cases on the pump come hell or high water. Charles Bailey did the same thing before his first successful mitral commissurotomy. People generally don't realize this.

I wonder if those stories are apocryphal or true. I'm not sure of the one about Gross.

> The one about Bailey, I am fairly sure is true, because on the afternoon of his first success in one hospital, he had just come from a morning operation at another hospital where he had lost the patient. As for Gross, by the way, and another first, I think he was resentful that, when he was planning a correction for coarctation of the aorta, CLARENCE CRAFOORD, who had visited him in Boston to learn from him, beat him to the punch when he got back to Sweden.

I think that was true.

> You had such a terrifically successful time at Mayo, about twenty-five years, and when it became Mayo Medical School, you were chosen to be its first chairman for the Department of Surgery. And you left. Why?

For a long time I never knew why I left. Even now, what I say about it may not be trustworthy. I just left. A new challenge? Something different? Perhaps it was like the time I was deciding which college to go to. All my friends were going to go to Dartmouth, Harvard, Princeton, and so forth. I went to the University of Minnesota. Why? Maybe just to be different.

At the time I left Mayo, people said, "Birmingham, Alabama? You've got to be crazy; there's blood in the streets!" And I suddenly found that all my friends were experts on blacks. They had never seen one; they didn't know anything about it. Again, it was maybe a repeat of why I went to the University of Minnesota instead of Harvard or Yale. I was just, maybe, different.

> **Not long ago, I met Dr. S. Richardson Hill, who was dean at the University of Alabama Medical School in Birmingham at the time, and he told me that the best thing he ever accomplished was getting you to come down on the pretext of just having you advise them on what the school needed to accomplish in surgery after the previous chairman, Champ Lyons, had died. Did you ever feel that you had been snookered?**

Who was kidding whom? I knew why I had come down. That was just a play they were making.

> **Let's now talk about some of your accomplishments in Birmingham. I understand that there are currently about two thousand university beds here. And I was especially impressed by the Kirklin Clinic, the outpatient facility. Could you comment on this?**

When I came down here, I joined academia, something, I suppose, that deep down in my heart I had always wanted to do. But, at that time, I found academia full of worms, and I saw a lot of things that I didn't like. One of them was the University of Alabama in Birmingham. It was my nature to try to improve it. To do this I developed the University of Alabama Health Services Foundation. No doubt it was a copy of the Mayo Foundation, but without some of the "pieces." For example, there was no salary committee, although I thought someday there might be. It was difficult but worth it, because I have high standards for myself, other people, *and* university medical centers. And, with all due respect, I don't think that many of them deserve their fame. Some do, and some don't.

At least I had the opportunity in a place that was "nothing," to see if I could make it into "something." And I figured that was what they wanted. So after a few years there was the University of Alabama Health Services Foundation, and JIM PITTMAN did the most to further this. When each new chairman came, Pittman said, "Of course, you will become part of the foundation." So, gradually, all the chairmen were in the foundation, but originally there was enormous faculty opposition to it; only surgery and anesthesiology were in at the beginning.

At one point, someone said to me, "You have no idea how terrible the practice conditions are." At the time, every doctor saw patients in his office, and the few patients that were seen that way were wealthy people in town—not blacks, of course. I take some pride that this hospital was the first one in the state of Alabama where a black could occupy a bed. I'm not an activist, particularly, but I thought that they were being screwed badly by the rest of the population.

Someone said that we would have to get all these guys together, and we decided that we would have to have a building. Why? Well, in a town which is fifty miles from Rochester was a famous little bank building; and it was famous because it was designed by Frank Lloyd Wright. So I figured, why not make Birmingham famous by having I. M. Pei build a building? People said he was the world's greatest architect, and he said, "I'll do it."

Then I had a bitter argument with the fellow who was president of UAB, and this made me quit as president of the foundation. Following this, he insisted, "The building has got to be named after you, sir." So that's the way that building came about.

Another of your accomplishments I want to mention is your textbook on cardiovascular surgery, which you cowrote with BRIAN BARRATT-BOYES. You and he were both at Mayo at one time. Did this proximity lead to your doing the book together?

No. We were on a bus in Buenos Aires, he with his wife, and I with mine. We were coming back from some meeting, and he said, "You know, I'm writing a book." I said, "That's funny; I am too." So I suggested to him that we write it together and make it twice as good. So, reluctantly, I think, he agreed. There were some problems about "the book" with Brian's second wife, but we got it done, and it was a wonderful experience for me and Brian, too, although he, perhaps, wouldn't admit it. He has had two reoperations for coronary bypass grafting, but he's a very talented guy. Sitting down there in Auckland, New Zealand, he made the world come to him because of his raw talent. He was a great surgeon and a great thinker.

> What I like especially about the book are the historical sections beginning each chapter on various subjects.

How can you understand the world if you don't know what happened in it?

> EUGENE BLACKSTONE worked with you for a number of years. Would you comment on this relationship?

Yes, I'd be happy to. I had been in Birmingham for a relatively short time, and a guy walks into my office one day, sits down, and says, "I'm Gene Blackstone. I want an internship here." I told him that there was a national committee he had to go through, the matching program and all that. He replied that he was not eligible for that. I thought that here is another guy who failed in medical school, went to some off-shore school or something like that. I was about to lose interest when he added that he had graduated three years earlier from the University of Chicago. I asked him what he had been doing since then, and he mentioned some names of some famous people with whom he had worked. So I thought that this was a kind of unusual kid and took him on as an intern. And he was unusual. We worked together for about twenty years, but UAB didn't understand his value and let the Cleveland Clinic "buy him." This was about two or three years ago.

> Moving on to your personal life: I know you married a physician, as I did. I thought this wise because only another physician can really understand the craziness of your life as such. Did you have the same felicitous experience?

Yes and no. It's true I married a physician, and I would do it again. She's still alive, I'm happy to say, and I'm still in love with her. There's an interesting aspect to that story. When I was at Mayo for all those years, they didn't want her to work as a doctor. They were afraid of some kind of precedent. When I came to Alabama, she did work for several years and did some very good things, in my opinion.

Maybe she understood when I came home at ten o'clock instead of five like most other men. But actually, I think my life with her was with her as a woman and not a woman doctor.

You had three children, and one has become a transplant surgeon. How is that working out?

That was my second one, Jim. I guess he's good.

Has he suffered at all from being the son of "the great John Kirklin"?

I don't know. Probably not; he doesn't give a damn about it. He went to Harvard; he took his residency at the MGH [Massachusetts General Hospital], a paragon of a place, I suppose. I called him a few weeks ago, and for the first time ever I said this to him: "Jim, is there some way I can help you?" I did this because he gets home at ten or eleven every night, and half the nights after he gets home, he has to get up again. That's no way to live. I can tell him that because I lived that way myself for a while.

He said, "Yeah. You could help me with my book." So I'm doing that.

Since you came to Alabama, you have assumed many more administrative burdens than you had at Mayo. Did that detract at all from your surgical work?

I have no way of knowing, because I have nothing to compare it with. The Mayo Clinic is, of course, a terribly interesting place even today. Alabama is also terribly interesting, but the two are terribly different. Jim, you may or may not know, recently had an opportunity to go the Mayo Clinic in Scottsdale, Arizona, but turned it down after investigating it thoroughly.

How old were you when you stopped doing surgery, and why did you stop?

I was about seventy. I always knew that I needed to stop. There was a surgeon I knew in Brazil who kept on operating long after everybody knew he should have quit. And I didn't want that to happen to me; but I wasn't quite ready to quit when it came time to retire from chairmanship of the Department of Surgery and the Division of Thoracic Surgery. So after this, I operated for a while and then quit before the world said, "That guy should have quit a long time ago.

Do you have any regrets about any things in the past?

Hundreds of things!

I always ask that question at the end of an interview, and there are two standard answers: the subject either has many regrets or has none at all. No one ever says "a few." Would you like to name a couple of your regrets?

I wish I had made a lot more money.

What are your current projects?

I now have two since I agreed to help Jim with his book. This is on heart transplantation, which is not "my bag," but I know a little bit about it because we were very interested in the damaging effects of cardiopulmonary bypass, which have a lot to do with the immune system. So that's one thing I'm doing.

About five years ago, for certain reasons, I began to have an interest in computerized patient records. I believe that, five years from now, an institution that does not have computerized patient records will be in the doghouse. The ally in this effort over the past five years has been the federal government.

As I reviewed your very extensive bibliography, I frequently came upon your contributions to symposia on the advances in cardiovascular surgery. As I read this material I got the impression that you are continually turning up at the end to remind us that every silver lining happens to have a cloud along with it. "Things are not quite as good as you think they are." Is that an accurate observation?

I think it is. It's a way of stimulating people.

Well then, what about the future?

Since I'm enjoying talking to you, I'll do my best to answer the question. Otherwise, I probably wouldn't. I am not an admirer of the present world. The one "journal" I read every day is the *Wall Street Journal*, so it colors my thinking a little.

My relations with the computer world also color my thinking a little. I think there must be a terrible time coming when people will have to begin to work again. I believe that the current era in health care, worldwide, as I view it, is—to say the least—temporary, tempestuous, and what will follow it I don't know.

In cardiac surgery I am impressed by the fact that people are now going for gimmicks: doing heart surgery without cardiopulmonary bypass, for example. There are instrument companies that are basing their entire financial future on developing instruments to operate through little keyholes. Maybe those trends are highly important; I don't know. They haven't swept the world. Some of the people I know and talk to who have experience with these procedures think them a little phony. So if I were a kid today, I probably would not become a cardiac surgeon. It's old hat now.

Is there anything else you would like to get into the record?

A million things. One is in regard to the second edition of the book by Kirklin and Barrett-Boyes, which was really written by Kirklin. It said all I had to say about cardiac surgery and said it in a carefully constructed and thoughtful way in spite of the predictions that there would never be a second edition.

Why did people make that prediction?

You would have to ask the people who said it. I suppose it was because the first edition was unique. BILL ROBERTS, for example, predicted that there would never be a second edition, because, I think, he thought the first edition was great—and so did I—partly because it involved Barratt-Boyes, from another part of the world. Yet I was a little constrained by that relationship, so I knew there would have to be a second edition, and there was. Judging by the reports from the publisher, it has been bought mostly, in the last few years, by cardiologists.

Well, this has been great. You have been so generous of your time . . .

I haven't told you anything.

Oh yes you have!

7

ARTHUR C. GUYTON, M.D.
(1919–   )

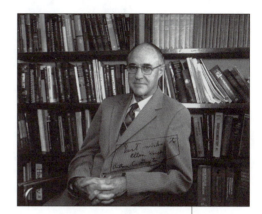

During the administration of President Lyndon Johnson, the notion of targeted or mission-oriented research became a dominant one on the Washington scene. Scientists of all stripes, however, realized how often it was that basic, undirected research often resulted in what might eventually be termed practical payoffs in terms of scientific advances. In response to the prevailing Washington bureaucratic view, JULIUS H. COMROE, JR. and Robert D. Dripps, in 1974, authored what has become something of a classic in its expression of research philosophy. The article was titled "Ben Franklin and Open Heart Surgery."[1]

They began by taking a poll of physicians and surgeons, asking them to select the most important *clinical* advance since 1945 that *directly* benefited their patients. The list of the top ten that resulted was headed by open-heart surgery. With this as a starting point, Comroe and Dripps then posed the question: was this "a giant leap" up to the top of the mountain by the cardiac surgeon, or did the surgeon have to take a number of steps up the back of the mountain before this great advance could be made? The illustration they used in posing this question is reproduced here (Fig. 7-1).

Among the many scientific disciplines contributing along the way, perhaps most notable was physiology. Without the basic knowledge of how the normal—and abnormal—circulations worked, this magnificent feat of medical science would never have been achieved.

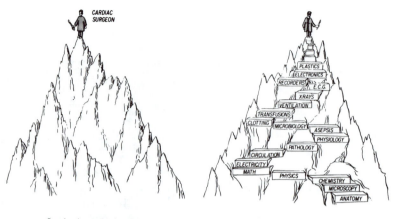

One giant leap to the pinnacle?   *Or did he climb the steps up the back of the mountain?*

FIGURE 7-1. Figure from J. H. Comroe and R. D. Dripps, Ben Franklin and open heart surgery, *Circ Res* 1974; 35:661–669.

(Reproduced by permission of Williams and Wilkins.)

One of the circulatory physiologists who distinguished himself during this period of investigative ferment was Arthur C. Guyton at the University of Mississippi. Graduating with a medical degree from Harvard, he directed his initial efforts toward surgery, cardiac surgery in particular. This potential career was stopped in its tracks when Guyton was struck down with paralytic polio while still a surgical resident at the Massachusetts General Hospital.

He refused, however, to become a victim. From the time of his boyhood days Guyton had demonstrated an aptitude for mechanics and electronics; he was also remarkably good at building things. Then, even as a medical student and house officer, he began to demonstrate an interest in medical science far different and sophisticated from that of most surgical residents. After surviving the initial onslaught of his disease, although still severely physically incapacitated, he drew upon these talents and, with the steadfast support of his wife, began a new life for himself in the field of physiology at the University of Mississippi School of Medicine, finally becoming chairman of the department in 1948. It was a post he would hold for forty-one years.

During this time, in addition to building an outstanding department, he carried on an enormous amount of basic research on the cardiovascular system and published a superb text in physiology, one that has gone through numerous editions, in many languages, and has been popular throughout the world.[2] His story is one of the most successful and inspiring in all of medicine.

———

Jackson, Mississippi
March 25, 1999

———

If I were to use three words to define "physiology" to a layperson, I would say it's about "how things work."

That's exactly how I would put it.

Now you have devoted your life to answering questions pertaining to this, and I think it is important for people to recognize the contributions of basic science to all the advances in the diagnosis and treatment of heart disease over the last eighty or ninety years. Your interests have been so far-ranging; I wonder if you could begin by telling us about some of the things you did as a boy that got you started on all this.

As I boy, I lived with my family in a small town, Oxford, Mississippi, and it still is a small town. The university is located there. We had a good deal of land around our house when I was a very small boy, and there was a pasture around the back where we kept a horse, and had a chicken yard with chicken houses, and so forth. By the time I got to be about four, five, or six years old, we gave up most of that, and I turned one of those chicken houses into a shop. So beginning at the age of seven or eight, I always had a shop.

You were always building things, weren't you?

Yes, I liked to make things. At first it was all woodworking. Later on, I had access to some metalworking tools, and still later on, when I got into medical school, I worked all through on a student fellowship in the biochemistry department with DR. [A. BAIRD] HASTINGS.

Before you even got to medical school, while you were growing up, you had to make a decision: would it be a career in physics, medicine, or even electrical engineering? What was it that turned you toward medicine? Was it the influence of your father, who was a physician?

I presume it was my father who influenced me that way, but he never tried to put obvious pressure on me. He would say something like, "If you're going to be a physicist, how are you going to make a living?" But physics was the one field that I enjoyed the most, that and mathematics, and physical types of chemistry.

You did your undergraduate work at "Ole Miss," the University of Mississippi, and then went to Harvard for medical school. How did that come about?

I went to Harvard principally because my older brother had gone there before me. He was five years older than I. After graduating from Harvard, he went to Johns Hopkins for ophthalmology. My father had been a specialist in eye, ears, nose, and throat. That was a usual combination back in those days, but my brother was strictly an ophthalmologist. He stayed on at Johns Hopkins after his residency, on the faculty, but he died at an early age and never had a chance to do too much. He was only in his thirties. I don't know exactly what happened, but I heard that he had had some cardiac symptoms of some sort.

Was it much of a culture shock, going from Mississippi to Boston?

No, but it was different. I had had mainly a physics and mathematics type of background, with very few courses requiring memorizing, at the University of Mississippi. I enjoyed that very much. I had very close relationships with the teachers because in those particular subjects there were not many students in the classes. In one class, I recall, there were only four of us. In another, there were not even that many who signed up so that it became a study program class, working back and forth with the teacher twenty or thirty minutes every week. I had a math course taught by the previous chancellor of the university with only eight students. It was a beautiful experience, going through the University of Mississippi.

When I got to Harvard, the "culture shock" was all the memorizing. We had anatomy right off the bat, and at that time, anatomy was just pure memorizing, quite a different story from what I had known before.

There were some outstanding people at Harvard while you were there, WALTER B. CANNON and others . . .

I didn't have much contact with Walter Cannon because he was at the retirement age at that time, and he came to work only a few hours a week, giving some lectures; but he wasn't too active. I had the most contact with Baird Hastings, in all respects. He was head of the Department of Biochemistry. He was also a physical chemist and interested in the physicochemical aspects of the body fluids and membrane transport. That was what attracted me to him. I worked with him on electrolytes and electrical methods for analyzing electrolytes.

In 1943 you became a surgical intern at the Massachusetts General Hospital. There seems to be a tradition among many surgeons and surgical programs that the work goes on endlessly, with no time for study or reflection. This seemed to bother you.

That was very true. It was during wartime, and the training program in the surgical department was really just a "workfest." The average day would be sixteen hours, and you would be worn out all the time. This may have changed somewhat. I have watched my own children go through surgical programs; they're hard but not to the point of continual total exhaustion. The problem that I found with that routine was that if you did find something you wanted to study specially, they didn't give you the time for it.

You still found time to develop a gastrointestinal suction machine, though, while you were at Mass. General.

Yes, but that wasn't introduced until after the war when I returned from military service. During the war, I worked in bacterial warfare at Camp Dietrich in Maryland, but while there I could do anything I wanted to in my spare time. I used this time to work on a tubular device that had pulsatile suction to keep those long Miller-Abbott tubes opened up. While I was a surgical house officer, I had found that if you put these ten-foot-long tubes down the GI tract, they always got blocked on the way down, and you or the nurse had to go back every fifteen minutes, half hour, or hour to open them up. So I put this pulsatile vacuum on them, which kept them clean and open. When I got back to the Mass. General, I brought several of these with me and sent some to Johns Hopkins as well. At Hopkins, they put them on patients and began to use them; they worked quite well. And, eventually, they put many of them on the service after I returned to Mass. General.

> Tell me about your work with Dr. Reginald H. Smithwick. What was he like?

I was with the last group at the beginning of the war that went through a full surgical internship—a full year, rather than a nine-month period, which came later when the war was on. All in our group went into the navy or the army. While at Mass. General, I worked quite closely with Dr. Smithwick, who was a "fine country boy." I think he was from western New York.

> I once assisted at one of those Smithwick operations, severing the sympathetic chain to treat hypertension. This was pretty impressive until all the drugs came out that could work equally well.

I helped him with about forty or fifty of them. Every time he would get a resident, the resident would help for a few weeks; then Smithwick would say, "Open up for me," and he would come in about fifteen minutes later; and still later on, he would let you take out part of the sympathetic chain yourself. (During World War II, I did a lot of these operations on dogs and studied the hemodynamics with and without the sympathetic nervous system.)

When I got out of the navy, Dr. Smithwick, who had moved by that time to Boston University from the Mass. General, asked me to join him. However, he was doing mostly sympathectomies, while Dr. [Edward] Churchill, the chief at Mass. General, wanted to develop cardiovascular surgery, which was my interest. So when Dr. Churchill told me he had a place for me, I went back there. He also gave me my own laboratory in his own suite there, and I would work up there in the evening.

> Tell me about the polio.

I had been back at the Mass. General about five or six months when I got polio. I got it at the end of October, and at first I just felt rather weak, still seeing patients. But there was such a heavy work schedule for the residents that you just didn't turn in sick; as long as you could move around, you kept on. If I had turned myself in when I first became ill, I probably would not have gotten as severe a case of polio as I did.

> DR. SABIN once told me that the more you exercised muscles while you were coming down with the disease, the worse they would later be affected. Maybe if you were a medical resident you would not have been so severely incapacitated!

Maybe, but I was working sixteen hours a day, and, after doing that day after day, seeing all the patients, busy all the time, feverish with a temperature of about 101, suddenly I was just too weak to walk anymore. I turned myself into the emergency ward, got a little sleep, and the next morning when I woke up and tried to reach my arm over my body, I couldn't do it.

When I got ill, it was not the usual time of year for a polio epidemic, so they thought at first that it was something other than polio. I had just come off neurosurgery ten days or two weeks before, and had treated a few patients with tuberculous meningitis and others with tuberculosis of the spinal cord, so these were possibilities. It turned out that I was one of the first new cases of a new polio epidemic in Boston, which became apparent a few weeks later. I was convinced, however, right from the beginning that I had contracted polio, although, at first, no one would believe me. But I made the diagnosis on myself, as it turned out.

I was hospitalized at the Mass. General for about four or five months before I was transferred to Warm Springs, Georgia.[3]

> It must have been a devastating experience for you, with a wife and children to support at the time.

You say to yourself, "How am I going to make a living? What's going to happen to them?" My father, being a doctor, felt the same way, and he was trying to make all sorts of arrangements for me right from the beginning. He even changed his will to set up a trust fund, mainly for my son and another child who was on the way.

What was the residual paralysis you wound up with?

For a time, I was virtually totally paralyzed in all the muscles of my body; about the only thing left was the ability to breathe. I couldn't turn over; I couldn't roll; I couldn't do anything. Then, about three weeks later, as well as I can recall these events of fifty-five years ago, I raised my left foot a little bit. The nurse came running, and I began to move the left foot to demonstrate. During the next few days, the muscles gradually got better in the left leg. I got a little more movement back in my left thigh, my right arm, and the trunk, but both shoulders were badly affected—the left shoulder is still totally paralyzed and the right severely limited so that I cannot raise either arm at the shoulder. I can flex the right arm at the elbow and can squeeze some with my right hand. Nothing is left in my left arm or forearm and nothing in the right leg from the hip down, and weakness is everywhere else. It was five or six months before I could barely push myself to the upright position, using my right arm and left leg.

You were at Warm Springs about six months and then returned to Mississippi, but, even before you left, you developed a couple of inventions for polio patients.

I couldn't build either of these devices, because I had no place to build them, but I could do all the drawing I wanted to do, so I drew designs for a "walking" leg brace and a motor-powered wheelchair. Later, I changed my big, long brace into a device that had a ratchet at the knee in such a way that, after I swung my right foot forward, the knee ratchet would lock, and then I could put my weight on the leg without any fear of it giving way, so I could walk on it. And then, when I was ready to take another step, the ratchet would unlock and I could swing that foot forward. Later on, when I left Warm Springs and went home, I decided to use a spring at the ankle instead of a jointed, solid brace to keep the foot from dropping. I made the one that I am still wearing today fifty years ago, and still using it.

I also designed a motorized type of wheelchair so that those who could not use their arms to move a chair could still get around.

> I have to note for the record the extent of your inventiveness, which may not be generally appreciated. We've already mentioned the suction device, the brace, and the wheelchair; but I've gone through your bibliography and found, among others: a square wave nerve stimulator, an apparatus for producing quantitative ischemia of the limb, an electrostatic particle counter, a method for continuous recording of hemoglobin, a technique for recording pulse pressure through the skin of dogs, a stereovectorcardiograph, an arteriovenous oxygen difference recorder, a method for continuous recording of pulmonary blood flow, a system for measuring capillary red cell velocity, and a method for measuring subcutaneous fluid pressure. I find it amazing that you were always able to devise the right instrumentation to provide answers to the physiological questions you were investigating.
>
> But now let's pick up on your life after Warm Springs, when you returned to Mississippi.

I went back to Mississippi more for a rest than anything else. I hoped to be able to do a bit of teaching and research. By that time they had gotten me up on crutches, and I could walk a little, with the crutches and a long leg brace.

I needed a job, some place to work, and fortunately, because of my medical degree and background in research, in 1947 the University of Mississippi Medical School gave me a position as an associate professor of pharmacology. I taught pharmacology to medical students and pharmacy students, mostly the latter. I also had a part-time position in physiology at the University of Tennessee, located sixty-five miles away in Memphis, Tennessee.

> How did you wind up as head of the Department of Physiology at Mississippi?

The head of our Department of Physiology at the University of Mississippi Medical School was given a position as dean of another medical school, and this left the physiology department with nobody to teach the course. He had had only one person there with him before he left, a trainee, so I just applied for the job when it became available. They were desperate, so they told me they would give me a try, figuring that I wouldn't be able to get up and around enough to handle the job. But it turned out that it was easier to be head of a department than just a teacher in a department; because then you could tell people what to do instead of just asking, "Would you please do this?"

By that time, I had already received a research grant from the NIH to study pulmonary edema and the physiology of this type of edema resulting from different types of heart disease. That research began to pay off quickly, with papers being published and so forth, so that, actually, I had more research going than anyone else in the school. It all worked out well, and I was free to lecture about material that I liked to study. With the NIH opening up more grant opportunities, we were able to get more grants, and before you knew it, we had more money for research there than our medical school had ever known.

Then I was given the position of acting head of the physiology department. They tried me out for about twenty months before they gave me the full title.

> I figured out that you were twenty-nine when you became head of the department and that when you retired, it was forty-one years later, 1948 to 1989. I think this must be some kind of a record. I recalled some other "long timers" including CARL J. WIGGERS at Western Reserve, who headed that department for thirty-five years; and OWEN H. WANGENSTEEN at the University of Minnesota, who headed the Department of Surgery there for thirty-seven years. I can't think of anyone who has beaten your record; can you?

I think that if you go back in history, around the turn of the century, you might find a different story, because they were all at work the same way I was at the time. For example, [ERNEST] STARLING, in England, probably had a very long period as the head of a department.[4]

> You once made a remark to the effect that if you wanted to learn about something, you had to do it by yourself, but still I'm sure that there must have been some people in physiology whom you looked up to, who were your models. Who were they?

None of them at Harvard because the department was in decline at the time, with Walter Cannon so ill with a chronic terminal illness, and on the scene so little of the time. It was the subject of physiology per se that enticed me. At about the time of my own appointment, Dr. Richard Bing was getting started at Johns Hopkins. He gave some lectures in physiology, although he was actually in the Department of Surgery under [ALFRED] BLALOCK. I was interested in some of his writings and visited his laboratory, although I don't think he knew who I was at the time. I had not yet begun to publish on circulatory physiology, although I did have some publications on some of the physical chemistry aspects of body fluids.

What influenced me mainly was the reading I did. The papers that I liked most were those of Blalock, who had done research at the University of Alabama before going to Johns Hopkins. I also read A. Rosenbleuth's and Cannon's work at Harvard, but I guess the papers that intrigued me most were those of Starling; I read virtually everything he had written and decided that that was the kind of research I wanted to do.

> There are a number of aspects of your research that I, as a cardiologist, would like to go into: your studies on interstitial fluid, hypertension, pulmonary edema, for example; but time does not permit. I would, however, like you to discuss your ideas on the control of the cardiac output. I recall a symposium on this topic in *Physiological Reviews* back in 1955, where your paper[5] was positioned among articles by STANLEY J. SARNOFF, DONALD E. GREGG, LOUIS N. KATZ, and ROBERT F. RUSHMER—some pretty heavy hitters in the field. Each of their labs had its own take on this; your own seemed derived right from Starling.

Actually, my thoughts on this didn't derive from Starling. Starling did the heart part, only. As I recall, he did mention venous return in one paper, but very little about venous return being a controller of cardiac output. He did show that you could stimulate the nerves to the heart and make it stronger or weaker, and, more or less, identified the nervous system as the real controller of heart activity and cardiac output by making the heart [muscle] stronger or weaker. That is, you could have a normal venous return, but then the heart could be made stronger or weaker and thereby modify the cardiac output. But what we showed very quickly was that we could make the heart weaker, then stronger, then weaker, then still stronger, and all these changes wouldn't significantly change the cardiac output. They did change the pumping activity of the heart *like mad,* but what would happen is that the heart would pump itself dry and become very much smaller without the cardiac output increasing significantly along with increase of heart muscle activity.

We realized that something else was involved. We decided that if you were designing a heart, you would design it in such a way that the needs for blood flow by all the tissues would be added up, and *that* would be what controlled the cardiac output. That is, every time a tissue lets a bit of blood flow through it, that increases the venous return; and the more active the tissues, the more the venous return increases. Therefore, the heart functions like a sump pump: whenever extra blood comes into it, it pumps it. So we just called the heart a "sump pump," although people didn't like this because it sounded too much like a sewerage system.

I tried to emphasize that control of cardiac output results from a balance between the heart *and* the venous system; that normally the heart acts as a sump pump, and venous return is the main controlling factor.

> At this point, I would like to move on to the subject of your textbook, which I think may be your crowning achievement for the scientific public at large. In 1956 you came out with your first edition. At that time, even in a more constrained area of interest, such as cardiology, the days of the single-authored text were just about over. CHARLES FRIEDBERG published his book in 1949, and PAUL H. WOOD, in England, published his in 1950. Thereafter, no one had the temerity to hold himself forth as expert enough in all of cardiology to produce a text on his own; multiauthorship became the norm, and still is.

In physiology, Wiggers wrote a single-authored book that was probably the last that was widely used, and there were some others in England.

> Shortly before your book came out in 1956, the one by CHARLES H. BEST and Norman B. Taylor (*The Physiological Bases of Medical Practice*) was

favored by many American students in 1955, as I recall. By 1961, the then-current edition of their book included about twenty-eight authors. However, starting from your first edition in 1956, every five years you produced a new edition, and not until your ninth edition, in 1996, did you have someone assist you on this, John Hall. My question is: how did you do it? Physiology covers so many areas; how did you manage to write about all of these on your own for so many years?

Well, I didn't mean to, but by working at a small school in the early years, I had few students in each class, only about thirty. But we had two sessions a year in physiology, because we admitted a new class every six months. We did this for almost ten years, while we were still a two-year school. I was the only person giving lectures in physiology, so I had to study it along with the students at first. I would lecture on one subject and then immediately go and start studying for the next.

The overhead-type classroom projectors had just come out, where you could write on or draw on clear plastic film and project it on a screen. At night, at home, preceding each upcoming lecture, I would draw pictures on plastic stencils covering different subjects I wanted to talk about the next day. I would literally spend six or eight hours straight, first reading what Best and Taylor would say or what Wiggers or others would have to say on that field, and get as much information as I could from these different books. Then I would leave myself about three hours to collect my thoughts and make an outline of the lecture. Next, I would use another hour to make eight or ten drawings, so that I could project these for the lecture. This worked fairly well; I did this every six months as each new class arrived. After about ten of those series, I realized that there was no book to which the students could refer. For this reason, I began to dictate summaries of my lectures after having delivered them, and I gave them to our secretaries to transcribe. That was another two hours of work. It made a pretty full day—sixteen or seventeen hours. That went on for a total of ninety days, the duration of the course, and those dictations constituted the first edition of the text.

We were fortunate to have an excellent secretarial pool at the time, and the secretaries were able to transcribe the dictations without requiring much correcting on my part. We were usually able to get the summaries to the students within a day or two—certainly before the time of their examination on each subject.

Then I found that the next class already had these notes handed down from the previous class, and the students wouldn't read the text-book at all. I thought to myself, "Well, if they're going to do it that way, I had better dictate this much more fully." So this procedure turned out to be a good way of preparing future lectures and editions of the book.

As you went through succeeding editions, how did you keep up with all the various areas, those that you were not personally working on?

You find good teachers in every area. So I would always study what the experts in each area had to say. I could usually determine the experts from review articles they had written. When it came to the necessity for fine details, I would look up individual papers. Naturally, over the years, the selected experts changed as time went on.

In teaching students, it is important to recognize that, in general, most of what they need to learn is covered in the basic reviews on the various subjects. But if you tried to cover all the details, you'd have to have a physiology course that was five years long. The problem with having many different authors is that each author often writes in detail. Each one wants to explain his own ideas very forcefully, and the book gets too big; then, too, it gets beyond the depth of the students.

In the book about your life and career by Brinson and Quinn,[6] the authors include the following quote: a student says, "I didn't understand that at all until I read Guyton." I thought this was just a bit of hyperbole until I told my son, who had just graduated from veterinary school, that I was going to visit with you and interview you. His immediate comment was, "Arthur Guyton? Boy, whenever we really wanted to know about something in physiology, that's where we went." I accept this as coming from the horse's mouth.

Incidentally, do you think being an M.D. rather than a Ph.D. in a basic science department was an advantage, a disadvantage, or a mixture of both?

It's a combination. It's a tremendous advantage in teaching medical students because their goal is to become a doctor. And if you can use medical examples in your teaching, it makes a great difference to them; they sit up and listen much more. It was a disadvantage in that, during my training as a physician, it gave me less time to study the many fine details of physiology. As the years went on, however, I had enough time to do that anyway.

> At the beginning of each edition of your textbook, starting with the first and running right through the most current edition, you have a dedication which reads: "To my father for the uncompromising principles that guided his life; My mother for leading her children into intellectual pursuits; My wife for her magnificent devotion to her family; My children for making everything worthwhile."
>
> I want to concentrate on your children at this point, because it is really fascinating to me how they turned out. I don't know whether anyone has ever done a statistical analysis of this, but it is my impression that surgeons have more children than any other specialists. In this sense you were very much like a surgeon. In addition, every one of your ten children went into medicine, and, apparently willingly, almost all of them graduated from Harvard Medical School. How did you manage it? The cost alone must have been staggering.

My wife had a terrific love for young children, the babies; and I loved small children from three, four, or five right through high school and even college, as they were growing up. It turned out that being in a wheelchair was an advantage, because instead of doing things for them all the time, you tell them how to do it. So I had a very close relationship with all the children, and, by having that close relationship and such a terrific fondness for them, I always said I would have as many as my wife wanted.

As for support of their education, all the boys went to undergraduate school at the University of Mississippi tuition-free, or practically free. They got a very good background there, they all had top grades at "Ole Miss," and they all got into Harvard Medical School. All through history, you know, Harvard has had one of the lowest medical school tuitions. When I went there, I paid four hundred dollars a year, and at that time at Johns Hopkins and the University of Pennsylvania, I believe, it was six hundred dollars. But Harvard Medical School always had a principle of not letting tuition be one of the factors in the choice of school for potential students.

Were your children able to get loans as well?

Some of them did have student scholarships, but by the time they got into Harvard, I was just beginning to make some money from the textbook, so that virtually all the money that came from the textbook in those early years went into their education.

I think it's remarkable that all of them seem to have turned out so well. Harper Hellems (former chairman of the Department of Medicine at the University of Mississippi) once told me that if any of your children ever came home with a grade less than an A, it was an occasion for mourning in the family. Is this true?

I think my wife would ask them, "What's wrong?" if they came home with a grade less than an A. She would say, "What's wrong with you?" or something like that. It's true; we let them know from the beginning that we expected them to be at the top of the class. But we did something else, too. Part of what we would do with the kids was at night, when my wife or I would read to them. And I would give *them* reading to do themselves; and later on ask them questions on what they had learned.

What kind of books did you read, and what kind of reading did you give them on their own?

What I would read to them would usually be some boys' or girls' novel. Then, I would give them a semiscientific publication to read: something like *Popular Mechanics.* After they had read it, I would quiz them on what they had read. When they got to high school, I would go up the scale and give them something like *Science News* and the like.

There's a common syndrome, which I have chosen to give the name "The Great Man's Child's Syndrome." It occurs when a son—it is usually a son—wilts in the shadow of his father's great reputation. It could just as well involve daughters and fathers, or even mothers, for that matter. The child finds it impossible to emerge as his or her own person in such a setting. Did this ever occur with any of your own children? Were there

**any that really did not want to go into medicine but felt they were com-
pelled to do so?**

We might have had a bit of that. One of our sons, after he had started
medical school, decided for a short time that this was not for him and
took a leave of absence from Harvard, after talking to the dean. I don't
remember the details at all. He came home, and we asked him what he
was going to do. He said he didn't know. I found out that what he *was*
doing was lying in bed and sleeping every morning. I told him, "You
can stay here as long as you want, providing you get up the same time
we do and find something to do."

He looked around at the jobs that were available, and they involved
things like delivering ice. You know what I mean? I told him he could
go into any area that interested him. I suggested electrical engineering
and gave him a two-volume set I had on the subject. I suggested he start
studying this and began to ask him questions each night on what he
had learned. After a while he discovered, "Well electrical engineers have
it hard, too." And within two months that boy decided that he had had
it pretty good up at Harvard. He really did. He went back, and we never
heard another word of complaint.

**I would like to talk about something else now. There seems to be a grow-
ing tendency to combine pharmacology and physiology within the same
department. I look upon this as a step backward; it took years for pharmacology to break loose as an independent discipline, and now some
places—including my own institution (the New Jersey Medical School)—
are reverting to the old format. What are your thoughts on this subject?**

This problem used to be much more widespread than it is now. A
tremendous amount of pharmacology is taught when you teach physiology; and a tremendous amount of physiology is involved in the
teaching of pharmacology. But that's also true in the discipline of medicine, which includes much physiology. In some medical schools, physiology is taught by the Department of Medicine, and in several schools
physiology has been taught in the discipline of surgery when the chiefs
of surgery were physiologically oriented. But, almost invariably, it has
been found that enough basic physiology was not being taught when

combined with medicine or surgery or pharmacology. Physiology was being treated like a second fiddle.

> **But when they combine physiology and pharmacology, isn't it pharmacology that gets short shrift? Usually the combined department is headed by a physiologist, right?**

Physiology is usually taught first, since the students have no previous background, so under those conditions, pharmacology does get short shrift. I would like all these departments to be separated and with separate courses. Then, when they teach medicine, revisit physiology and pharmacology and show how they are applicable to each area within medicine: the heart, the brain, the gastrointestinal system, and so on. Not only in medical school do I think this important, but during internship and residency years the trainee still needs didactic programs in the basics.

If I had my way, I would give medical students a very quick survey of the whole field of medical education during the first three to five months of medical school. Then I would cover the basic sciences as we do now; and finally go into the specialty fields such as medicine, surgery, neurosurgery, cardiac medicine, et cetera. But as the students do each of these fractions, I would make sure they learn each of the pieces from which the clinical units are built: physiology, pharmacology, anatomy, biochemistry . . . all of them.

About one in ten entering medical students has had the experience of a year or a few months of working in a hospital, where they have observed a good deal of clinical medicine. This makes a big difference to them in studying medicine, making these connections. That's why I would like to expose students to some clinical medicine right from the beginning; then come to the basic work; and then back to the clinical specialties in real detail. At the University of Mississippi, the Department of Family Medicine has tried to do this to some extent.

> **There's just one last thing. Did you ever read the book *Creative Malady*, by GEORGE PICKERING?[7] It is a fascinating book that I recommend to you. In it he describes several prominent people—Charles Darwin, Sigmund Freud, Florence Nightingale, Marcel Proust, among them—who were**

plagued by some illness for a good portion of their lives. What Pickering reveals about them, however, is how they turned their handicaps to their advantage in accomplishing whatever it was that made them famous. As I was coming to meet you, I began to wonder: if you had not had polio, and had become a cardiac surgeon, would you have wound up accomplishing as much in your life as you have as a physiologist?

I have no thoughts on that. The reason is because what I have accomplished in physiology came about spontaneously, mainly, and not by some conscious design. I like physiology, so I did physiology; I like making devices, so I made devices for different research purposes; I like physics and physical engineering, so I liked using their principles in understanding the basic principles of physiology. In other words, everything came about very spontaneously. If I hadn't contracted polio, what spontaneous things would have come forth? I'm sure I would have played with all the different types of cardiovascular operations. Probably every time someone would do a new operative procedure, I would try to do it myself—just for the fun of it.

In other words, just to see "how it works."

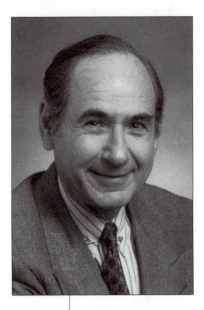

8

ALBERT STARR, M.D.
(1926–   )

In the course of conversation, Dr. Albert Starr is liable to comment on how lucky he has been in his professional life. But although luck is often a contributing factor in the success of any individual, in Albert Starr's case a neutral observer would have to conclude that it was not a major one.

It is a long journey from the doors of James Madison High School in Brooklyn, New York, to the highest echelons of cardiac surgery. As the surgeon responsible for introducing the first successful artificial heart valve, he has been recognized as one of the leading innovators in an era characterized by many lifesaving innovations. First the background:

Although only a first step in valve surgery upon the heart, the "finger fracturing" technique of the stenotic mitral valve, as introduced by Charles Bailey, DWIGHT HARKEN, and RUSSELL BROCK, dispelled forever the previous concept that the clinical problem in rheumatic heart disease resided primarily in the heart muscle (see Bailey interview). Clearly, the mechanical obstruction in mitral stenosis was the primary factor in the pathogenesis of this disorder. Yet even though this closed-heart procedure was a major advance, the fact that it was performed blindly, without actually viewing the valve, presented a major shortcoming.

In some cases, the valve might not have been opened sufficiently at the time of surgery; in others, progress of the disease would cause restenosis, requiring a second operation. In some patients the diseased valve was so calcified that it resisted all efforts by the surgeon to open it up. On the other hand, a surgeon who was too aggressive in attempting to open the valve might convert a stenotic valve into a seriously regurgitant (leaking) one, thereby substituting one debilitating valve defect for another. Of course, in those patients whose diseased valves were defective both in opening and closing, with mitral stenosis and regurgitation, the operation might be contraindicated for fear of increasing the degree of regurgitation to a dangerous degree. In patients with isolated mitral regurgitation accounting for these patients' symptoms, the operation was useless. Adding to the problems for clinicians treating patients with valve disease was the realization that for many patients presenting with valve problems, either on a rheumatic or other basis, it was the aortic valve that was the major problem, either in combination with mitral disease or by itself. Numerous previous attempts to approach the aortic valve with closed-heart surgery had been unsuccessful, and it was only with the introduction of open-heart surgery with cardiopulmonary bypass that surgery upon diseased heart valves could be conducted under direct vision.

Dr. Starr took his undergraduate and medical degrees at Columbia University. He began his surgical career as an intern at Johns Hopkins, where he worked and became friendly with DENTON A. COOLEY, then completing a surgical residency under ALFRED BLALOCK, famed for the "blue baby" operation he had introduced with HELEN B. TAUSSIG. Although there was no room for Starr in Blalock's cardiac surgery program, with the recommendation of Cooley, Starr received Blalock's support to be accepted for training in cardiac surgery back at Columbia-Presbyterian in New York. Two years later, Starr received an invitation to head cardiac surgery at the University of Oregon in Portland, where the program had been faltering badly.

Although Dr. Starr deserves credit for other innovations as well as building an outstanding heart surgery program at his adopted institution, he will be remembered primarily for the introduction of the Starr-Edwards valve, a caged-ball device that proved to be the first successful mechanical prosthesis used in valve surgery. While previous efforts had been made to construct various types of artificial valves, all of them had essentially floundered, including Dr. Dwight Harken's attempts to use a caged-ball valve in the aortic position.

It was the persistence of Starr and the engineer Miles Lowell Edwards, who approached him shortly after his arrival in Portland, to perfect their own caged-ball valve, first in the mitral position and then in the aortic position, that resulted in its widespread success and adoption elsewhere. Even though many other types of valves, made from a wide variety of materials, have since been introduced, the Starr-Edwards valve, unchanged since modifications introduced in 1965, has continued to be the standard against which all others must be judged.[1]

Because of space limitations at the medical school, in 1986 Dr. Starr moved his clinical activities to St. Vincent Hospital, where he heads the Heart Institute while still maintaining his position as chief of cardiopulmonary surgery at the Oregon Health Sciences University.

Portland, Oregon
April 18, 2000

In 1995, I attended a surgical historical symposium at the annual meeting of the American College of Cardiology, at which you were one of the speakers. At that time you said something to the effect that, on a trip from New York to Oregon, you learned about open-heart surgery by spending a week with John Kirklin and a week with C. WALTON LILLEHEI. I wonder if you would expand on that.

When I finished my surgical residency, open-heart surgery was just in its infancy. This was at the end of June in 1957. At that time New York was pretty well "behind the curve" in terms of open-heart surgery. We were just doing a few atrial septal defects; nothing really complicated. So I had an odyssey to the West, stopping off first in Cleveland, where I met FRED CROSS and looked at the disc oxygenator, and EARLE KAY, who worked closely with him in a very active practice. I also knew the fellow at Western Reserve, Jay Ankeny, who eventually became president of the Society of Thoracic Surgery. He finished his surgical residency at Columbia-Presbyterian three or four years before I did, so we had known each other as residents, a pretty tight bond. He was repairing some ventricular septal defects using the [RICHARD] DeWALL bubble oxygenator and the rotator-disc oxygenator as well. So I also spent some time with him. But the main drag was at the University of Minnesota and the Mayo Clinic. This was in July that I visited both places, and it was hot as hell, so my wife would stay at the hotel while I would go to the hospital and hang out to observe what was done.

At Minnesota Lillehei and his associate, [RICHARD] VARCO, were very friendly. There were always five or six guys hanging around at any one time, and I watched operations on complicated ventricular septal defects and Tetralogy [of Fallot] operations and observed the kids post-operatively. DeWall was a resident then and had designed the bubble oxygenator. Lillehei was always ready to answer any questions and make sure that we understood what he was doing. I was really impressed with his openness and willingness to transmit information to younger people.

At Rochester, things were much more structured; they seemed more businesslike; they did not take a lot of time out to talk. But the operations were more disciplined and very precise. This was a reflection of Kirklin's personality. He was very well organized and everything was very precise in the operating room: his manners, his emotions very tightly engineered but really very excellent. There I observed them using the Mayo-Gibbon oxygenator. From this trip, I decided to use the rotating-disc oxygenator developed by Kay and Cross in Cleveland as our first oxygenator here in Oregon. It was manufactured in Cleveland, and it was a pretty primitive device; we had to take the discs out, wash them, and reassemble them, silicoating them. But it seemed simpler than the stationary-screen oxygenator, and that influenced our choosing it to start off.

What was it about you that made you such an attractive candidate to start the open-heart surgical program in Oregon? After all, you were in a pretty junior position at that time.

I was very junior. I think Westerners put a tremendous emphasis on Ivy League breeding. So the fact that I was from Columbia was a very important consideration, and even to this day, you know, if a recruit is from the MGH [Massachusetts General Hospital] or Harvard, it carries a lot of weight.

> It seems that, at the time you went West, there had been a sort of decline at Hopkins after the ALFRED BLALOCK years. When I was a young man in the sixties, Columbia also seemed to be "behind the curve," as you put it. This was before the arrival of JAMES R. MALM at Columbia.

Malm was one of my classmates at college, and we were exactly of the same generation. He was in the V-12 Navy program going to Columbia's medical school while I was a civilian student, deferred from the World War II draft based upon my young age at the time. I started medical school before the age of eighteen.

The Blalock story is very interesting because you ask yourself, "How does a service decline?" And "What can a chief do to perpetuate the service?" The fact is that, in medicine, we don't have a good method for this. In industry, for example, if you have a great company, most of the time you can orchestrate the departure of a CEO and the arrival of a new one by a board that is carefully focused on that problem. In a medical school the chips fall where they may, and so there is not the kind of management that you would have in a for-profit corporation with a board of directors that has clout and shareholders who count. So it is sort of left to chance. And most of the time it isn't possible for even the most powerful chief to orchestrate events after his own departure.

What happens is that a powerful individual creates counter-reactions in the rest of the faculty. And although Blalock was revered in the surgical world, his own colleagues in other disciplines at Hopkins viewed the preponderance of cardiac surgery at that institution as an uncomfortable "nuisance," and so I don't think it was by chance alone that the program faltered after his retirement. They didn't want one of his cronies to become chief.

> That's always the story with cardiac surgery. It becomes the tail wagging the dog of any medical school. Everyone else resents cardiac surgery becoming so predominant.

Exactly. The cardiac surgeon becomes so predominant that it creates resentment, and you don't have any mechanisms in place to overcome that.

Were you doing open-heart surgery before you came to Oregon?

Only as an assistant. In Oregon they had attempted a few cases before I came but with disastrous results.

Of course the major event of your professional life was the development of the mitral valve prosthesis. Had you this idea in mind before you came to Portland? Where did it all begin? What was Edward's role?

From a very early age, what I feared most in life was not death but anonymity. So that was a really driving force in my makeup. For some reason—I don't know exactly why —I wanted to be recognized. I was always thinking about how I might achieve that. I thought that perhaps through an inventive process might be the way, even before I went to medical school. I set this idea aside to learn medicine and practice surgery, and then one day this guy who wanted to accomplish this early goal just walked through the door. Immediately everything clicked with Edwards; that developing an artificial mitral valve would be the way to do it.

I always wondered precisely what it was that led surgeons like you to develop the early heart valves. It seemed to me that CHARLES HUFNAGEL was the patron saint of all this.

Hufnagel was my hero!

Why was it that a good mitral valve prosthesis got developed before an aortic valve substitute? After all, Hufnagel began with the aortic regurgitation problem, putting his device in the descending aorta with closed-heart surgery before you could even replace the native aortic valve with open-heart surgery.

I addressed that with Edwards. What he wanted to work on was an artificial heart. I told him that we couldn't do that; we didn't even have artificial valves yet. So I told him that we had to do a valve first and that we had our choice between a mitral valve or an aortic valve. In regard to the aortic valve there was, at the time, a glimmering of hope with the artificial individual leaflets that Hufnagel had developed, finally building the leaflets into a composite three-leaflet valve made of Silastic. [Henry] Bahnson had also been working on textile leaflets in the aortic position then.

Going back to Hufnagel's valve that he placed in the aorta, the contribution there was the demonstration that you could have a valve whose opening and closing could be controlled by the systolic and diastolic blood flow phases of the pumping of blood from the heart into the aorta. It's of interest that, in regard to the development of this, when Hufnagel was working in [Robert] Gross's lab, he was not working on valvular prostheses; he was working on the problem of coarctation of the aorta (see Fig 3-1). And he developed the acrylic tube as a way of excising the coarctation and replacing it with this tube. It was only later that he figured, "Now that I have experience with putting this acrylic tube in the aorta, why don't I put a ball valve in it to treat aortic regurgitation?"

> When the ball valve was in place, it could be quite audible. This calls to mind a story, which may be apocryphal: It seems that one of Hufnagel's patients, who was an inveterate poker player, would sit in the ward, recovering from the operation, and play poker with a few other patients. Every time he got a really good hand, even though his facial expression would not change, his excitement was given away as his audible heart rate would speed up, tipping off the other players.

It was a very noisy valve and also subject to thrombosis, so we sometimes had to take them out for acute occlusion of the aorta. It also sometimes caused hemolysis.

So the reason for going to the mitral valve was that we already had what might have been a partial answer to the aortic valve replacement problem with no answer to the mitral problem. Therefore, if we wanted to do something important, then the development of an artificial mitral valve, I could assure Edwards, would be it, because it had not yet been done.

> As a cardiologist who was responsible for sending patients with mitral stenosis to surgery for closed mitral commissurotomies, I was always

> worried, as were all of us, that following the commissurotomy, a patient with little or no mitral regurgitation preop might end up with a real problem of mitral regurgitation. Only the development of a good valve replacement could solve this dilemma.

There was a real clinical need for a mitral valve for those patients and those presenting initially with a problem primarily of mitral regurgitation.

> Of course, a lot of elderly patients had just as great a need for valve replacement for aortic stenosis.

That wasn't as obvious to us at the time. We did not have a clear demographic idea of the need for artificial valves, the magnitude of the need. When Edwards asked me, "How many of these valves do you think will be installed?" I said, "A couple of hundred," thinking in terms of worldwide needs. I didn't realize that it would be hundreds of thousands.

> Talk about epidemiology! Before your 1961 publication came out, there was some work on artificial valves reported by Ellis and Bulbulian at Mayo and also a report from NINA S. BRAUNWALD and others at the NIH. Could you place these in context?

Ellis had various approaches to mitral valve replacement, and either he or one of his colleagues at the clinic did have a ball-type valve. They also had a flap-type valve, hinged at one end. Both of those valves thrombosed very rapidly after implantation, causing them to give up on the ball valve very early while they continued with the other type, perhaps even trying to implant a few clinically before they finally gave up on this as well because of thrombosis. At Oregon we failed with many different types of leaflet valves but went back to a ball-type valve even with the knowledge that Ellis had already failed with the ball-type valve. We did this because we felt his failure was due to problems with the design and construction of his valve rather than failure of the basic concept of a ball valve.[2]

The Braunwald valve was a cloth-type valve with two leaflets and artificial chordae tendinae; a replica of the normal valve. The problem was that this was not a fully engineered package you could just sew in, but one in which you had to adjust the length of the artificial chords and connect them to the existing papillary muscles in various ways, trying to make them work physiologically. Then the cloth would get a neo-intima [lining], which would thicken and stiffen and become nonfunctional over the long term.

> I've done a lot of dog work, as I'm sure you have too, and you always assume that what works in dogs will work in humans. But your experience with using the valve in dogs was different in terms of thrombosis, wasn't it?

It was a very different situation in that, whereas all the dogs that had other types of valves died within two or three days—because dogs have a more active thrombosing system than humans do—with the ball valve we were very lucky in that our first dog lived a long time. After that, all of the subsequent dogs receiving the standard ball valve died from valve thrombosis, but this time, instead of dying within two or three days, they would live for three or four weeks. So it was obvious this was a better-designed ball valve in the dog than had previously been used, but we still could not get long-term survival until we used the shielded valve. The shielded valve allowed reproducible mitral valve replacement because in the area where the clot usually formed the Silastic barrier prevented this from happening.

> If you were so concerned about thrombosis, why didn't you just anti-coagulate the dogs?

It was a lot of trouble! It was a lot of trouble just to get the dogs, let alone being able to operate on them. We had no procurement system.

> Really? Back in Utah where I was a fellow, we could get dogs for three dollars each from guys who would pick strays up from all over the place.

That was the problem. Guys would pick up various breeds from all over the place. They were all kinds of breeds, and some of them were sick, some were malnourished, some of them were stolen pets. It wasn't until the middle of the sixties that we had an organized dog farm breeding dogs for laboratory use.

Behind the scenes the medical people have a lot of control of what you
can do because they are the ones who refer the patients to the surgeons
for treatment. Sometimes they can hold back surgical progress, but in
your case it was quite different. Could you tell me about this?

[Herbert] Griswold was the chief of cardiology, and incidentally he was
the first full-time chief of cardiology at the new university hospital of
the University of Oregon in Portland, which opened in 1956, the year
before I came. He was young and very open-minded and controlled the
major cardiological source of patients within the state. A lot of patients
came in with mitral stenosis, mitral regurgitation, or mixed lesions. A
number of them were in oxygen tents on the medical floor and in
severe heart failure.

In 1959 he came to visit our lab, this being after we had started to
use the shielded valve in the dogs. He saw, literally, a kennel full of dogs
at various stages after operation, all happy and jumping up in their
cages, licking his hands, and whatnot. He said, "You know what, Al? I
have some seriously ill patients in oxygen tents, and I think you should
use the valve in them."

I thought it would take at least another two or three years to vali-
date the valve because what I wanted to do was to establish that long-
term healing took place. Remember, we had no idea whether or not you
could obtain permanent fixation following implantation of these valves
in a moving heart. Would the valve implant heal, or would it be eventually dislodged? How would you design a sewing ring to prevent leaks
around the valve and future separation of the valve? So, to me it was a
long-term project, but Griswold had a lot more clinical experience than
I did, and he had a lot of sick patients who needed *something* or otherwise they were going to be dead. So his chief of medicine, Howard
Lewis, was very supportive of him, and, between the two of them, they
prevailed upon our surgical department to have me do this. Dr. Burt
Dunphy was chief of the department of surgery, and he was also very
supportive in carrying out early clinical trials and was solidly behind
the effort. And he made sure that at the first presentation of the work
at the American Surgical Association, the most prestigious organization, that Michael DeBakey, whom he called before the meeting, would

discuss the paper covering our first eight cases.[3] DeBakey was reluctant, for some reason, but Dunphy really twisted his arm to do it. In his discussion, which was favorable, DeBakey said he didn't have very much to add, although he said that if he were on a committee deciding whether to award a grant for this work, he would not have given the money. In other words, he would not have expected the results that we achieved.

> **Did you have any problems with your medical colleagues when you lost your first patient to an air embolism? Sometimes a tragic outcome of a new surgical procedure like this will turn off the medical people, and it's hard to proceed thereafter.**

I did not have any problems with them at all. I remember the patient very well. After the operation the cardiologist, Griswold, came in and listened to the valve, and he felt it was a historic occasion: this was the first intracardiac mechanical valve functioning in a patient who had a good circulation. And then Howard Lewis came down, and he listened to the patient. Then, when this patient, who was near death before the operation, died, they simply accepted the complication because they now knew that the valve could work, that Starr could put it in. They recognized that we had to work out some of the surgical details but that the death was not due to valve failure itself.

> **There's an old expression, "If it ain't broke, don't fix it." It seems to me that, with all the new valves that have come out, you stuck with the same valve all these years, even though there were some modifications.**

Well, it really wasn't the same valve we started out with; it went through a lot of changes, and the changes were significant. The initial valve we put in was handmade and constructed from acrylic. It was bulky. Then we went to stainless steel but found that stainless steel could corrode when exposed to the circulation for some time. So we searched for a better material, finally settling on Stellite 21, a very strong nonferrous material that could be machined and core cast. And we had to develop a production line to mass-produce these valves when there had never been such an operation before. How to do it? What kinds of workers?

What kinds of skills were needed? What kind of environment? Everything had to be improvised.

Regarding the valve itself, we had to determine the optimal shape for the sewing ring. It took us five years before we reached that point. We also had to work on thinning the struts down to the greatest possible extent without weakening them to reduce the amount of foreign material exposed to the blood. We had to fine-tune the ball-to-orifice ratio: if the ball was too small in relation to the orifice, it could stick in the orifice; if the ball was too big, then the cage would be too bulky. We had to find the optimal relationship. After five years, by 1965, we felt we had as perfect a ball valve as you could construct, and we stopped modifying it at that point. And the valve being produced by Edwards Life Sciences right now is the same as the one we had arrived at in 1965.

You once wrote a paper that reminded me of Eisenhower's term, "the military-industrial complex." The title of your paper was "The Thoracic Surgical Industrial Complex," which actually was a very favorable paper on the subject.[4] You pointed out that surgeons really had to work very closely with engineers in order to get these advances introduced to medicine.

Now even more so.

What do you think of the newspaper reports we have been seeing about "scandals" involving the intrusion of engineers and technicians in the operating room and elsewhere performing the doctor's functions? My own opinion is that, in the pacemaker area, for example, without taking anything away from the doctors, the company technical people actually know a hell of a lot more about the electronics and are really needed.

I have nothing against the close collaboration with industry. The first thing industry provides is venture capital, and that's an enormous advantage. Instead of going to some government agency and hoping that the establishment people sitting around the table will allow something to be done, you get the venture capital people to do it. They know how to take risks; that's their business. In addition to providing the capital, they provide the engineering expertise. Not every hospital is blessed with a bioengineering department. As a matter of fact, in the past there were no bioengineering departments; there were no degrees in bioengineering! So these companies provided the necessary technological support. Finally, they develop methods of manufacturing and distribution; and then education became a very important part of the distribution system.

Over all these years, have you been able to maintain your independence as a surgical professional despite all these tie-ins with industry? That is, without any "taint" accruing to this commercial involvement?

I don't think I've been injured in any way by my relationship with Edwards and then Baxter [Laboratories]. The first thing I did after Edwards told me that he wanted to form a company to manufacture this valve was to go to the chief of surgery, Dr. Dunphy, and tell him, "Dr. Dunphy, these guys are forming a company and have offered me the possibility to become a shareholder. What should I do? I have a long surgical career ahead of me, and I am interested in surgery and not in becoming an entrepreneur."

He said, "Al, the future involves a very close relationship between the two entities. Being a consultant to industry is fine. I happen to be a consultant to Ethicon, for example. So if you want to be a consultant to Edwards Laboratories, feel free to do so."

But you weren't an owner . . .

No, I was a consultant to Edwards Laboratories, which later became Baxter Laboratories. Then the question of royalties arose. How do royalties shape up in the medical field? That was really hard to do. We went to the Ethics Committee of the American Medical Association, and they stated that they did not want to have taken from a doctor the rights of his intellectual property. They did not feel that a doctor should have to give up his or her intellectual property, and therefore there was no reason why a doctor should not benefit from royalties derived from patents. So that's what we did.

Did you share the patent with Edwards, then?

Yes, because the patent would not be valid if people who had made a substantial contribution to the patent were not on the patent. Otherwise there would always be a cloud over the patent, and some person could one day claim that *they* were improperly deprived of their intellectual property. So the best thing to do is to have the patent as inclusive as possible. Edwards was a professional inventor with many other inventions to his credit, and he had a high-powered patent attorney in town. The attorney insisted that Starr be on the patent on this co-invention, and that it would be tainted if all the inventors involved were not on it.

With the increasing problems with financing that many medical schools are having and have had in the past, I wonder if the University of Oregon benefited in any way from this.

No, and that's an interesting story. I went to the chief financial officer of the university, Bill Zimmerman, and said, "Bill, you know I've been working on this valve with Edwards, and he wants to patent it. Now what role does the university play in any patentable inventions that have been developed on your campus by your faculty?"

He said, "We don't have a role. We've never encountered this before."

"Well, what do you want to do?"

"I'll let you know." And after a few weeks he told me, "Al, we don't want to get involved." Now that was before the days when places like Stanford had faculty involved with surrounding industries and this became an important source of their income. The situation now has completely changed. We have agreements in place now, at this hospital [St. Vincent], for example, where half the benefits of any invention of our full-time people belong to the hospital.

What are your comments on the other valves that have been developed following the introduction of your own valve in the sixties?

You may recall the ball valve became the gold standard, and from 1960 to about 1970 or 1971 it was overwhelmingly the predominant valve. Then DON SHILEY developed the next step. He had initially worked for Edwards here in Oregon, and Don was his chief engineer. Shiley had actually designed the ball valve for the aortic configuration; Edwards, after having done the mitral valve prosthetic design, had assigned the aortic to Shiley. Edwards had him work with me to develop any modifications needed for a valve in the aortic position. So Shiley became quite knowledgeable about valvular heart disease and artificial valves. He decided to leave Edwards and form his own company for the purpose of making other medical devices but also for making what became known as the Kay-Shiley valve, a Silastic disc moving up and down in a cage. It was not a good valve and was eventually abandoned. But it was a start for Shiley, who then developed a valve using the tilting-disc concept.

He tells the story that one Sunday afternoon he was watching an NFL ballgame on television, and his mind began to wander, and he thought, "I've got to get out of this disc thing. The edges are wearing out on the Kay-Shiley valve, and I've got to think of some other way of doing this." And then he thought of tossing a disc back and forth with a kind of stop on the outflow and another on the inflow, letting the disc tilt instead of just moving parallel to the orifice. He told me that he just leaped out of his chair, made some notes, made a little drawing, and went right to the lab and started making one. Then he went to DENTON COOLEY and asked if he was interested in working with him. Denton was not interested, so he then went to [VIKING] BJÖRK.

Now Björk was one of the earliest users of the ball valve, but he had some complaints about it. In a few instances, especially in patients with small aortic roots, he noted significant gradients across the valve and felt that in some patients the ball valve was unsuitable for this reason. This would be in cases not only with small aortic roots but those which reduce in diameter at the tubobulbar junction in relation to the size of the annulus. The problem wasn't confined only to Sweden but relates specifically to this anatomic variant of the aortic root which may be present in a small minority of patients. For these reasons Björk worked with Shiley on the Björk- Shiley valve, although it was really Shiley who developed it.

The ball valve does not have an obstructive element built into it, but obviously the larger the orifice, the larger must be the ball and the larger must be the cage. For most circumstances it allows very satisfactory hemodynamic function, especially for mitral valve replacement. In the aortic position, however, depending upon anatomical features, there could be a systolic gradient as high as 25 to 30 mm Hg.

The original tilting valves had problems with struts cracking, but currently the tilting-disc monostrut and the Medtronic Hall tilting-disc valves are excellent. In addition, the St. Jude valve has proven to be an excellent prosthesis with long durability. All of these nonball valves, however, carry with them the risk of thrombotic stenosis around the inside of the rim between it and the disc. Then disc entrapment can occur with potentially catastrophic results. This type of failure mode does not occur abruptly with the ball valve prosthesis, where there is discontinuity between the prosthetic orifice and the closing mechanism, and is extremely rare or absent with bioprostheses.

As far as we can tell, there are no clinical differences in patients who have ball valve replacement versus other newer types of prostheses. The ball valve continues to be used by us as well as others in many parts of the world because, unlike with other mechanical prostheses, catastrophic acute malfunction due to thrombus is less likely to occur in patients whose anticoagulation might not be adequate from time to time.[5]

> **Something else I find interesting is that you just went and developed these valves without any Food and Drug Administration approval. I don't think medical innovators can even go to the bathroom today without FDA approval.**

Well, the FDA was not involved with devices until the late sixties or early seventies. If we had to get their approval, we would never have been able to do this work.

> **Something else I would like you to comment on is the effect of patient status or selection upon the success or failure of a new surgical procedure.**

Patient variables are very important, and I owe a lot to Gary Grunkemeier, our statistician, in recognizing this. What Gary really showed is that if you divide the patient population into various subsets according to certain risk factors, using the same prosthesis in each group with the same surgical team, the results could be extremely different, varying from a 10 percent survival rate to a 90 percent survival rate at the end of five years. So critical patient characteristics were very important in the results of the operation.

But if I may be the devil's advocate for a moment: there's always this tug of war between the surgeons and the medical people; the surgeons always want the better candidates, and the medical people are always holding off until they feel that the patient really needs the operation.

Yes, and what the cardiologists have gradually learned on their own is that the earlier the surgery is performed, the better the result, a cycle heading in the right direction. It could also be a cycle heading in the wrong direction; that is when they give you worse and worse patients, resulting in progressively poorer surgical outcomes as a result.

Tell me about your contributions to congenital heart surgery.

My contribution here was in introducing to Oregon the advances in total correction of Tetralogy of Fallot that John Kirklin, for example, had done shortly before at the Mayo Clinic, as well as other congenital defects. In Tetralogy, I believe I helped emphasize that it was a *progressive* disease and that earlier operations for it were important.

Have you been involved in cardiac transplantation?

I initiated the transplantation program in Oregon. It has a great future, and at the moment it is the best treatment of end-stage heart disease. It has enabled us to put patients on temporary devices before transplantation, and these devices are so good that some of the patients are clinging to them as permanent devices. So all this is leading to implantable artificial hearts. Meanwhile immunosuppressive treatment for patients with transplants has improved greatly, and we anticipate even greater improvement possibly to the point at which even animal hearts can be used instead of human ones in the future.

Of course, human heart transplantation has the problem of supply and demand.

That's what I mean. You might have only 2,500 hearts available annually for the whole country, with as many as 100,000 or more patients who may need cardiac replacement.

> **You have been involved with cardiomyoplasty. What is it exactly, and how good is it in meeting the needs of patients with end-stage heart disease?**

Cardiomyoplasty is based on the principle that, with programmed stimulation, skeletal muscle can be converted to fatigue-resistant cardiac muscle–type metabolism. [ALAIN] CARPENTIER used this discovery to explore the use of skeletal muscle in various configurations to add energy to the circulation. One of these configurations is to take the latisimus dorsi muscle and wrap it around the heart and then repetitively stimulate the nervous supply to that muscle in synchrony with the heart rate. Within six weeks or so the muscle becomes fatigue resistant, and in some patients it has offered considerable improvement, but not *predictably,* and such improvement that has occurred has not been massive.

> **It seems to me that the left ventricular assist devices have been improving all the time and coming to play a major role now in the treatment of advanced heart failure. Has this been your experience?**

They are good and last at least for three to five years, perhaps longer. What surprises me about the assist devices is that it has taken so long for them to become a clinical reality. And in this case I believe there has been active intervention in slowing down the clinical deployment of these devices. Now I'm not a paranoid person by any means; I'm the least paranoid of any surgeon I know, but I believe that financial considerations have resulted in a concerted effort to delay the introduction of these devices in clinical application. And this relates to the government, which does not want to foot the bill. In my opinion the role of government needs to be limited as much as possible, consistent with a free market economy and adequate patient safety.

> **Where do we stand now with the possibility of a totally implantable artificial heart? Has anyone come up with a solution to the propensity for blood clot formation within them?**

I think that the direction where all this is going is that you don't need a total artificial heart with four chambers. What you need is an implantable left ventricular assist device that will last at least five years, and we have them. They're very practical, very effective, and in about 20 to 30 percent of cases, patients can be weaned from them after their natural hearts have had a chance to recover after six months or a year. If not, they can receive a transplant or another artificial device.

What I find peculiar is that this treatment is not more widely used. But the field is so heavily regulated, for example, that I cannot put one of these devices in at this hospital because we don't have a transplant program here at St. Vincent. So right now, no hospital without a transplantation program can use this method of treatment, and such centers are limited in number. Now does this make sense? One of these devices may cost fifty thousand dollars, but many papers have been presented now showing that, even despite this initial outlay, the overall cost of treating end-stage heart disease is greatly reduced by having one of these devices implanted because the number of hospitalizations for congestive heart failure is greatly reduced.

> **At the end of these sessions, I always ask the question "Do you have any regrets?" In your case I am almost reluctant to do so; you seem to me to be about one of the sunniest personalities I have met in medicine, either in or out of the operating room!**

Regrets? Oh no. It isn't that I haven't had opportunities to go elsewhere as chief of surgery, New York or Los Angeles, for example; but I've been happy here in Portland. Perhaps if I had another life, I might try one of these other routes just to see what would happen, but you just can't have multiple lives.

Actually, I have been very lucky all my life. I came from a very modest background, a graduate of James Madison, a public high school in Brooklyn. I applied to this Ivy League school, Columbia, and although anything but Ivy League, I tried to appear a bit that way when I appeared for my interview, and they accepted me. I was fortunate to be accepted to Columbia's medical school as well and had skipped so many grades in primary school that by the time I entered medical school I was too young to be drafted. So I never was called to serve in World War II, where some of my former Brooklyn classmates were probably killed. I did later serve in Korea during that war, first as a battalion surgeon and then as a surgeon in a MASH unit.

Following medical school, I was fortunate to get a surgical internship at Hopkins, where Blalock was still active. While I was at Hopkins, I was befriended by Denton Cooley, so that when I failed to get a spot on Blalock's cardiac surgical team as a resident, thanks to Denton's recommendation, Dr. Blalock called the chief at Presbyterian and got me a residency back there at Bellevue-Presbyterian. Then, with not much more than a surgical residency behind me and really very little in the way of cardiac surgical experience, I was offered the chance to head such a program at the University of Oregon. After I arrived there, Edwards showed up with the chance to really do something significant in the field of cardiac surgery, and it all worked out. So there certainly is no reason for regrets. I have been an unusually lucky man.

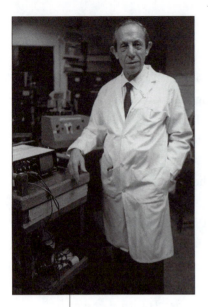

9

PAUL M. ZOLL, M.D.
(1911–1999)

The heart is frequently referred to as a pump, which it obviously is. However, it is a pump that, to work properly, depends on an exquisitely designed electrical system to ensure that each part of the heart performs its pumping function in a coordinated way and at rates that are optimal for proper functioning of the organism under varying conditions. Each part of the heart has its own intrinsic or characteristic rate, and that portion with the most rapid one, the sino-atrial node in the upper portion of the right atrium, determines the overall heart rate as its signal spreads through the atria and then through the major conducting bundle (of His) to the ventricles, the major pumping chambers of the heart (see Fig. 3-1).

In some patients this electrical connection between the upper and lower chambers is disrupted, and, as a result, without any more rapidly occurring signals from above, the ventricles begin beating at their own rather slow intrinsic rate, about thirty to fifty beats per minute. In complete heart block the rate may drop even lower than this, even with periods of complete pause. When this occurs, the output of the heart is insufficient to supply adequate blood flow to the brain, and unconsciousness, occasionally accompanied by convulsions, ensues. These Stokes-Adams attacks, named for the nineteenth-century Dublin physicians who independently described patients suffering from them, are almost always harbingers of imminent death.

There is another, quite different and even more common and lethal electrical malfunction of the heart, one that occurs primarily in patients with coronary heart disease either during an acute myocardial infarction or at other times when the patient is ambulatory and unaware of this threat that lies in wait. An underlying electrical instability of the myocardial tissue leads to a complete disruption of the ordinary cardiac contraction. This is replaced by a mass of uncoordinated small muscle bundle contractions, which are unable to combine for effective pumping of blood, often described as the "bag of worms" appearance of ventricular fibrillation. Near the middle of the twentieth century, when the incidence of coronary heart disease appeared to be reaching epidemic proportions in the United States, in-hospital deaths from acute myocardial infarction stood at about 30 percent, many of them as a result of this electrical complication of the disease.

Paul Zoll committed just about the entire span of his medical career to the treatment of these entities.[1] Following his service overseas during World War II, he came to Beth Israel Hospital in Boston, where he worked under the great HERRMAN L. BLUMGART, assisting him and the pathologist MONROE J. SCHLESINGER in pathological studies of the coronary circulation in patients dying from coronary disease. While engaged in this work, as well as carrying on the private practice of medicine, Zoll became interested in the treatment of complete heart block and Stokes-Adams disease. His efforts included the introduction of more rational methods of infusing medications for this; but more important was his introduction of a means to stimulate the heart with external shocks administered to the chest to stimulate cardiac contractions.[2]

Following Zoll's lead, other researchers introduced transvenous pacemakers for temporary pacing. These and pacemaker wires directly connected to the heart during thoracotomy were attached to permanent implantable batteries for long-term management of patients with heart block by Zoll and others. Newer devices appeared later, making these pacemakers longer lasting, able to work on demand (i.e., only when heart rates fell below a certain rate), and more responsive to the varying metabolic demands of the body. Finally, in his later years, Dr. Zoll and his group developed a temporary external pacemaker in the form of a vest that could be applied to patients assessed to be not in heart block but with the potential of developing it. This new model does not cause the painful chest contractions induced by Zoll's initial device, and by avoiding use in patients not clearly needing such pacemakers, the discomfort and possible complications of invasive procedures can now be avoided.

Following the work on the external pacemaker for heart block, Zoll realized that patients with ventricular fibrillation might also be candidates for externally applied electrical shocks to restore normal cardiac rhythm. The overall concept was not a new one; as far back as 1899, shocks directly applied to the fibrillating hearts of dogs had been shown to convert them to normal sinus rhythm.[3] In more recent times (1947), surgeon CLAUDE S. BECK at Western Reserve in Cleveland had performed the first successful human defibrillation by opening the chest of a postoperative patient, massaging the heart, and applying paddles directly to the heart.[4] WILLIAM B. KOUWENHOVEN, an engineer at Johns Hopkins, had been working on this problem for some time. However, it was Zoll who in 1955 performed the first successful defibrillation using externally applied paddles.[5]

After the successful demonstration of external defibrillation, other methods were applied to make such therapy more efficient: the use of bedside monitors with alarms and the establishment of coronary care units. The mortality rate for acute myocardial infarction in-hospital fell from 30 to 15 percent. Finally, the introduction of external cardiac massage by the Johns Hopkins group demonstrated that the circulation could be adequately maintained in the period between the onset of cardiac arrest and the reversion to normal rhythm by defibrillation.[6]

It also became apparent that externally applied electrical shocks could be effective in a variety of other disorders of the heartbeat, and "cardioversion" became an extremely useful means of reversing them. The DC defibrillator of BERNARD LOWN gradually replaced the AC defibrillator of Zoll out of fear that the AC unit would convert such arrhythmias to ventricular fibrillation (a view about which Zoll maintained serious reservations), but it was Zoll who had shown the way.

The next great leap forward would be the rescue of those patients with coronary and other heart disease at risk for sudden unexpected death out-of-hospital when simply going about their business without any warning before ventricular fibrillation occurred. It was the automatic implantable cardioverter-defibrillator (AICD) introduced by MICHEL MIROWSKI that effectively addressed this problem.

Although future improvements in such technology will undoubtedly come, when one looks back on the whole story of electrotherapy for cardiac disease it is Paul Zoll who will be recognized as the single most important contributor to these developments. His intelligence, dedication, modesty, and good humor were all very much in evidence at the breakfast meeting we had in Anaheim, California, at the annual scientific meeting of the American Heart Association in 1987.

Anaheim, California
November 17, 1987

How did you get into cardiac pacing?

I got interested in cardiac pacing before it had a name, really, because I had observed DWIGHT HARKEN do surgery during the war in removal of bone fragments and foreign bodies from in and around the heart.[7]

Were you in the same unit with him?

Yes. We had been classmates at Harvard, and we got put into the same unit in England at the time I was taken out of a field unit and moved to this station hospital in England.

And, although you were an internist, you assisted him at surgery?

No, I didn't do any surgery. I did all the electrocardiography and made observations during surgery. I was a cardiologist at the station hospital, which was a pretty big installation. During these operations, I observed the close relation of the heart to the esophagus, which I had remembered from medical school, and I observed him fishing out foreign bodies from the heart. He did actual cardiotomies to pick them out. So it was a gift; it was a bold, adventurous, and somewhat dangerous business with Dwight Harken. I credit him greatly for having the courage to stand up to his convictions. If you know him, he is a really redheaded surgeon and a very strong personality. Harken's work came after the Mass General Unit in Italy had tried doing some of these extractions and came up with a dictum that stated: Nobody should do this anymore; it's too dangerous. And yet Harken went ahead and got permission to do it; and it was successful and saved lots of lives.

I thought that was a marvelous procedure, the way he did it, and, to the point I am making, I observed how sensitive the heart is to mechanical stimulation—it just goes up in a flurry of ectopic beats. That was in the back of my mind, and for years I thought that maybe we could do something about cardiac arrest, but I never pursued this. I was too busy doing other things on coronary artery disease with HERRMAN BLUMGART and MONROE SCHLESINGER in that injection-dissection study.[8] I also had a busy practice. Our system was one of the part-time private-practice type so that you could get to see what the real issues were in medical practice.

Then I had a patient referred to me who had a new onset of Stokes-Adams disease. This was a sixty-year-old woman who had been perfectly well, and then, for no obvious reason, she began to have heart block and seizures. I had seen an occasional patient with varying heart block but never anything like this. I went to Herrman Blumgart for help, and he called everybody he knew in the United States who was anybody in cardiology, and we had all kinds of suggestions. But this poor woman went on; her heart rate got slower; her seizures became more frequent; and she died after three weeks. There was nothing else wrong with her, and that was so damned frustrating. In the first place, I was upset since she was such a very nice lady; and in the second place, it was aggravating and frustrating. It just wasn't right, that with an organ so sensitive and responsive to mechanical stimulation, that she should die under our hands with nothing else wrong with her. So that was the motivation.

When I was a medical student, I became aware of Albert Hyman in Brooklyn, New York, and his efforts at cardiac stimulation.[9] I had read his reports with considerable interest, but it seemed to me that his approach was an awful way to go. In 1932 he published a paper in which he described passing a long needle through the chest wall directed toward the right atrium. Later on, I thought, "What the hell would you want to stimulate the atrium for in a patient with heart block? You want to stimulate the ventricle." That's pretty obvious.

Hyman had an electromechanical device that you pumped up; you then turned a wheel to make an electrical charge, and it would put out a stimulus for eight to ten minutes or something like that. I don't remember the details. The only thing that I could find in the article was that he had stimulated the atrium of a rabbit, and he had a tracing showing P waves in a rabbit he had so stimulated. I didn't know at the time, and I'm not sure now that he ever tried this in patients, but he never published anything to indicate that he had. I learned that, locally, there had been an outcry about him suggesting doing things like this that weren't "right."

So I was aware of Hyman's work, and that was all I had looked into beforehand, concluding that this was not the way to go. It became very clear to me, watching this poor woman, that you needed a means of pacing that is safe and nontraumatic; that's the primary thing. You cannot go to a patient with Stokes-Adams disease and subject him or her to a thoracotomy to stimulate the heart and then pull out and have the whole thing recur two days later. It's just not feasible. At the time I didn't realize that other kinds of cardiac arrest [ventricular fibrillation] may have the same problem, but that became obvious later on. We used the word "external" to describe the type of pacing we proposed. It had to be safe; and it had to be quickly applied before brain damage occurred, which was within three or four minutes, as everybody knew. This had been emphasized by CLAUDE BECK, who, in 1947, had successfully resuscitated a patient with ventricular fibrillation.[10]

He was at Western Reserve in Cleveland, and a real pioneer in cardiac surgery.

Right. In 1947, he reported saving a fourteen-year-old boy with open-chest cardiac massage after the patient had postoperative ventricular fibrillation. He opened the chest, massaged the heart, and then used defibrillating paddles he got from CARL WIGGERS's laboratory. Wiggers was head of the Department of Physiology.

And Claude Beck put out the fiat: in the presence of cardiac arrest or suspected cardiac arrest, you cut the chest open promptly to do cardiac massage, and then you get somebody to do something about it.

> I recall all the surgeons running around with penknives looking for chests to open up. We used to joke about not falling asleep in conferences or in the halls for fear of getting a thoracotomy from one of our surgeons.

It was not only the chest and general surgeons but everybody, including the ophthalmologists, and they were scared silly. There were necktie parties, which meant that the medical resident always wore a necktie while everybody else did not wear any tie at all, or, at most, a bow tie. And if there was a cardiac arrest, the medical resident was advised to be careful, or he would have his necktie cut off while he stood watching the surgeon resuscitate. That was the atmosphere at that time, that you did an immediate reflex thoracotomy for cardiac arrest.

Well, let me get back to pacing for heart block. After that nice lady had died, I did some exploratory things. We even built a small pacemaker, which did not work. It was much too weak; it didn't have sufficient output. I really didn't understand electronics at all. So I made a few tentative efforts, which failed. Then, in 1950, [JOHN] CALLAGHAN and [WILFRED] BIGELOW from Canada came to speak at the Boston Surgical Society. One of the surgeons, Howard Frank, was a friend of mine and asked if I was interested in attending because Callaghan was going to talk about cardiac stimulation for application during hypothermia. They were working on hypothermia as a method for prolonging the duration of cardiac arrest for open-heart surgery for congenital heart disease. With hypothermia the body's metabolism is lowered so you can extend the operative time without inducing organ damage. But with hypothermia, cardiac arrest could occur, and they had tried to stimulate the heart electrically to treat this. They showed some slides, demonstrating how they would pass a catheter electrode down the jugular vein into the heart near the sino-atrial node in the dog.

This was so narrow-minded! Such exact placement wasn't necessary. They had observed during surgery just what I had: that the [entire] heart was very responsive to stimuli. All you had to do was flip it with your finger or knife blade. It was very sensitive to mechanical as well as electrical stimuli. This had been in the physiological literature for years.

After the lecture, I went up to Callaghan and asked, "What kind of a pacemaker did you use?" He hesitated a minute and then told me that there was a commercially available one made by the Grass Instrument Company, the Grass Physiological Stimulator, and that it was used in physiology laboratories. So I thanked him and went back to speak with Karl Kreyar, who was head of the Department of Pharmacology, and asked him if he had a Grass Physiological Stimulator I could borrow. He gave me one and said, "Send it back when you're through with it." I never returned it. We used it for years until someone stole it from my lab.

Before we go on, there is something about Callaghan and Bigelow I want to tell you about. I've already told you how they came. And I gave credit to Callaghan for telling me about the Grass stimulator. Well, Bigelow, who was a big wheel in thoracic surgery, published a book of reminiscences in which he discussed how their interest in hypothermia led them to the development of a cardiac pacemaker. In the book, he said that I had badgered Callaghan at the time of the visit to Boston as to what kind of a pacemaker they were using. He wrote that they had built the pacemaker themselves with the help of an engineer, named something like Hopps, and that they had never gotten credit for developing the first pacemaker because I had stolen it from them. He said that when they got back to Toronto, there was a letter from me to Callaghan demanding to know the circuitry of the pacemaker. I don't remember ever writing such a letter. I looked through my files and couldn't find it. I spoke to my associates to ask if they ever got any help from Hopps, and they told me they did not.

There was a short paper published in *Pace* by Callaghan showing the pacemaker that Hopps had built for them, with a photograph of the instrument. Using a magnifying glass to look carefully at the unit, we saw that the amplitudes provided by it were totally inadequate for external cardiac pacing, so I couldn't have borrowed his unit for my own work.

To get back to my own story: With access to a Grass stimulator, I could do things on my own as long as it didn't interfere with my primary research, which was working on a series that eventually totaled about twelve hundred hearts that had been injected by the Schlesinger technique in which, with Blumgart as the head of the project, we made many clinical-pathological correlations in coronary heart disease. That was very important work, and for years I thought it much more important than this foolishness that I was doing with electrical stimulation.

Nevertheless, we started doing some experiments. First off, I took a big, thick electrical wire and insulated it, put a glob of solder on the end, and connected it to our old Grass stimulator. We passed it down the esophagus of an unconscious dog which was in normal sinus rhythm. We used this first as an exploring electrode to let us know whether we were behind the atrium or ventricle. Then we stimulated it with a strong enough current to produce an ectopic beat. To record this, I ran an electrocardiogram on the dog, but the pacing stimulus was so strong that it wiped out the ECG tracing and we couldn't see anything. Later on, we were able to use a different version of the electrocardiograph machine with a different transformer coupling, one that didn't result in such a tremendous artifact, but it was still difficult to record. Sanborn helped us with a special machine that had a "viseo" apparatus, or some such thing, that included a fluorescent drum that rotated, and, although you couldn't record the ECG on paper with stimuli, by looking through a hood in the dark room you could see that, on the ECG recording, our stimulator had produced a ventricular extrasystole. I said, "We have solved the problem of cardiac arrest." That was a little excessive, but I was very excited. I called everybody to the basement in the research building at Beth Israel, where we were working, to come and look at what we had found.

We then had to prove that the electrical beat was accompanied by a mechanical contraction. We felt the irregular pulse produced by the extrasystole and went on from there. After a while, however, I was still not too happy with pacing from an esophageal site because, in an unconscious patient, quickly passing an esophageal wire down was not the easiest thing in the world. You would have to have a pretty stiff wire, and this might also be traumatic. Then we realized that the dogs have triangular chests; you could actually see the cardiac impulses on both sides of the chest. So the "brilliant" idea came to me: why not put leads on both sides of the heart externally without putting one down the esophagus? And we found that, with this new arrangement, you could still pace the hearts at about the same thresholds as before, with the esophageal electrode.

We continued to make other improvements in our techniques and waited for a patient. The patients didn't come until finally, in the summer of 1952, just about two years after Callaghan's visit, we got our first patient. He was the father of a neighbor of mine, in fact, who had come to the emergency room at Beth Israel Hospital with Stokes-Adams attacks. I had left word that we were looking for such a patient, and by the time we saw him, it was clear that he was going to die, so that it would not be unethical to attempt to stimulate him by a method that, in itself, might kill him for all we knew. And this poor eighty-year-old man came in, and after his being in the Emergency Room with repeated seizures over a period of four or five hours, someone remembered that, down in the basement, there was some guy who wanted to see a patient like this. They called me, and I ran up the four flights of stairs with my big black box and attached it to the patient. For twenty minutes we drove his heart. He stopped having seizures, and by feeling the pulse in his groin, I was satisfied that we were producing effective heartbeats. I got an electrocardiogram, but it was a lousy one. Nonetheless, it was the first electrocardiogram of effective pacemaking in man.

We reported this in the *New England Journal of Medicine*,[11] and although the tracing baseline moved up and down with each stimulus, you could see in the figure published, in my view at any rate, that we were demonstrating a stimulus followed by a QRS complex on the ECG. After twenty minutes he died. On autopsy, it was revealed that he died from cardiac tamponade. During those four or five hours, he had had about thirty chest punctures to administer intracardiac epinephrine to keep his heart beating, and one of the needles had hit a large vein causing bleeding into the pericardial sac, the immediate cause of his death. But at least we had a demonstration that our device worked.

Almost exactly a month later, we had another patient come in with Stokes-Adams attacks and repeated seizures. But these attacks were intermittent; they would come and go. So now we had a chance for a real success; the patient was alive and in fairly good condition. So we put the pacemaker on him and we stimulated him, and it worked. Again, I had a terrible time getting a good ECG recording. Then I put my finger on his pulse and had the photography department come in to take photographs of my finger moving up and down to prove that we had an effective response to our pacing. This wasn't very good evidence, but it was the best we could get at the time. Later on, with various manipulations of leads, et cetera, we were finally able to get visible recordings.

We stimulated him on and off, interrupting our pacing to see if he might pick up a normal rhythm on his own. We did this for forty-eight hours, with someone at his bedside constantly, but his heart did not pick up on its own. Then people began to get nervous. "What are you going to do? You can't let go. You've got to keep going." And we didn't know what to do. Even my cardiac fellow said, "Maybe we shouldn't be doing this. Maybe you're tampering with 'the will of God' or something."

What we finally did, after forty-eight hours, was to start giving him intramuscular ephedrine, and, after three more hours or so, after one of our pacemaker interruptions, he began to come back on his own. He finally recovered and was fine. And the interesting thing about this guy that was so unusual was that he didn't have any pain from the stimulating shocks. With external pacing you get this enormous contraction of the chest wall muscles. The dogs had never complained about this; they were anesthetized. But neither did this patient. He ate, he slept, he talked, he complained about having to be in a hospital. He even joked with us. The chest wall contractions never bothered him.

I saw a couple of patients just jump off the bed with each stimulus.

Yes, and that's what happens with most patients. This first one put us off the track because of his tolerance of the pacing. Later on, we recognized what a problem this would be. But there were other problems. First you had to restore an effective heartbeat, which is the primary emergency thing. Once you do that, you're in the clear and can go about taking your good old time thinking about what to do next. The next thing was to wait for the return of effective intrinsic cardiac rhythmicity. It took forty-eight hours to do it in this man, but we finally learned that it was not too difficult if you sort of weaned a patient off the pacemaker by giving him a sympathomimetic amine. We started with ephedrine because I thought it was the mildest.

It worked in the hospital. The patient went home but died six months later after another Stokes-Adams attack. And this brings us to the third problem: once you have handled the initial attack when you first see the patient, how do you prevent this all from happening again? What you needed was a reliable, long-term pacemaker.

In the meantime, I began to get calls from all over Boston after the publication of our initial papers. And there were a considerable number of these cases. Early on in this work, I was told that I was wasting my time working on this very rare condition. Nothing would come of it. This did not prove to be the case at all, and while others suggested I do something else, Herrman Blumgart never did.

At about this time, I joined up with another fellow in the department, Arthur Linenthal, to develop a new technique for intravenous drug therapy to increase the heart rate. We found that the trick here was to use these powerful sympathomimetic drugs like epinephrine or isoproterenol in very dilute solutions. Before this, people had been administering these drugs from undiluted ampoules rapidly intravenously, and getting all kinds of dangerous arrhythmias. The dictum became that you did not use sympathomimetic drugs because they were too dangerous. Of course they were too dangerous if you were administering gross overdosages. What we did was dilute the drugs and control administration drip by drip to get the desired effects. Arthur and I went all over Boston at all times of the night, counting the rate of administration by drops per minute. And that was the trick; you had to be absolutely meticulous about it. We wrote a long and very detailed paper on this.[12] That was long before you had mechanized drop counters which took over the chore.

Meanwhile, we were working over the years trying to develop a proper electrode that, connected to an implanted pacemaker, could stimulate the heart effectively over a long period of time and without problems. Shortly after the publication in 1952 of our pacemaker paper, we had a visit from Louis Goodman, who represented a small company, Electrodyne, that wanted to get into the medical instrument field. Goodman was the president, and his partners were Alan Belgard, an engineer, and a third, very nice fellow named Norman Simon. They had been working for Gillette on a project regarding the testing of razor blade sharpness but had gotten wind that Gillette was about to have this done in-house. Having seen something about our work in the newspapers, Goodman came to me and said, "Can we work with you on this? We would like to get where we can build pacemakers."

I told him that we needed something new. The Grass stimulator was just too big, cumbersome, and complicated. We needed a small pacemaker, which could be implanted, and we would have to work out all of its required electrical characteristics in the laboratory. I told him that I didn't know anything, electrically speaking, and would have to rely on them. Goodman soon quit the project, believing that it wasn't going anywhere, but Belgard and Simon came into the laboratory for a year or more and, for years afterwards, continued to work for me. Belgard still is involved; Simon died of esophageal cancer a few years ago.

Belgard, especially, was a very bright guy. He knew his electronics very well. All I had to do was tell him something once about what we were doing with physiology and the medical implications, and he never forgot it. He tried to keep me informed about the electronics, but I couldn't remember it all, of course. We still have one or two of the old pacemakers left. We had a great relationship for many years.

A major problem that confronted us was the development of an adequate electrode. In the beginning, when we implanted an electrode in the heart of a dog, at first the stimulating threshold would be nice and low. However, within a few weeks, the threshold would rise and keep rising. Finally, it would get up so high that it would be at the same level that would be used if you were pacing externally. When we operated to remove the electrode from the dog, we would find a lot of tissue growth around it, but no signs of infection. We were blind at the time to the fact that this was a foreign body reaction. Because this kind of reaction was variable, we thought it might be related to the kind of metal used; and we tried all different kinds of metals. We finally got on to platinum-iridium, but increasing thresholds over time was still a problem, and it took us about ten years to solve it.

We weren't the only ones having problems. In Minnesota, the surgeon [C. WALTON] LILLEHEI was having trouble with heart block following repairs of ventricular septal defects. He began to put pacemaker wires into the heart at the time of surgery, but every one of them stopped working within seven to eight weeks. The threshold kept going up, but he wouldn't recognize that, and I thought that that was disgraceful. I still do.

We finally recognized the foreign body reaction as the cause of the problem, and the way to correct it was to clean the electrode thoroughly and then sterilize it without touching it after it was clean, microscopically clean. And that solved the problem. We published our first article on long-term pacing in 1961.[13] This was after [ÅKE] SENNING had reported the first long-term implantation in 1958, followed by [WILLIAM] CHARDACK.[14]

Of course Senning's pacemaker broke down rather quickly, and they had to replace it. I waited to put ours in because I didn't think it ethical to go ahead until we could be sure of our results.

I always thought Chardack was the first to put in a long-term implantable pacemaker. Did he know about Senning?

I don't know.

What about the development of the intravenously introduced pacemaker wires for long-term pacing, so that you didn't have to subject the patient to a thoracotomy?

The problem with the original external pacemaker was that it hurt too much. Some people couldn't tolerate it, and they had to be sedated heavily. Wire fracture was another major problem after thoracotomy and implantation, and it was a nightmare. So when endocardial pacemaking via the transvenous route was introduced by SEYMOUR FURMAN,[15] everybody went to that and abandoned external pacing, claiming that it never worked, which was crazy, because it's obvious that it did. I'm sensitive on that point.

But there were problems with the pulse generators, even with the transvenous pacemakers. They became unreliable, with an unacceptable failure rate. It took years to recognize that the major problem was that fluid would seep into the pacemaker because the casing was not impermeable. The mercury zinc oxide cell that was used in the early pulse generators manufactures hydrogen in its electrochemical process, and the hydrogen had to go somewhere. That's why the casing was semipermeable. It let hydrogen out, but water would come in and kill the circuitry in a year or so. We were lucky if these pacemakers lasted two years. Pacing would stop abruptly, and the patients would die. It was a nightmare for years.

Finally, we caught on to the idea that we needed an impermeable casing that could hold the hydrogen in under pressure, and we could figure out the life span of this before the casing would break open, and before the battery would die from exhaustion. And nobody listened. Well, the problem was solved in the seventies with the introduction of the lithium cells, which don't make anything. That was a major development.

So much for pacing. Let's go on now to the defibrillation story. I looked up some history on this involving William Kouwenhoven, who, back in the twenties, started work on this problem for an electric company, which was having its linemen electrocuted.

Let me tell you how we got to that. After 1952, while we were working on implanting pacemakers, we had other problems. One of them was that we had to have pulse generators on the patient, set and ready to go at the proper voltage. It had to be made as simple as possible, with as few knobs as possible, so that all the attendant had to do was turn it on when the patient had a Stokes-Adams seizure. But this wasn't good enough. Patients could have special nurses around the clock, and the nurse would go out to make arrangements for lunch, or go to the ladies' room and come back and find the patient dead. It was as if Stokes-Adams disease was a malignant, intelligent being; it would happen at the worst times. It soon became clear that you had to have some sensing electrical instrument that was more reliable than a human being. You can't expect a human being to sit there, day after day, week after week, with nothing happening, and then you had to flip it on. I even found some nurses sitting at the bedside, thinking everything was fine, and the patients were dead!

So you needed a monitor. It didn't take much imagination to realize that what you needed to monitor was the ECG response, the QRS complex. This was a big, unmistakable signal; and you had to have audible sounds with each beat; and when things went wrong, you had to have a loud, unpleasant audible alarm, in case you weren't listening to the beeps, so that when pacing started, this noise would alert you to the fact that pacing had begun. By checking the patient, you could then see what the situation was—whether it was a true or false alarm, et cetera—and then act accordingly. So that's where the first Electrodyne monitors came from. They were described in a 1956 article that had "Unexpected Arrest" in the title.[16] "Unexpected" was the key word. Questions then came up whether external pacing could be used for other kinds of arrest, other than Stokes-Adams disease, and we collected cases showing that it could be used for asystole without seizures or severe bradycardias. But then the question came up: what about the patients who had ventricular fibrillation?

Obviously, the next natural problem to tackle.

Obviously. Now Wiggers had written way back in 1938, or perhaps as late as 1950, that according to his calculations of the energy required to defibrillate, it could not be done externally. Fortunately, although I had read that years before, I had forgotten it by the time we were addressing the problem ourselves, so I went ahead, not knowing any better. And I thought, "For Christ's sake, here is a problem, the termination of ventricular fibrillation, whose solution is similar to that which we used for exciting heartbeats in Stokes-Adams disease." And instead of applying electrodes directly to the surface of the heart after thoracotomy, which is inconvenient and clinically inappropriate, we would apply external charges as we did for emergency standstill. This would be much more appropriate for clinical fibrillation than having the surgeons open the chest to apply paddles directly to the heart, then close the chest, then have the whole thing repeated again when fibrillation recurred. There was one patient reported who was opened seventeen times this way for recurrent fibrillation. Obviously, I thought that was not practical. Even the most accomplished cardiac surgeon might get tired of it, even if the patient didn't.

But what you suggested wasn't what Beck was advocating.

No. The atmosphere at the time, promoted by Beck, was that you did reflex thoracotomy. He would say, "If a resident of mine hesitates, and loses any of those three seconds you have available, I'd kick him out right away." I recall one time in Cleveland, Beck and I were on the same program, with him to follow me. My job at this particular meeting was to talk about external pacing and resuscitation. I stated that it only takes fifteen to twenty seconds to put the pacemaker leads on and turn it on, and it either worked or it didn't. If it did not, it was too late; the heart was anoxic and unresponsive. Beck followed and just wiped up the floor with me. He said this was absolutely wrong; that he would never tolerate such a thing; that you can't waste even ten or fifteen seconds and all that stuff.

Nonetheless, we proceeded with our attempts to develop external defibrillation. Alan Belgard was the guy who really did all this. I just asked him to build me one, and, eventually, he did.

While you were working on this, were you aware that Kouwenhoven and his associates were working on cardiac resuscitation around the same time?

At the beginning, I was not aware of him. In 1954 he and a cardiologist from Johns Hopkins by the name of Milnor visited our lab.[17] We discussed the problem and agreed on it. By that time, I believe we had already done one patient. There were three groups working on this around the same time. The third was [Arthur] Guyton in Mississippi. I'm not sure about the temporal sequence.

It wasn't until 1955, I think, after we had done a number of patients in whom we had stopped the fibrillation but who had died, that we had our first patient who survived.

When I was an intern, there was a big controversy over whether to use the AC or DC defibrillators. Tell me about this.

Alan Belgard said that there were two ways to produce a charge adequate for external defibrillation. One was with alternating current (AC), and one was with direct current (DC). We developed the AC defibrillator, reducing it to a practical size, and figuring out the proper pulse duration and so on after a period of study and experimentation. The other way to go was with direct current. But for this, you needed larger capacitors or "condensers," as they were called in those days, and he said that to build one that would work you would need a room full of paper capacitors. It was just impractical at the time. That's why we went to AC step-up transformers. Within the next few years, however, the technology of capacitors grew and improved. They came out with capacitors that were big but reasonable in size, and that's what [BERNARD] LOWN went to. He worked with an engineer originally from Czechoslovakia by the name of Berkowitz, I believe, who was with American Optical.

They came out with the DC defibrillator in 1961 or 1962,[18] and Lown presented this as if it were a brand-new thing, and no one had ever been defibrillated before. He is a marvelous man with language, really superb and a genius in what he says. He either doesn't care what he says, or (perhaps) he *does* care. He got up and said, "The age of

WENCKEBACH has ended." Very dramatic. Although he didn't say, "We are now in the Lown era," that's what he meant. And Zoll never existed.

By that time, we had external pacemakers that were often successful but had real flaws, and I recognized them. Endocardial pacemakers, introduced transvenously, had come in, and, although it took some time, I began to agree that this was the way to go. So we had pacemakers, we had monitors, and we had defibrillators. This is where Hughes Day comes in. He was from Bethany, Kansas, and visited us upon his return from a trip to England. During our talk, he said, "Why don't you build a special unit where you combine monitors, pacemakers, defibrillators, and people who know how to use them for patients coming in with myocardial infarctions, and who may be at risk for cardiac arrest?"

I said that that would be a great idea and wanted to do it, but Beth Israel didn't have the resources to set it up, and others on the staff might be against it. Blumgart felt that we couldn't do it. Day asked me if I minded if he did it, and I told him, "Go ahead and good luck." I felt it would be great because you could finally demonstrate how effective external pacemaking [or defibrillation] really was, while some people still doubted it in those days. So, on his return to Bethany, Day got financial support from a charitable foundation to set up a system, complete with tape recorder to record every event, and he demonstrated within a year that you can resuscitate patients with acute myocardial infarction and cardiac arrest [standstill or fibrillation] with a high probability of success if you did it properly, with the proper equipment, and proper people on hand.[19] Mortality was cut in half right away from about 30 percent to approximately 16 percent. That was the beginning of the cardiac care unit; it was marvelous, and I like to feel I was a part of it.

How did you finally solve the problem of excessive muscular twitching and pain with the externally applied electrodes, a relatively recent development?

Eventually, everybody was using the transvenous endocardial approach for temporary purposes as well as long-term pacing. That upset me because, in many cases, I knew it was wrong. Much of the time a patient will come in with a myocardial infarction and a partial block that may or may not ultimately become complete and require pacing. You then have an agonizing decision of whether or not to submit him to the risks and trauma of an invasive surgical procedure [pacemaker insertion] in anticipation of this possibly happening. Or else you can wait to see if heart block occurs and then attempt to treat it. [Doris] Escher says she can put in a transvenous pacemaker in four minutes, but I said that was too long. To get away from these unnecessary transvenous pacemaker insertions, we had to develop an external pacemaker that was painless as well as effective. You could have it on the chest, ready to go if necessary, but atraumatic and easily removable if pacing was shown to be unnecessary. My son, Ross, who came to work with me at this time, was instrumental in this.

He is a physicist. He had decided not to become a doctor. Herrman Blumgart was chairman of the Admissions Committee at Harvard. One day, he said to me, "Isn't Ross in his last year at Harvard College now? How come he hasn't come to ask me about being admitted to the medical school? Have him call me for an appointment." I did, and Ross went to see him. Pardon my fatherly pleasure in this little story that's really not to the point, but afterward Blumgart called me and said, "Do you know what your son said to me? We had a very pleasant talk for a bit, and I asked him if he was interested in going to medical school because he had the qualifications. But he said that he would rather be a physicist if he could be a good physicist. If he failed at being a good physicist, then he would go into medicine!"*

> That's funny. BARUCH BLUMBERG told me a similar story about himself. He felt he wasn't smart enough to be a mathematician, so he became a doctor.

To get back to pacemakers, Ross, Belgard, and I got together to discuss the problem of pain, of which there were two types: one due to skeletal muscle contraction, and another due to superficial stinging and burning of the skin. The obvious thing was to disburse the current, to use a

---

* Ross Zoll eventually obtained an M.D. degree and is a practicing anesthesiologist.

large electrode instead of the small metal discs originally used. We had to develop an electrode that was not only big enough to reduce current density, but uniform in its conductivity so that there would not be any hot spots. We also thought that high impedance would be necessary, so that it would take a larger voltage, but with a current that would be more uniform.

Ross suggested that we also prolong the pulse duration, so that we could go farther out on the strength-duration curve so that the threshold would be lower. I said that you couldn't do that, being prejudiced from what I had read from Wiggers. According to him, if you used a longer strength-duration curve, you would risk the danger of ventricular fibrillation. That was a myth propagated in the literature ever since Wiggers's work, that you would produce fibrillation because you got into the relative refractory period, the vulnerable phase. That turned out not to be exactly true. At any rate, Ross did not believe it and suggested we try prolonging the pulse duration in the laboratory to see the effect for ourselves. So we did careful studies of the threshold for single responses on the strength-duration curve versus the threshold for repetitive responses for fibrillation, and the ratio stayed about the same. It didn't matter how long the stimulus was; you did not increase the risk of fibrillation. This was later confirmed by a study performed by some people at Purdue.

We eventually determined that if you used a 40 msec pulse or even a 20 msec pulse duration instead of something below 4 msec (as previously felt required), you would get a lower current amplitude for threshold and, thereby, put in a smaller, less painful stimulus. It reduces the strength of muscular contraction and gets below the skin threshold for pain.

> There's still one loose end here. It was claimed that the AC defibrillator could occasionally cause ventricular fibrillation whereas the DC defibrillator did not.

Yes.

> But, on the other hand, if you fibrillated patients with the AC defibrillator, you could always give them another shock and get them out of it.

Exactly.

But why run the risk of fibrillating them in the first place?

The answer to that, again, is that if you want to avoid fibrillating with an AC defibrillator, you simply put in a timing circuit. That's all there is to it. If a patient is already in fibrillation, it doesn't make any difference where you put in the shock; if a patient is being shocked to terminate a tachycardia, the proper timing of the impulse will avoid fibrillation.

Let's go back to your early influences. You came in contact with so many giants of medicine. As a student, you spent six months with Soma Weiss.

I had an elective with him at Boston City Hospital. He was great, a real showman. One study involved looking up all the patients with alcoholism who died, looking for alcoholic myocarditis, and I found four cases of beri-beri.

Isn't it amazing? I work with Tim Regan, and he really made us aware of how common alcoholic cardiomyopathy really was. Before that we must have been missing alcoholic heart disease left and right.
The story goes that Weiss died from a subarachnoid hemorrhage he diagnosed in himself.

That's true. We had several cases of subarachnoid hemorrhages on the wards when I was with him, and he always spotted them. I also went on rounds with [George] Minot and William Castle, but it was the pathologist Monroe Schlesinger who influenced me more than anybody else. He was an absolute perfectionist, with a very questioning mind. You couldn't say anything to him without him pointing out all the opposing factors involved. With him I learned to be critical. He, Blumgart, and I would sit down going over case after case in that dissection-injection study and evaluate the pathologic findings for correlation with the clinical story. Then we would decide into which category that patient fell.

I understand that there was a lot of resistance to your initial pacing work.

There was a lot of resistance, but Blumgart was very supportive. He told me to do what I had to do, and that he would take care of me for the next thirty years. I also got support from an unexpected quarter. There was talk about our interfering with "God's will" from time to time, and I had a patient who was a monsignor. He heard about our work, and not long after that, an editorial came out in the Catholic weekly magazine *The Pilot*. It stated that there had been some unusual activity in one of the Boston hospitals about resuscitating people from arrests with new techniques. He wrote, "We should not discourage this sort of thing. God works in many wondrous ways, and it is not impossible that he chose this doctor as his instrument."

10

MICHAEL E. DEBAKEY, M.D.
(1908–   )

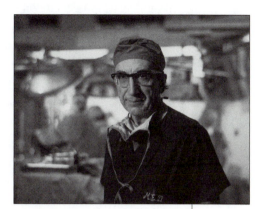

This chapter on Dr. DeBakey could have been placed in any part of this book and fit well, so pervasive and dominant has been his influence in the entire field of twentieth-century cardiovascular surgery. To begin with, he remains one of the few practicing surgeons who, like his medical counterpart, William Dock, began his career early enough to include the almost obligatory visit to European research centers, an important kind of exposure for those who wished to learn of the very latest developments in their chosen field, and who contemplated an academic research career back in the United States.

Although he will be remembered primarily for his work on the repair of aortic aneurysms and aortic dissections (the classification of the latter's types bears his name), his interests have extended to all portions of the arterial tree. Early on, he recognized the segmental nature of vascular disease, which resulted in his pioneering efforts with carotid endarterectomy to prevent or treat strokes. In 1964, with his associate H. EDWARD GARRETT, he performed one of the earliest attempts at coronary bypass surgery. Relatively early in his career he developed a pump for purposes of blood transfusion that was then adapted by JOHN H. GIBBON, JR. to make the first heart-lung machine for cardiopulmonary bypass surgery operable. He has maintained a long-term research interest in development of the total artificial heart as well as left ventricular assist devices and cardiac transplantation. A whole school of outstanding cardio-vascular surgeons has emerged from the crucible of DeBakey's surgical training program at the Methodist Hospital in Houston.

Although often recognized by the public as an influential medical figure, frequently called upon by the U.S. government and other nations for his guidance, DeBakey has also played an important role in medical academic affairs by, among other accomplishments, establishing a first-rate medical school at Baylor in Houston, where he has served as departmental chairman, then president, and then chancellor. His organizational abilities have proved invaluable to the military, where his efforts to mobilize surgical resources finally led to the well-known MASH (Mobile Army Surgical Hospital) units, responsible for the saving of so many servicemen's live in time of war.

Of primary value to medical historians and other scholars was his pivotal role in the establishment of the National Library of Medicine following World War II. This library has become one of the greatest repositories of medical knowledge in the world.

It can easily be argued that no other figure in the history of twentieth-century cardiovascular surgery has had such a widespread and permanent impact on advances in the field, public health policy, and the preservation and extension of medical knowledge. He has also been responsible for the training of other surgeons—over a thousand of them—to follow in his footsteps.

Houston, Texas
November 18, 1997

I am a professor of medicine who is easing off about forty years after my graduation, but you have been out of medical school about sixty-five years and are still going strong. So reviewing your very busy and successful professional life is quite a tall order. I hope we can get through it all in this conversation, at least covering the high points. Let's start off with your family: you came from Lebanon?

My father and mother came to the United States as children because of the opportunities America offered to honest, industrious citizens. I and all my siblings were born in this country.

Why did they pick Louisiana?

Because they spoke French, common to both Louisiana and Lebanon.

Although you were raised during the Great Depression, you and your siblings did not actually suffer through it as many others did.

That's true. My father was an astute and very successful businessman. He owned several pharmacies, farms, and ranches, built a number of buildings on the main street, and had other investments and real estate. It was rare for students in college at that time to have an automobile, but my parents gave me one.

You were also fortunate in another way, becoming a fast matriculator, which was also unusual for those times.

When I entered college, my goal was to go to medical school. At the same time, I wanted to get my bachelor of science degree. At the end of my sophomore year at college, I had enough credits to be admitted to medical school and was accepted, but I still wanted to get my bachelor's degree. So I asked my various professors to recommend me for the required courses for that degree while I was in medical school. That had never been done before, and they advised me against it. But I was persistent, and they liked me, so they allowed me to do it. I had worked as a student-instructor for the professor of zoology for two years, and he had asked me to remain in zoology. By the time I finished my sophomore year in medical school, I had all the credits I needed for my bachelor's degree, so I graduated with my undergraduate college class four years after I had begun.

Probably the earliest thing you did in cardiovascular research involved the bypass pump. Could you tell me about that?

When I developed the pump, I had no idea of using it for the heart-lung machine. I was working as a research assistant while in medical school. One medical faculty member there was a young man doing research on the arterial pulse wave, and he needed a pump to do this in vitro work. He wanted to modify the wave in conducting this research, and my assignment was to find a pump for that purpose. I went to the medical library to find out as much as I could about pumps. I didn't find a great deal in the medical library, but one of my college classmates whom I knew well was studying engineering. When I asked him, "Do you fellows know much about pumps?" he said, "Oh yes, we have a good background in pumping."

I told him what I was trying to do, and he suggested that I go to the engineering school library, which I did, and there I found a wealth of material on pumps, going back to Archimedes and his screw pump for irrigation purposes. I also found some literature relating to some newer developments after the introduction of rubber tubing in the mid–nineteenth century. Some experimental work had been reported showing that compressing a rubber tube could cause fluid to flow out of it. That led me to work on various ways of compressing a rubber tube to make fluid flow out, and that led to my designing the roller pump.

That publication came out in 1934.[1] What was the purpose of it then?

The reason that article was published in 1934 was that I was then using it for direct blood transfusion (from patient to patient), and I became sort of a local blood transfusion expert. I went all around town giving blood transfusions using the pump, even though it was initially developed as a research device.

It became incorporated into the heart-lung machine after I attended a medical meeting where JOHN GIBBON had an exhibit. As he was talking to me about it, he mentioned that he was still having trouble with the pump. At that time, he was using a sigmamotor pump to compress the tubing. I told him about my pump, which I thought might work better, and I sent him a model of it. He then incorporated it into his heart-lung machine, and, of course, everyone working on these machines used it after that.[2]

> **When you were at Tulane, you came very much under the wing of ALTON OCHSNER. When you think of clinics, you think of his along with the other prominent clinics that were developed—Mayo, Lahey, and so on. What was Ochsner like, and what was it about him that created such an impression in the medical community?**

He was a rather charismatic character who had great influence. He was a workaholic, and so was I. The professor and medical student were therefore naturally attracted. When I was a senior student, he asked me to work in his laboratory as a technician. He said, "You ought to be a surgeon," and that's how our association began. From then on, he treated me like a son. He was extremely kind and considerate, and, in fact, after I graduated and finished my internship and residency in surgery, he arranged for me to receive further training abroad, which my parents supported financially. When I returned, I worked as an assistant in his department for a time and wrote many scientific papers with him. Dr. Ochsner was my mentor.

> While you were still a medical student, there was another influence in your career, RUDOLPH MATAS. Photographs of him, portly with that white mustache and goatee, always remind me of that Kentucky Fried Chicken colonel in the ads, but he was quite a prominent surgeon and really a pioneer in vascular work.[3]

I did come under his influence to some extent because he was still practicing even in his later years. The way I came to know him is interesting. As a medical student, I was able to read the French and German literature. When faculty members discovered I could, they asked me to translate articles for them because back in the thirties some of the most advanced work was published in foreign journals. I would look for those journals in the medical school library, but most of the foreign journals were only in Matas's personal library. The librarian would send Dr. Matas the list of journals I had requested, and he would send them over. On one occasion, the librarian told me that Dr. Matas wanted to meet me, and asked that I go to his home to get the books myself. He wanted to see who this person was who was reading all his journals. When I went to his home on St. Charles Avenue, he met me at the door and was very gracious. He invited me in and started asking about my family, my upbringing, and the like. He offered me a glass of port wine, which I sipped only to be polite, since I don't drink alcohol. After that, he invited me to borrow the books from his library any time I needed them. He said, "You come personally to get whatever you want; this library is yours."

Dr. Matas's entire house was a library. He had books stacked all over the living room, upstairs, everywhere. In fact he had to prop up the residence because the books had created such a weight. When the Mardi Gras parade went by his house, the king always stopped and toasted him, and he invited me to join him on the veranda on those occasions. We became very close; and he asked me to complete one of his articles on the history of medicine in Louisiana. He then brought out a steamer trunk just filled with documents and said, "I probably will never finish this, but I would like you to take it over."

By this time, however, I had gotten an appointment to come to Baylor, and I explained to him that I was very busy developing the department. I promised him that I would get in touch with him as soon as I had a chance, but he died in the meantime. I never did get around to it.

Well, you're only eighty-eight; perhaps you will find some spare time one of these days. Did you relate to Matas in any other way?

Dr. Matas, who was getting on in years, would refer to Dr. Ochsner any patients he saw in his office who needed surgical treatment, and I would assist Dr. Ochsner with the operations on them.

Ever since World War II, when Europe was devastated and no scientific work could be done there, most of the cardiovascular research has occurred in the United States. So people tend to forget that during the prewar years such work took place mainly in Europe. People forget that.

That's true. Before the war, if you wanted a postgraduate education and wanted to advance academically, you had to go to Europe.

Did Ochsner advise you to do this? And tell me about RENÉ LERICHE and others you met there.

Dr. Ochsner did advise me to go to Europe, and I went to Leriche in Strasbourg because Matas recommended him to Dr. Ochsner. Dr. Ochsner was German-trained and did not know much about the French people. But I had heard of Leriche and read some of his articles. At that time he was one of the foremost surgeons interested in vascular diseases, and he had developed procedures like sympathectomy and arterectomy, which were then new. Some of this later work did not have much clinical utility, but he was very innovative and that interested me.

When Dr. Ochsner asked Dr. Matas about Leriche, Dr. Matas, who knew Leriche well, sent him a letter of recommendation, upon which Leriche accepted me as *assistant étrangée.* So I spent a year with Leriche, who was very kind to me.

What was he like?

He looked very much like Mozart. He was very charismatic and dynamic, but rather philosophic. He was really an intellectual with a great background in history, literature, and music. Even in his lectures he would touch on historical and literary characters. On one occasion when he was talking about a kidney problem, he reminded the audience that the man who described this condition had once approached Napoleon about some necessary sanitation measures when they were traveling together, and Napoleon approved his suggestion. He was always injecting stories like that in his lectures.

Leriche was a meticulous surgeon in technique for something like a sympathectomy, which he was especially interested in, but when he got into the abdomen to do a gastrectomy, a procedure he didn't have any particular interest in, he was not a good technician. What he liked to do he did well. He described Leriche's syndrome precisely without having an arteriogram; and he stated exactly where the occlusion was, at the bifurcation of the abdominal aorta and iliac arteries. He also described it as a localized lesion and even proposed the surgical treatment, recommending resection and homograft replacement, although he knew that this was not possible in 1926. But it's interesting that JACQUES OUDOT did perform exactly what he had recommended some thirty years later, in the fifties. So Leriche was a visionary, and if you read his articles about pain, for instance, you are aware of his philosophical approach.

How about your experiences with MARTIN KIRSCHNER?

After spending a year with Leriche, I went directly from Strasbourg to

Heidelberg. And the contrast was obvious as soon as I got there. The German system was very precise and structured, whereas in Leriche's clinic there was a sort of looseness about the organization, and to some extent it was not as precise as it might have been. When I arrived in Heidelberg, I noticed that the hospital was spic and span and well organized. For example, Kirschner was a great believer in postoperative exercises, and every day a man would come to the wards, including the orthopedic wards, and if the patient could move anything, even an arm or a leg, he was encouraged to do it to the sound of martial music.

> **I guess that kept the incidence of postoperative pulmonary embolism down.**

Yes it did. Kirschner was a great technician, particularly in his abdominal surgery, a lot of which he did under local anesthesia. He was also very kind to me; I had dinner at his home at least once a month.

> **Were you there as an observer, or did you actually operate?**

I didn't operate on my own, but I assisted with operations performed.

> **We will get back to some of these surgical techniques, but I want to focus now on your return to Tulane, where your were on the faculty for a few years, and then during World War II you were instrumental in starting up what came to be called MASH (Mobile Auxiliary Surgical Hospital) units. Could you tell me how this got started?**

We had a severe shortage of well-trained personnel, particularly in board-certified surgeons or even experienced surgeons who would have been so qualified had they taken their boards at the time. There was a paucity of such people. And there wasn't a single board-certified surgeon in the regular U.S. Army, except for the surgeon general himself, Norman Kirk, who was certified in orthopedic surgery. This was also true for other medical disciplines. Full-time army physicians were primarily general practitioners, with limited training in the specialties.

So the surgical work had to be done by the civilian personnel who had been called to duty. Many were volunteers, but a good number of highly trained professors and surgeons came in through special units, such as the MGH (Massachusetts General Hospital) Unit, the Emory Unit, and others, sponsored by various schools. I was going to go with the Tulane Unit, but Dr. Ochsner tried to hold me as "essential" to the medical school. I made such a fuss about going that he finally relented, and when Fred Rankin [chief surgical consultant, Surgeon General's Office] learned that I was going to be admitted into the service, he insisted on bringing me to Washington to join his staff. So I became part of his surgical consultative division. We participated in planning all the surgical staff work that had to be done for the army, and we were eager to develop the concept that the wounded should be treated as early as possible after injury. So we set up these so-called field hospitals near the front, where before little more than first aid had been available. By putting in a surgical unit, we were able to treat the wounded right away, even if they had chest or abdominal injuries. So we developed what we called "Auxiliary Surgical Units." The M (for mobile) units came later, in Korea. The units we organized in World War II consisted of a surgeon, an assistant, an anesthesiologist, an operating room nurse, with perhaps one other nurse and a technician—maybe five, six, or seven people in the unit who could be moved from a major hospital in the center to one of the mobile units at the front as they were needed. They then became very mobile and proved to be extremely effective. We collected data to show how effective they were in reducing the mortality rate, and even restoring normal activity in patients at the end. From that standpoint, this was a new concept in military medicine so that during the Korean War, they actually established mobile auxiliary surgical hospitals, and that's where the term "MASH" originated.

At the risk of skipping over some of your military experiences, since you were involved with the U.S. Army for five years, from 1942 through 1946, I want to turn to something else that is very dear to my heart as a writer and medical historian. And that is the National Library of Medicine.

This is how the National Library of Medicine came about. I had to write a number of military orders without any background in military medicine, so I had to do a considerable amount of library research. When I went to the surgeon general's library to do that research, I was impressed with its extensive scope, but the building that housed the collection was very old. The roof leaked; they had to put tarpaulins over the books when it rained. And they even had to use an outhouse for toilet facilities because there were none in the building. It was incredible!

At the end of the war, I made a strong point about these deficiencies. I told the surgeon general, "This library is a national treasure, and it ought to be better housed." I was told that they had been trying to get a new building for thirty years but could never compete with tanks and the like. Then it suddenly occurred to me: this doesn't belong in the army; this is a national library and belongs to the country. So I began a movement to get it out of the army by writing several "white papers" and making some presentations to a group of civilian library consultants.

Now, you have to understand that this wasn't a very popular idea because the army really thought it was their treasure, and it was. They had started it and felt obligated to maintain it. But, in my opinion, it had developed beyond them, and that is why I made such an issue about it. They tried to retain it by changing its name to "The Armed Forces Medical Library," representing all the armed forces, but what finally moved it out was the Hoover Commission. Tracy S. Voorhees, one of "Hoover's men," served as chairman of the Medical Task Force of the commission to reorganize the government. He asked me to work on this project full-time. By this time, I had returned to Tulane from the army but was able to get a leave of absence and went to Washington, where I spent eight or nine months working on the project.

When I finally wrote the report, Mr. Voorhees asked me to go with him to brief Mr. Hoover on our report. Mr. Hoover had an apartment at the Waldorf-Astoria in New York. We had lunch with him, and Hoover, after thumbing impatiently through the report, finally turned to Voorhees and said, "Tracy, do you know how many task forces I have? I have about fifty. Suppose every one of them had some thirty-five or so recommendations as you have here, who would read the report? So tell me, what is the *single* most important one?"

Before Voorhees could say anything, I jumped in with "the library," and it struck a sympathetic chord with Hoover because he was interested in libraries. Remember, he gave a library to Stanford. So that became a prominent medical recommendation, and Congress adopted it quickly.

But you had trouble getting it through Congress.

Yes. At the time, Senator Lister Hill was one of its leading advocates, and I worked with his staff in developing the legislation. One day he called me and said, "Mike, we have the votes to pass this legislation, but the problem is your Speaker of the House [Sam Rayburn of Texas]." Hill told me, "Rayburn has tabled it and won't let it come up for a vote."

The reason was that the American Medical Association, which was located in Chicago, wanted the library located there. And we, of course, wanted the library to be part of the NIH [National Institutes of Health]. Senator Hill asked me if I knew anyone in Houston who had any influence on Rayburn. By that time I had already left Tulane and was now at Baylor in Houston. Since I had only recently arrived in Houston, I didn't yet know anyone with that kind of influence. I did call Ovita Culp Hobby, who had been head of the WACs [Women's Army Corps] in Washington during the war, and became a very good friend of mine when I moved to Houston. She said that she didn't think that there was anyone in Houston with any influence on Rayburn. But when I realized that this was a political matter, and that Rayburn didn't want to offend anyone in Chicago, where the Democratic Convention was to be held, it triggered the idea of calling on the secretary of the Democratic Party, whose husband I had operated on.

At that time her name was Dorothy Vredenberg, and after I operated on Mr. Vredenberg for an aneurysm of the abdominal aorta, I came to know them well. I called her and said, "Dorothy, you could do a great service to the country by getting Rayburn to let the library bill come up in Congress. We have the votes to pass it." She said, "Mike, let me see what I can do." The next day she called me with the good news that Rayburn was going to let it go through. Then Lister Hill called me and said, "Mike, I don't know what you did, but whatever it was, we're going to get that bill through." And that's how it passed.

> And we are all indebted to you for that. There's not just military medicine in the library but all of medicine.

It's critical to all of us, and the whole world has access to it and uses it.[4]

> Now I would like to move on to something else, surgery of the aorta, because if you had done nothing else in your career, this alone would guarantee you a place in some kind of pantheon of cardiovascular surgery. You began the bulk of this work in the fifties, and I wonder if you could tell us how you worked your way up from the abdominal aorta to the thoracic aorta to the aortic arch and root.[5]

I was at a meeting in Chicago around 1949 or 1950, when [ROBERT] GROSS and [CHARLES] HUFNAGEL presented their experimental work with the use of homografts to bridge the defect in coarctation of the aorta. They showed that in animal experiments it could be done. That suggested to me the possibility of using homografts for aneurysms. I had become interested in aneurysms long before, including Matas's description of aneurysmorrhaphy, and we had actually done some of that in New Orleans, mostly for peripheral aneurysms affecting the femoral and popliteal arteries. It seemed to me an ideal way of dealing with this if a homograft could be used to bridge a defect.

I had the good fortune of being able to do all the autopsies at the old Jefferson Davis Hospital here in Houston—the city/county hospital that's now called the Ben Taub. And although that's another story, we at Baylor had taken over that hospital, and the coroner was very cooperative. From my standpoint, autopsies were an important teaching experience for the residents, and when I offered to do the autopsies for him, he accepted. I would do the autopsies with the residents, and that gave me the opportunity to obtain aortic homografts from the younger people who had died as the result of auto accidents and the like.

How did you preserve them?

At that time we simply preserved them in sterile saline because they were fresh. Later, antibodies were added to the solution. Finally, in 1952, I had a patient who had a large aneurysm of the abdominal aorta, and I said, "Let's use a homograft on him," and we did. The fresh homograft worked beautifully. At that time, I didn't know that CHARLES DUBOST in Paris had done one some months before we did; we found out about it later.

We quickly developed quite a series of cases, and at the American Surgical Association meeting in 1952, we presented our first two cases in a discussion of a paper by Dr. Arthur Blakemore. Dr. Blakemore's presentation was concerned with treatment of aneurysms of the abdominal aorta by inserting a wire through a needle into the aneurysm, and using a machine to provide an electrical impulse in the wire to form a thrombus. As you know, historically, creation of a thrombus in the aorta was one of the methods used to treat aortic aneurysms. When Dr. Blakemore rose to close the discussion of his paper, he concluded that our report was interesting, but he doubted whether this could be used in most cases. The following year, we published a report in *Surgery, Gynecology, and Obstetrics* on our results in twelve patients successfully treated by this surgical method.

Shortly after that, a patient from Arkansas was referred to me, and he had an aneurysm of the lower part of the descending thoracic aorta, causing severe pain. I concluded that it was syphilitic because it was eroding the body of the vertebra, which was characteristic of syphilitic aneurysms, and that was the cause of the severe pain. I told the patient that although we had never repaired an aneurysm in the chest, we had done enough repairs of abdominal aortic aneurysms to feel confident that it could also be done there. He was in such severe pain, I think, that he was willing to take any chance, and, fortunately, the operation was successful. He lived about twelve or thirteen years and returned periodically to see me. Finally, he came here for a checkup after all that time, but by then he had cancer of the lung; he was a smoker. I resected the lung, but he died a few years later from metastasis to his brain. That success triggered my interest in aneurysms of the descending thoracic aorta.

Most arteriosclerotic aneurysms of the aorta are located in the upper segment of the thoracic aorta. At that time, we weren't aware of the possibility of development of spinal cord ischemia [from interruption of the blood supply to the spinal cord] as a result of repairing thoracic aneurysms. We were aware that in repair of coarctations of the aorta, spinal cord ischemia could occur occasionally, but the collateral circulation that developed as a result of the coarctation usually, but not always, prevented this complication. We did four or five cases of thoracic aneurysmal repair before we had a patient in whom paresis of the legs developed. That's what led us to develop that atrial-femoral bypass [left atrium to femoral artery] to prevent this complication, and we still use it today. This reduced the incidence of paralysis significantly, but it can still occur occasionally.

The next problem was aneurysms of the ascending aorta. In 1953, we had our first patient. By this time, we had the heart-lung machine that we had developed in our laboratory, similar to John Gibbon's. We put the patient on the heart-lung machine, and the operation was a success. It is always important for that first case to be successful! Then, the next thing was aneurysm of the aortic arch, and in 1954 I performed the first successful case of resection and homograft replacement for this condition. Also in 1954, we had a patient with a dissecting aneurysm, which, at that time, was always fatal. It was fortunately a type III, which is in the descending thoracic aorta and easier to approach than those higher up. The operation was successful. This stimulated our interest in other dissecting aneurysms, and as time went on, we successfully tackled types I and II, which involve more proximal parts of the aorta.

Do you still think that medical treatment of type III is still the preferred treatment as opposed to the other types of aortic dissection?

Definitely, but in very old people, especially if there is no sign of progression, we treat them medically. Other patients with dissecting aneurysms who are treated medically ultimately require surgery because the disease progresses, and even if their blood pressure is controlled, two or three years later you find that you have to operate.

What led you away from homografts and into Dacron?

This is an example of how previous work can inspire you. A New York surgeon by the name of A. B. Voorhees, Jr., who has since died, presented a paper on experimental work with what was then called "vinyon N cloth." That paper suggested to me the possibility of doing some experimental work on our own on the use of some other plastic materials. I went downtown to get some nylon cloth. The store was out of nylon, but the clerk showed me a new material called Dacron. I looked at it, felt it, and I liked it, so I bought a yard, and we started doing some experimental work with it. Actually, I would take two sheets, cut them in the diameter I wanted, and then sew the edges on each side with my wife's sewing machine to form a tube. After a year or two of experimental work in the laboratory on dogs, I became convinced that this Dacron graft could be used on human beings.

In those days we didn't have human research committees; we relied on our own ethical conduct. But I was convinced that the Dacron graft could be successful, so in 1954, when I had a patient with an aneurysm of the abdominal aorta, I decided to use it. I made this Dacron bifurcation tube on my wife's sewing machine, sterilized it, and used it. It was successful, and that was the important point. Then I began to work on a way to knit these tubes into desired shapes.

A patient on whom I had operated for an abdominal aortic aneurysm, and in whom I had used an aortic homograft, helped me considerably with this problem. He was head of Stuart Pharmaceutical Company, one of the largest in California. He was a very wealthy man, and he became interested in what we were doing. He had a half-interest in a socks-knitting factory in Reading, Pennsylvania. He suggested that I visit it, which I did. The person I spoke with there told me the socks-knitting machine wouldn't work for my purpose, but referred me to a Swiss immigrant, Thomas Edman, at the Franklin Textile Institute in Philadelphia, who was an expert in this field. I went to Philadelphia to meet him, and although he had been working there full-time, he finally came to work for us. The executive from Stuart Pharmaceuticals provided a grant of twenty-five thousand dollars for a machine for this purpose, which Mr. Edman developed. He would send these seamless Dacron tubes to me, and I would put them on a stent and create a crimping, to permit flexibility without collapsing them. I would then put them in an oven and bake them to fix memory into the crimped form.

I used these Dacron grafts on patients and even sent some to my colleagues who were also interested in working in the field. Ultimately, one of the companies in Philadelphia, I believe, bought the machine that Mr. Edman had developed, and that became the grandfather of all the knitting machines we have today.

> There is often a great time lag between the discovery of something in medicine and the actual application of it—which I call the "long P-R interval." One example, of course, is the discovery of penicillin by ALEXANDER FLEMING; it took twelve years before HOWARD FLOREY actually used penicillin successfully in patients. Another example is HENRY SOUTTAR's use of the closed mitral commissurotomy years before Bailey, BROCK, and HARKEN.
>
> Now there are two instances in your own career where you were first in the door, and then there was that long interval. The first was the carotid endarterectomy, which you had performed many years before this procedure actually became popular in the prevention of strokes. And it was only when you reported a nineteen-year follow-up on your first patient that this became well known.[6]

That's right; I did that first operation in 1953, and I reported on a series of twelve or thirteen patients at a neurological meeting in New York. What kept me from publishing it sooner was the strong criticism that ensued. As a result, I realized that I had to accumulate some convincing data. This first patient was from Lake Charles, Louisiana, my hometown, and that, I believe, is why he agreed to be operated on. I told him that this procedure had never been done before.

Was it your work in the aorta that led you into this new area?

No, it was more than that; it was again the influence of previous studies. The neurological group at the Massachusetts General Hospital had done a thorough investigation of patients who had died of strokes and who had lesions at the bifurcation of the carotid artery. These neurologists virtually indicated that such lesions caused strokes in these patients, and that their removal might prevent the stroke from developing. But nobody had done this operation, and when my patient from Lake Charles appeared in my office, I put all the facts together and concluded that his carotid disease was causing his TIA's [transient ischemic attacks in the brain]. He was a bus driver, and he had to stop working from time to time because his arm and his right leg would become transiently paralyzed. It was a classical case.

We did an arteriogram, which showed the location of the block in his carotid artery, and when I suggested the operation, he consented; as I said, he was from Lake Charles and knew my family. When he came back many years later, he was perfectly fine, but I told him I needed an arteriogram to be sure everything was all right. He consented, and the test showed that all was well.

> **The other instance of the "long P-R interval" is the coronary bypass operation. Most people think that René Favaloro and his associates at the Cleveland Clinic were the first, but you had actually performed a bypass well before them.[7]**

That's true, but you must remember that we were not the first. I was stimulated by the work of DAVE SABISTON, who had done the first coronary bypass operation. What Favaloro had done was use interposition grafts; this involved removing the blocked segment and replacing it with a vein graft. In the coronary bypass operation, as it evolved, the blocked segment is left alone, and a saphenous vein graft is attached to the ascending aorta proximally and is attached distally to the coronary artery beyond the obstruction.

If you really want to go back in time, the truth of the matter is that ALEXIS CARREL, in 1913, performed the first coronary bypass operation on a dog, using a carotid artery homograft attached to the descending thoracic aorta and to what he called a branch of the left coronary artery. He described this procedure in great detail; the dog lived four hours, and although it died, he believed that this was the way to deal with a blocked artery. We performed the first successful coronary bypass on our patient in 1964, but Dave Sabiston did his in 1962. I was impressed with the article he wrote in the *Johns Hopkins Medical Journal*.[8] His patient died of a stroke a few days after the operation, not as a result of failure of the coronary bypass.

A great deal of experimental work was going on in the years before the first bypass operation on a human. A whole series of articles on coronary bypass operations on animals had been published, and in our own laboratory, as we reported in 1961, three years before our first patient's operation, we demonstrated a patency rate of about 50 percent in dogs at six months, but we thought we needed to improve that rate before we performed the operation on a human.

> **One thing struck me about your doing a saphenous bypass on that patient. Under today's rules of informed consent, you would not have been able to do that, right? But when you got in there and found the artery so botched up that all you could do was a bypass, you couldn't very well have awakened the patient and said, "Excuse me, sir, but now we'd like to try something a little different. . . ."**

Of course not. And those rules were not in effect then; you were expected to observe ethical codes voluntarily. When we scheduled this patient for surgery, it was for an endarterectomy, but we were determined to save his life after we virtually destroyed his artery in attempting this procedure. But life has become more and more complicated now, and as we do more and more, we have to have some kind of structured means to determine how and when to do them. I don't object to this, but they do hinder innovations somewhat. You have to balance it all to avoid any ethical violations.

> **Was there a fear in the early days that the vein grafts would not hold up under arterial pressures, which were much higher than those that existed in the venous system?**

Experimental work showed they did, but we didn't know that after time they would deteriorate and obstructions would develop after the initial bypass was performed.

> **Do you see on the horizon the possibility of preventing these late obstructions from occurring?**

On the basis of experimental work we published on this complication, there is some reason to believe that the way the vein graft is prepared will help reduce the incidence of this problem, but it still doesn't completely eliminate it.

> **You have also been a pioneer in the use of left ventricular assist devices.**

That's also an interesting story. I became interested in the artificial heart in the early fifties, and what triggered my interest in left ventricular assist devices was their potential in extending the time that you could use the heart-lung machine. Our experience with the heart-lung machine had shown us that it was difficult to wean some patients off it after you completed the operation. We also found that if you could support the heart for an hour or two after the operation, you could wean some of them off successfully.

This led me to think that if you could extend use of the heart-lung machine to beyond two hours, you might be able to wean more patients off the heart-lung machine. But you couldn't use the heart-lung machine beyond several hours, so we began some experimental work in the laboratory on use of a ventricular device for longer-term support after the patient had been disconnected from the heart-lung machine. The first device we developed we had occasion to use in 1963 in a patient of my associate, Dr. Stanley Crawford. He had replaced one aortic valve in this patient, and on the next day, cardiac arrest developed. We used the device on the patient, but although we did not realize it at first, brain damage occurred, and he died from that. Before this, however, hypotension and severe pulmonary edema had developed, owing to heart failure, and we decided to perform a left-atrium-to-descending-thoracic-aorta conduit using the pump, and within hours the pulmonary edema cleared up and remained so for several days during the ventricular assistance until his death several days later. It was very impressive and supported the validity of this concept.

We went back to the laboratory to improve the pump, and finally in 1966, we used it for the first time on a Mexican lady with severe heart failure on whom we had performed aortic and mitral valve replacement. After completion of the aortic and mitral valve replacements, we were unable to wean her off the heart-lung machine. We then used our ventricular assist device with inflow from the left atrium and outflow to the right axillary artery. With a pump flow of 3,000 ml/min. we were able to wean her off the heart-lung machine. We supported her heart for ten days, after which her heart recovered. She later resumed normal activities and was tragically killed in an automobile accident six years after the operation.[9]

> To turn to something else: I have always been impressed by the fact that the head of every surgical program becomes, in effect, a father figure. This is true in medicine in general but especially, I think, in surgery: WILLIAM HALSTED had his people, then Robert Gross, ALFRED BLALOCK, and so on. And you actually descended from the line of Matas and Ochsner. Who are your heirs? Who are the people of whom you are the most proud? There must be dozens you have developed over the years.

For example, the surgeon who operated on President Boris Yeltsin, Dr. Renat Akchurin, was trained here by me. I consider him to be the top cardiovascular surgeon in Russia, and he is regarded as the most prestigious one there. A number of other people whom I have trained have become department heads at medical schools: Bob Wallace at George Washington University, Edward Garrett in Tennessee, William Blaisdale in Davis, California, and Lazar Greenfield at the University of Michigan. In the early days, during the sixties and seventies, my department was one of the basic training grounds for cardiovascular surgeons. At that time, we had as many as eight or ten foreign doctors in training with us who subsequently returned home to become heads of their own training centers in Japan, Belgium, Russia, Scotland, Greece, France, England, Italy, South America, and Asia. The two major Italian cardiovascular surgeons in Rome and Milan trained here with us. Some years ago, our trainees formed a society called the Michael E. DeBakey International Surgical Society.

> There's one trainee you had who names you with Brock and Blalock as one of his three primary mentors, and that is DENTON COOLEY. He spent twenty years with you here before he left. The separation must have been very painful for you.

Not particularly. What happened that led to the separation—and I don't know why he did this, but he admitted it to the investigating committee—was his improper use of the total artificial heart that was developed in our laboratory. I was out of town at the time this happened. According to his own testimony, [Domingo] Liotta, an Argentinean physician who had been working with us as a research fellow in our laboratory, offered to use it in a patient of Cooley's, and Cooley accepted the offer. Now, Cooley had never done any work on this device in the laboratory; in fact he rather disdained laboratory work. He was a good clinician and surgeon. According to Liotta, he went to Cooley because I refused to use the total artificial heart on a human being. My reason was that the data we had did not justify human implantation. Up to then, no animal in which we had implanted the heart had survived beyond forty-eight hours.

This human experimentation with our covertly taken device was a violation of our agreement with the NIH, the sponsors of the research, and I was the principal investigator. Before the device could be used in a patient, it was necessary to get approval from our institutional research committee as well as the NIH. Approval for this operation had been granted by neither, and I refused to ask for it because we didn't have the data to support it. So what Cooley and Liotta did created a real problem for the college, because we then had to explain to the NIH how this happened. The board of trustees of Baylor College of Medicine established a committee to investigate the matter, and both Liotta and Cooley appeared before the committee. Cooley's justification was that he was trying to save a patient's life. Before the committee was about to present their findings to the board of trustees of Baylor College of Medicine, one of the members of the board advised Cooley to resign, and he did.

The NIH accepted the college's report, and they recognized that the violation was not our fault, but that this had been done secretly, and they allowed us to continue our work.[10]

Did Cooley ever apologize to you over this?

He just resigned and left. The episode was a disappointment, not painful but certainly a disappointment, because I certainly had respected his surgical capabilities. Perhaps he was somewhat naive to do what he did; I don't know what his motives were.

Are your current relations with him cordial?

He works at St. Luke's, and I have no contact there. Regarding this whole issue, I refer to this issue in a recent article I published about the ventricular assist device, so it is in the public domain.[11]

The artificial heart: what is the future for it, with all the past problems of clot formation in the JARVIK heart and so on?

Jarvik with [WILLIAM] DeVRIES sat in this room with me and tried to persuade me to join with them when they got approval to do ten patients. They wanted me to do five of them at this institution, but I explained to them that I couldn't ask our human research committee to approve the procedure unless I had data to support the use. I showed them a paper about our own artificial heart and said, "This is essentially similar to your artificial heart." Jarvik expressed amazement to see that it was so similar to his own model. He said he would supply us with experimental data about the feasibility of using it, but I never received any, even after I sent my associate, George Noon, who was working with me on the artificial heart, to Utah. When he couldn't get it, I told Jarvik, "I can't join you."

When the Food and Drug Administration consulted me for my opinion about it, I recommended that they *not* approve it, but they approved it anyway. And, of course, as you know, it was a disaster, and they never completed the ten cases, stopping after the seventh, I believe. It never should have been done, and even today the artificial heart has extreme limitations, although it has been improved a good deal. Still, none of them can be considered permanent implantations.

From our own experience with the total artificial heart, I became convinced that work in this field should be directed toward ventricular assistance. Consequently, I began concentrating on a ventricular assistance device. I had the good fortune to do a heart transplant on a NASA engineer who became interested in what we were doing. I asked him one day if any of his engineers might be interested in helping us. He thought they would and arranged for me to go out to the Johnson Space Center, where I met with five or six of them and showed them some of the artificial hearts we had developed in the laboratory. They started working with us informally at first, and later formally. As a consequence, we have developed a ventricular assist device about the size of an AA battery that we have been using in animals and expect sometime this coming year to go into clinical trials with it.

What do you think about the Batista operation?*

I don't know. He visited me here in Houston a few months ago, discussing his work with me for an hour and a half or two hours. I asked him, "What are your follow-up results?" He had very little data but believed that about 60 percent of his patients had good results at the end of the year. I asked if this was really any better than medical therapy, and he thought his patients could "do more." And that's about all he had.

More recently, my colleagues at the Cleveland Clinic and Buffalo tell me that they may get the best results by also repairing the mitral valve in conjunction with removal of the myocardial wall. It's hard to say.

Something else that is of interest is the role of infection in heart disease. Of course with AIDS and other infectious agents implicated, infection is becoming more and more of a general medical problem, but you published something about Chlamydia and aortic valve disease. Where does that stand now?

Here, again, is an example of the importance of previous work; rarely is something developed de novo. It is well established that Marek's disease in chicks is caused by a virus that produces lesions in the arteries and kills the chicks. When you look at these lesions postmortem, they look like atherosclerosis. This gave me the idea that human atherosclerosis might be due to a virus, particularly when you think about retroviruses. So I talked with JOE MELNICK, one of the world's authorities on viruses, and he offered to test this theory. I provided him with specimens I removed from patients operated on for occlusive disease of

---

* A procedure for advanced, intractable heart failure introduced by Brazilian surgeon R. Batista; it involves partial left ventricular resection to reduce the size of the ventricle and thus the tension developed during systolic contraction to improve cardiac performance.

the arteries, and there was no question in his mind that a virus is associated with the lesion; all the imprints are there. Dr. Melnick thinks it belongs to the herpetic family, although the virus has not yet been identified. Five or six laboratories in other parts of the country and abroad have confirmed our observations, and some more recent studies have suggested a possible bacterial etiology.

> To be continued. . . . Although we're focusing here mainly on American medicine, as an international figure, you are particularly well placed to identify some of the non-American cardiac surgeons who have made important contributions during the twentieth century. I came up with a few names on my own: Brock, BRIAN BARRATT-BOYES, VIKING O. BJÖRK, ALAIN CARPENTIER . . . . Who were some of the other prominent cardiologists and cardiovascular surgeons, foreign-born, who impressed you?

Among the foreign cardiovascular surgeons, there are only a few: in Stockholm, Björk's mentor, CLARENCE CRAFOORD, who performed the first aortic coarctation repair; in Paris Dubost and Carpentier; Barratt-Boyes in New Zealand; Brock in England.

> Let me get back to your personal life now. Is your brother still living and practicing surgery? And what about the rest of the family?

My brother, Ernest, an excellent surgeon, practiced general and thoracic surgery in Mobile, Alabama, and still lives there. My two sisters, Selma and Lois, are still active in scientific writing, editing, and publishing.

> You had four sons from your first marriage before your wife's tragic death, and a daughter from your second marriage. Although none of your sons have gone into medicine, is there a chance that your daughter will?

She is a sophomore at Southwestern University now, and her major is biology. She is taking all the premedical sciences so she may go into medicine. She hasn't declared herself but she certainly is interested in biology as a career.

> Are you at all disappointed that your sons have not followed in your footsteps, so to speak?

No. That doesn't disappoint me at all. I always wanted them to do what they wanted to do, and I supported their educational development toward those ends. They all did well, and they are all good citizens. That's the most important thing.

Let's get back to you, personally: are you still operating?

I'm not operating as extensively as I used to, and to be perfectly honest, I try to avoid it because the postoperative responsibilities usurp a great deal of time. If you operate on a patient, you've got to take care of him, and right now I am focused in the laboratory, to advance this ventricular assist device; and I am analyzing the sixty thousand patients I have in my data bank. I'm working on an article concerning twelve thousand of these patients with a 95 percent follow-up of up to thirty years, analyzing the risk factors for the four major arterial beds that we operate on: the coronary bed; the branches of the aortic arch including the carotids; the abdominal visceral branches, particularly the renal arteries involved with hypertension; and the terminal aorta and its branches to the lower extremities. Of interest is the fact that, when you correlate the various risk factors with these diseases, each arterial bed behaves differently in terms of recurrence and survival, and this is highly statistically significant. The highest recurrence rates occur in the coronary arteries and the peripheral vascular beds, the lowest is in the renal, and the carotids are in between. Isn't that interesting? The question is, "Why?" And the survival expectancy is also different for each one.

Well, you certainly have kept busy, and you obviously have taken good care of yourself. Looking at you, I would never guess that you are in your late eighties. "FRANNY" [FRANCIS D.] MOORE used to say that surgery was an athletic experience and has talked about going in and "digging guys out of a hole" when they were too old to operate and insisted on continuing. You know the story of FERDINAND SAUERBRUCH; they had to put him in a straitjacket to get him to stop.[12]

I would never do that; I can stop now. It doesn't bother me at all because there are so many other things I want to do, and operating reduces the time for these activities. Occasionally I am forced into operating by former patients of mine who beg me to do it. So I will do an abdominal aortic aneurysm or something like that, but the post-operative care requires so much of my time that I try to turn these patients over to my associates, who are capable of doing the operations.

"Been there; done that!"

Exactly.

One final question: is there anything in your past professional life that you regret?

If you look back at your life, there are always certain things you would have liked to do differently or better, but unfortunately, at that time you didn't have the experience and knowledge that you later acquired. But I have been blessed in my life. I have had great success in so many different areas; I've had wonderful relationships with friends all over the world; I have been treated well and enjoyed what I've done.

Well, I have one regret: I have written about the history of medicine and cardiology in the past, but your work in aortic disease was so prominent, something I grew up with as a medical student and beyond, that I tended to ignore all the other contributions you have made to the field.

People sometimes ask me, "What would you like to be remembered by?" and I must say that the aortic surgery that I pioneered was probably the most important thing, from a historical standpoint. If you look back to those earlier times, when I began, the aorta was almost inviolate from a surgical standpoint. Now we can operate on any part of the aorta we want to and do it successfully. That's most gratifying.

I also take pride in the many cardiovascular surgeons I have trained throughout the world who have gone on to become chairmen of their departments, have developed outstanding programs of medical education, research, and patient care, and are contributing to new medical knowledge through their research.

Finally, I am grateful to my parents, family, and colleagues for all the support they have always provided to enhance my career and fulfillment. I feel extremely privileged and blessed.

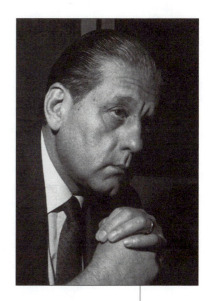

11

RENÉ G. FAVALORO, M.D.
(1923–2000)

At the beginning of the twentieth century, coronary artery disease
was not recognized as a major health problem; and it was believed
that, when it did occur, it was always suddenly fatal. Then, in 1912,
a Chicago physician, JAMES B. HERRICK, based on his own observations as well as that of others, reported on the clinical features of
sudden coronary obstruction, pointing out that sudden death did not
always result.[1] This landmark report took time to seep into the collective consciousness of the medical profession, aided by the development of electrocardiography, which began to reveal characteristic
patterns of acute coronary occlusion with myocardial infarction.

By midcentury, the United States and other industrialized
countries recognized that coronary disease represented a major
health concern; it was often referred to as an "epidemic" both in the
popular media and in medical journals. This realization spurred a
number of surgical attempts to address this problem, all of them of
questionable efficacy and/or safety. Included were procedures
such as "poudrage," the installation of irritating substances
between the heart and pericardium to stimulate the growth of new
vessels into the heart as part of the scarring process; the VINEBERG
procedure, in which a mammary artery was tunneled into the
ischemic myocardium to promote new vessel growth; and
endarterectomy, a reaming out of the obstructed vessel with or without a tissue patch to enlarge the opening and permit greater flow.[2]

It was not until the development of selective coronary cine-angiography by F. MASON SONES at the Cleveland Clinic in the early sixties, however, that the coronary circulation in living patients could be adequately visualized and evaluated.[3] Coinciding with this development was the arrival at the clinic of a new trainee in cardiac surgery, a South American who, at the overripe age of thirty-nine for such a position, had just emerged from twelve years of self-imposed exile in Argentina's pampas. It was the collaboration between Sones and René Favaloro, this new enthusiastic, energetic, and innovative character on the Cleveland Clinic scene, that led to the introduction of what has become the standard method of the surgical approach to coronary disease: bypassing the obstructed artery. This technique was new, but it had been suggested in the laboratory as early as 1910 by the father of all cardiovascular surgery, ALEXIS CARREL. In the dog laboratory, Carrel had performed an anastamosis between the aorta and a coronary artery, using a carotid segment to join the two arteries and suggesting that, sometime in the future, this technique might be used to restore flow to ischemic muscle beyond an obstructed coronary artery.[4] Although Favaloro was not the first to employ the bypass technique—using either vein graft or internal mammary artery—it was he who pursued it most vigorously and, with the support of the Cleveland Clinic's medical and surgical staff, made the "cabbage" (CABG, or coronary artery bypass graft) a reality.[5]

Some years ago, I was standing outside a conference center where an afternoon session of the annual meeting of the American Heart Association had just adjourned. There on the sidewalk, just a few yards away, I spied a tall, dark, immaculately tailored figure as seemingly oblivious of the unobservant young cardiologists rushing past him as they were of him. I recognized René Favaloro and couldn't fathom why, apparently, no one else in the vicinity did. I promised myself that if I ever resumed work on my oral history of twentieth-century cardiology, Dr. Favaloro would be included.

He struck me as an operatic figure—he could have passed for the older brother of the tenor Placido Domingo—and his passions about life, politics, people, and medical science fit this mold. Although he returned to Argentina in 1971 to create his institute for research and the training of South American surgeons, he eventually became a worldwide figure. One of his attachments was to the state of Israel, and in an address he gave in Tel Aviv, he crystallized his beliefs as follows: "I would like to ask especially of the younger people to understand that material things are temporary; only ideals last forever, and within this context, the battle cry should be: education and scientific development for a society in which social justice is the priority."

Unfortunately, he was unable to persist in this battle for perfection. Just less than a year after our meeting, depressed by the mountain of debt his institute had accumulated, and finding no relief for it, Dr. Favaloro took his own life. It was a tragedy greater and more deeply felt than any performance of any tragic opera.

New York, New York
August 2, 1999

I know that the least important goal in your life was becoming wealthy, but in the United States we would be tempted to call your story a journey from rags to riches, given your very modest beginnings back in Argentina. How did you ever manage to go to medical school in the first place?[6]

You know that in Argentina, even now, the universities are run by the government, even though they have complete autonomy; that is, they can make their own rules and regulations for education and administration. In other words, the government puts up the money for the universities but has nothing to do with how they are conducted. There is no tuition. But even though the universities are free, you have to survive; you have your living expenses.

I came from a family that I would not call poor, but lower middle class. My mother was a dressmaker, and my father was a carpenter. He was really an artist; he worked with only two or three assistants and did very fine carving with very delicately constructed pieces. But he really didn't make too much money; it was the art that was important to him. For this reason, my mother had to work as a dressmaker to make additional money. I began working with my father at the age of ten or twelve, mainly when I was on vacation and even, sometimes, during the year to help the family. I bet I could have made a living doing carving because I really liked doing that.

You became interested in chest surgery fairly early after completing medical school.

Yes. I finished medical school in 1948. As a consequence, there were only a few opportunities to perform chest surgery, given the state of surgery at this time. In Buenos Aires there was a famous surgical school run by the Finochietto brothers. Every Wednesday they held something like a postgraduate education course, starting at seven in the morning and running until eleven in the evening. La Plata, where I was working, was only about thirty miles from Buenos Aires, and therefore I was able to attend many of these sessions. Dr. Oscar Vaccarezza was doing some chest surgery, and another surgeon, Horacio Resano, was performing esophageal resections, mainly for esophageal cancer. I really became interested in chest surgery as I observed these operations, and, at the beginning, we did a few cases of carcinoma of the esophagus at our University Hospital in La Plata. We had many problems at first, but by attending that school in Buenos Aires, I was able to learn the small tricks that enabled us to begin in thoracic surgery.

Another influence on my career was DR. CLARENCE CRAFOORD, one of the fathers of cardiovascular surgery, who performed the first successful operation for coarctation of the aorta. In 1949, he visited Argentina, having been invited by the head professor, and I was lucky enough to be selected to assist him. I was really impressed, not only by his surgical technique but by his use of anesthesia. The patient was intubated, given high doses of curare, and then connected to a small respirator—and that was it. For us, it was unbelievable because we did not have at that time such facility in Argentina.

At one point you interrupted your pursuit of thoracic surgery, but it was for political reasons. What was that all about?

It's a long story. In 1943 we had a military coup; and our army was very much influenced by the German army. For many years our top military officers went to Germany for training. By 1945 or 1946, [Juan] Péron had become the most important military person within that military clique. There was no question that they were really on the far right; and remember that we were then in the middle of the Second World War. At the beginning it seemed that Hitler and Mussolini were winning everywhere, and they were supported by our military. The people in the street, on the contrary, were very democratic. But the military controlled everything, even the universities, by this time.

When I finished medical school, the director of the University Hospital called me in and told me, "You are number one in your class, and there is an open space for you on the staff of the hospital." He then handed me a card, on one side of which I had to write that I was not opposed to the government; the other side was to be signed by a politician in the government, attesting to this.

This was very difficult for me; I always believed in freedom. I went home to think this over, and the next day I told him, "If you think I am a good fellow, and was number one in my class, and worked day and night living in the hospital, how come I have to fill out that card?" I refused completely, and all doors were closed to me. As a consequence, I exiled myself inside the country, going to the southwest, to the dry pampas. It's an area that is very similar to the southwestern United States, Texas or Arizona. I spent twelve years there as a country doctor. At first I was alone, but then my brother, who was also a doctor, joined me; and after starting with only a small house, we were able to build up a small clinic with all the necessary facilities. We had good X-ray equipment, a room for surgery, an emergency room; we were really working day and night. We were doing everything you could imagine: gastric resections, colon resections, thyroidectomies; all types of general surgery and trauma surgery. However, all this time I was thinking of resuming my training in thoracic and cardiovascular surgery.

Finally, I went to my old professor, Jose Maria Mainetti, who is still alive at ninety-one, and asked him to look into a place in the United States where I could obtain the best training. Mainetti was one of the best surgeons I had ever met, and he was in close contact with many places in America with good surgical programs: the Lahey Clinic, the Mayo Clinic, the Cleveland Clinic; and he even operated in some of these places. When he was off on another trip to the United States in 1961, I asked him to look for a good place for me to be trained. On his return, he recommended the Cleveland Clinic, which was a very smart choice. In Argentina, we knew about the other famous places in the United States—the Lahey Clinic, Mayo, Johns Hopkins—but no one knew anything about the Cleveland Clinic. Mainetti was a very good friend of [George Jr.] "Barney" Crile, son of one of the founders of the Cleveland Clinic, George Crile, Sr., and told me, "Look, there is a fellow there named MASON SONES, who is working in the cardiac laboratory, and I'll bet you that he is ten years ahead of everybody else in the field." Mainetti had seen the beautiful coronary angiograms that Sones had been taking; they had an excellent research department under Willem Kolff; and they had a good thoracic surgeon in DONALD EFFLER. He told me, "This is the place for you," and that's why I went to the Cleveland Clinic.

> **Several people were very important to you during your experience in Cleveland, and I would like you to go down the list, giving your comments about them.**

George Crile was the head of the General Surgery Department. He was the first person I met at the Cleveland Clinic. We talked for about half an hour, me with my usual broken English, but I was able to communicate. He then put me in touch with Effler. Over the years, I became very close to George Crile, who was a tremendous fellow. You may recall that he was severely criticized at one time for his stand on the surgery for breast cancer when he said that you did not have to perform the radical mastectomy of [WILLIAM S.] HALSTED. Besides being an excellent surgeon, he was a very humanistic man and authored several books other than his medical work.

Tell me about Donald Effler.

The first time I met Effler, we talked for about half an hour, and then he told me that I had none of the certifications necessary for becoming a surgical fellow. I knew nothing about the ECFMG [Examination for Certification of Foreign Medical Graduates] or any of the other necessary steps to enter training in the United States. He told me that that did not matter; that I could initially come as an observer, and then I would have time to study for and pass the necessary examinations.

Effler was a born leader. Perhaps it was his Germanic background, but he knew how to manage a department. He was a very good surgeon. He did esophageal surgery and lung resections very well. He had been trained by Brian Blades, first becoming an excellent thoracic surgeon and then a vascular surgeon as well.

He was a very good speaker and also had an excellent sense of humor; a true leader. When I went to Cleveland, I was already thirty-nine years old, while all the Americans in training were very young. And I had the impression that Effler felt a little "lonesome" in his department. Dr. LARRY GROVES was his partner and an excellent surgeon, but he was a fellow who never talked. He rarely communicated with you. He mumbled a lot, and I remember once, after we had made rounds, I told Effler, "It is very difficult for me to understand Larry Groves."

"Don't worry," he said, "I have the same problem."

I don't know how, but we really matched. After three months, it seemed to be that we had known one another for many years. My wife was also close to his wife, Joanna, and the friendship grew.

What was WILLIAM PROUDFIT's role in the setup? He was a medical man.

Proudfit became head of the cardiology department. He is an extraordinary fellow. Besides medicine, he is very knowledgeable about history and art; a very humanistic approach in life. As head of the cardiology department, he was also responsible for some tremendous contributions. All our knowledge about the natural history of coronary artery disease was revealed by Proudfit, who reviewed thousands of patient records. He made important correlations between the clinical picture and the coronary arteriographic findings.[7] He was also an excellent clinician. It was Proudfit in the clinical area, Sones in the laboratory, and Effler and I, and all the others in the surgical department.

> I think the person you were closest to was Mason Sones.

No question about it.

> I knew him slightly. If you remember the old Andy Hardy movies with Mickey Rooney, he always seemed to me to be the Mickey Rooney of cardiology. He was always up to something, and he liked nothing better than to puncture the self-importance of other "experts," and the more public the setting, the better he seemed to like it. He never minced any words and was always very honest.

Extremely honest. We were like brothers. I suffered a lot when he died. He smoked heavily all his life. You know, he even smoked when he was doing heart catheterizations. He had a long pick-up clamp, half on the table and half outside, where a cigarette would be burning. During the study, he would take some pauses and use the pick-up to take a couple of puffs on the cigarette. Unbelievable! He died from lung cancer.

He didn't like to write and produced only a few papers, but he is the father of cineangiography. He had a room, working with the Phillips Company, and first developed cineangiography in Cleveland; and then coronary cineangiography. In the beginning it was congenital heart disease and later coronary artery disease. He worked day and night. He burned his eyes, later requiring cataract surgery.

> It was true he didn't write much, but when he did, it was important. That one short paper in *Modern Concepts in Cardiovascular Disease,* on coronary arteriography,[8] was probably more important than a dozen papers by other contemporaries in the field.

He dedicated his life to medicine. His first marriage was sacrificed to it. His health was affected. But every time we made an advance, he was so happy.

> You really made a study of all the coronary arteriograms he had taken, hundreds and hundreds of them. I don't believe that many people today take such pains to become expert, even when such important decisions are based upon them.

That is a big mistake. Today, with all the technological improvements, it is very easy to do a cineangiogram. To read it and have the right interpretation is another thing.

What was your relation to Kolff?

Kolff was in charge of the artificial organ department, and I spent many hours in his research department. When my surgical duties were over and I had any free time, I worked with him with the artificial heart, for example. We even did some lung transplants in dogs, if you can believe it, and this was as early as 1965 or 1967. We did many things with him. Kolff really is a philosopher, a man beyond science, and, in my broken English, it is impossible to describe him adequately. He had fellows from all over the world. I cannot understand why he never got the Nobel Prize.

> It's interesting that you should say that. I once put him up for that honor, getting DR. ARTHUR KORNBERG to sponsor him. In addition to inventing the first successful artificial kidney, he was responsible for so many other innovations, in cardiovascular disease and other medical fields. Unfortunately, his work was not on the molecular level, and any other kind of major accomplishment sort of rules out a Nobel these days. I believe multiple other efforts to get him recognized in this way have been unsuccessful.
>
> But let's get back to Dr. Favaloro. Before you got into all your important coronary work, you almost returned to Argentina in 1965.

In 1965 I finished my training in Cleveland as chief resident, and I went back to Argentina feeling that I was really prepared to start open-heart surgery there. But the conditions were not right. I spent two to three months looking for proper facilities, trying to get the government to cooperate. Meanwhile, Effler was sending me at least two letters a week urging me to come back to Cleveland, and I finally did come back.

> Historically, Cleveland was a special place in regard to surgery for coronary artery disease. CLAUDE Beck introduced his poudrage operation at Western Reserve, and after ARTHUR VINEBERG started doing his operation in Canada, you used that a good deal in your own work for a time. Sones showed that, eventually, the mammary implants advocated by Vineberg resulted in collaterals developing in the heart, but it took time, didn't it?

I am still convinced that the Vineberg operation was a good operation, if you had the proper indications. If a patient has diffuse disease with collaterals, the Vineberg is a good operation—the mammary implants can feed into these. With the direct approach, using a saphenous or mammary artery bypass, you have only one connection. With the Vineberg, if you make the tunnel in the proper place, I insist that in cases with diffuse disease and multiple collaterals, the arterial implant will grow noticeably within four or five months, and in ten months they will all be connected. And if the obstruction in the affected coronary artery becomes worse, the collaterals to this area will increase.

The problem was that we didn't have any other approach than this at first, and we were doing Vinebergs in left main coronary obstructions, proximal left anterior descending obstructions—conditions in which we could not wait six months or more for the collaterals to develop; the patient could infarct or die within this time. Once in a while, maybe two or three times a year, I still will combine a Vineberg with some of the bypasses. So it can be a useful operation, and now the new concept of "angiogenesis," promoting collateral development by injection of various genetically derived substances in the ischemic myocardium, is really a kind of Vineberg approach all over again.

We are working on angiogenesis in Argentina and have already done this in over fifty pigs. By next year, I bet you we will start this application in humans, with a slightly different approach than is now being done.

How long does it take for new vessels to develop with this technique? The Vineberg took months.

This happens very quickly, only a few weeks. When I started doing bypasses in 1967, there was a transitional period when we were doing bypasses and Vinebergs in the same patients: three bypasses with two Vinebergs in one patient; two bypasses and one Vineberg in another; many patients had the combined procedures. In 1965 or 1966, I operated on a cardiologist with severe unstable angina. I implanted two Vinebergs. Several years later he was restudied, and at this time, while the left coronary had become totally occluded, the entire left ventricle was perfused by the two Vinebergs. It would be interesting to go back and reevaluate many of these patients who had Vinebergs and establish the outcomes.

The operation that came into vogue after the Vineberg procedure was the patch graft.

Yes, for localized obstructions. The Vineberg was still used for diffuse disease. For the localized obstructions we would make a longitudinal incision over the area of obstruction with a pericardial patch placed on top to enlarge the lumen. But the longer the obstructions, the less well the patches worked, because the irregular areas within the lumen were still there and the arteries thrombosed.

Before the coronary bypass, there was the coronary interposition technique. Tell me about this.

First of all, the bypass was not a new concept. In the peripheral circulation we were doing a number of arterial bypasses. At the Cleveland Clinic there was a large hypertension clinic under the direction of IRVINE PAGE; and in patients with renal artery obstructions causing hypertension, [EUGENE] POUTASSE was doing bypass surgery in them.

Because of the favorable results in these patients, I thought that a saphenous vein might have a role to play in coronary revascularization. At the beginning of 1967, we first started with interposition. In a patient with a right coronary artery totally occluded but with the distal segment being perfused by collaterals from the left coronary artery, it was very easy to transect the artery and interpose a length of saphenous vein with proximal and distal anastamoses to reestablish flow in the artery, as demonstrated by coronary arteriography.

But you were very clever in your choice of this first patient, as you have written, because you knew in advance that there was good collateralization from the left coronary system and that, if the anastomosis was not successful, you had insurance against doing any damage.

Many times I was asked about the experimental work we did before these operations, but we never did any experimental animal work. We dealt with the patients' problems as we encountered them. But we soon learned that the interposition operation had limitations. So then we began to do coronary bypasses, first with the right coronary artery and then with the branches in the left coronary system. The year of development did not really come until 1968 because, at the beginning, Mason was very conservative. I was pushing to do more, while Mason was saying, "Wait, wait. Let's see what happens in four months, six months. We don't know what will happen. Suppose the grafts become obstructed by this time? We would be in real trouble."

As I just said, we started on the right coronary, which was technically easier. Then we approached left coronary obstructions. The left coronary had been a real tragedy for us when we tried to use the patch technique. When there were proximal left obstructions, the results had been terrible; there was about a 70 percent mortality. When we had the first successful bypass to the left anterior descending artery in a patient with left main obstruction, and I could see the whole left system fill postoperatively on angiography, I had a tremendous feeling of satisfaction.

In 1968 we were able to perform, in addition to bypasses, left ventricular reconstructions, because some of the patients had ventricular aneurysms or large scarred areas, which prevented normal ventricular function. We also did bypasses plus valve replacements. We even did the first case of a bypass in a patient with acute myocardial infarction.

Did you know at this time that SABISTON and GARRETT had done coronary bypasses?

No. Sabiston was the first one to call me and tell me that he had done a patient, but the patient died soon after surgery. And Garrett told me, when Effler and I saw him at a meeting of the American Association of Thoracic Surgeons, that he had done one patient in 1964. We pushed him to restudy that patient. If the graft was still functional, we would be able to gain three more years in demonstrating the patency of the grafts. He was a very good and honest fellow who had been with DeBakey at the time and later went to Arizona. He published a report of this in 1973, after thousands of bypasses had been done already.

You helped to introduce some innovations in the use of the mammary arteries, first with the Vineberg procedure and then with the coronary bypass, using the mammary arteries rather than the saphenous vein grafts.

With the original Vineberg operation, a left thoracotomy was performed, and this gave access only to the left internal mammary. In 1964 and 1965 we began to use for the first time a midline thoracotomy, which gave us access to both internal mammaries. To keep the operative field open in these procedures, I had to devise a retractor. When I visited Japan years later, the scrub nurses immediately knew who I was because my retractor was being used in their surgical suites.

The other thing I did with the mammaries involves their use in coronary bypassing rather than the Vineberg procedure. GEORGE GREEN in New York pioneered the use of the internal mammaries in coronary bypassing, first performed by [Vasily] Kolessov in 1966.[9] Green was using a microscopic technique to dissect out and connect the internal mammaries. I went to visit him and asked him how many hours I would need in the laboratory to learn how to employ the microscopic technique in the operating room. "Over one hundred hours," he told me. I went back to Cleveland and told my colleagues that this would never be practical if you had to spend 120 to 140 hours learning how to use it. And I was convinced that the microscope really wasn't necessary to perform the anastomosis. We used to have glasses with 2X to 3X magnification; and that was enough. In 1970 I performed the first mammary bypass without the use of a microscope, and after that it became obvious that the mammary bypasses were superior to the saphenous grafts, mainly in the follow-up after implantation. We have some patients studied as long as after twenty years or more, and their mammary implants are still open. The arterial bypasses are so good that, like the group in France headed by [ALAIN] CARPENTIER, we also are using radial arteries, provided that adequate circulation will remain to the hand after removal of these segments. We use them in conjunction with the mammaries, connecting them proximally to the mammary and distally to parts of the coronary circulation not covered by the mammary implant itself. We can also use a portion of the epigastric or gastroepiploic arteries to provide complete arterial revascularization of the heart. No question that this is the best current approach.

What about the "nontouch" technique?

At the beginning, we would try to completely dissect out the portion of the diseased coronary artery where the graft would be inserted. Now these are very small arteries, only 2 or 3 mm sometimes. This was a big mistake, because it was difficult to perform a good anastomosis. We found that all you had to do was expose the surface of the artery in its bed through a small incision, and after this, insertion of the graft would be much easier and more successful than had we dissected out the whole circumference of the recipient artery before. That is what we called the "nontouch" technique.

> I think it should be recalled that, at first, the surgical innovations at the Cleveland Clinic were not welcomed with open arms. A lot of the medical people were initially very skeptical.

All of them were friends of mine: GEORGE BURCH, WILLIAM LIKOFF, HENRY RUSSEK, CHARLES FRIEDBERG, HENRY MCINTOSH. But the only one who, at the beginning, felt that ours was a good approach was Willis Hurst; he was the first top cardiologist who recognized our work for what it was.

It's true that the meetings sometimes became very wild. One very important one was in 1970; it was the sixth World Congress in Cardiology in London. Friedberg and I were at a session to discuss coronary artery surgery, and he had a great sense of humor and was an excellent speaker. He began by saying that all cardiovascular surgeons are the same: "If the heart has a hole in it, they want to close it; if the heart doesn't have a hole, they make one." Everyone laughed, but when I presented our statistics from the Cleveland Clinic, the joking stopped, because Charley said he found it hard to believe that our mortality could have been so low. I stated that if anybody doubted our statistics, the doors of the Cleveland Clinic were open to anyone who wanted to come in and check them!

At another meeting, in San Francisco, I had come up from Argentina for the annual meeting of the American College of Cardiology. At one point, when I was involved with a discussion with Likoff, I believe, suddenly the chairman said, "Look. Your time is over."

My answer was, " Do you think that I flew over six thousand miles to have you tell me that my time is over?" So I kept on talking!

What has been the influence of PTCA* (percutaneous transluminal coronary angioplasty) on the surgical approach to the treatment of obstructive coronary artery disease?

PTCA is a very important contribution. I met DR. [ANDREAS] GRUENTZIG in Switzerland, where he first introduced this. PTCA and coronary bypass surgery are not two techniques in opposition to one another; each has its place. The big mistake comes when the interventional cardiologist wants to do PTCA in all his patients, and the cardiac surgeon wants to do bypass surgery in all his patients. There are three physicians with input to any of these decisions: the referring physician, the cardiologist who does the catheterization, and the cardiac surgeon. A combined decision, based on free discussion, should be made for each patient. At present, I see that in many hospitals all over the world, the decision is made alone by the cardiologists in the catheterization lab. They want to perform PTCA in the majority of patients. This is wrong. The most important thing, I tell my fellows, is that they should put themselves in the place of the patient and make a decision on what is best for *him or her.*

The big discussion now in multiple randomized studies, most of them performed incorrectly, is whether PTCA or surgery is preferable in patients with multiple vessel disease.

Your exhaustive review of these multiple studies must have taken a tremendous effort on your part.[10] But what I have concluded from my reading and personal experience, is that you can randomize thousands

---

* Insertion of a balloon catheter in a narrowed artery and expanding the balloon to enlarge the opening. Today, this procedure is frequently accompanied by the insertion of a stent, a distensible wire mesh tube, to keep the treated vessel from constricting again in the future.

of patients, but you cannot randomize one. Each patient is different and must be considered as such.

I agree. Each patient has different anatomy and different needs. PTCA is usually the better choice in a younger patient, say about fifty or less, who has one or two obstructions, with good indications for this procedure. Today this would be done with a stent, even though the stents may later occlude in 20 or 30 percent in time. And this is considerably higher in the smaller arteries; in those below 2 or 2.5 mm in diameter, the restenosis rate may be as high as 40 percent. In these, in older patients, those with previous PTCAs that have become stenosed, and other patients with complicated anatomy, bypass surgery may well be the best choice.

What is your opinion of mini-invasive surgery?[*]

We perform it at our institution, and it is a valid operation when you have the proper indications either for coronary or valve surgery. The patients love it; they get in and out of the hospital quicker, with fewer aftereffects of surgery. But the indications are for only few cases, and the number of these performed is coming down if you look at the data from various surgical centers.

It's hard to believe, but it is over twenty-five years since you returned to Argentina. You were still a young man when you went back after several incredibly productive years in Cleveland. With so many years still left to you at the time, did you ever regret not staying on in Cleveland?

No, although everybody else thought I was crazy. The one most difficult to convince about my decisions was Mason Sones. I told him, "You have only one choice. You can come with me to Buenos Aires!" I came to love the United States as my second country, but I loved Argentina and Latin America more. They had real problems, and I felt I had to return.

---

[*] Coronary bypass surgery performed through several small portals rather than the standard sternal-splitting incision and performed without cardiopulmonary bypass and cardiac arrest.

I actually planned my leaving Cleveland about ten months in advance. I sat down in my office and wrote my letter of resignation. No one said anything for about two weeks, but it hit everybody in the clinic like a bomb. I had become well known elsewhere in the United States, and when it became known that I was about to leave Cleveland, I got offers from all over the country. One of the hospitals in the Miami area, for example, offered me two million dollars tax-free! But money was not what decided me. My motivation was stated very clearly in my letter of resignation: I wanted to do surgery in my homeland and do teaching and research there, training future generations of heart surgeons throughout Latin America. And, I believe, we have accomplished that.

It's hard to say exactly, but as I visit Indonesia I find someone we have trained; the same in Thailand; the same in Japan; all over the world. In Latin America alone, we have trained over four hundred, and today there is not a single country in all of Latin America without fellows that have come out of our program. I would like to be remembered more as a teacher than as a surgeon. Teaching gives me the most satisfaction.

How old are you now? When are you going to stop?

I am seventy-six now and have already cut down the number of cases I do. I also have to cut down the amount of traveling I do; I am doing too much of that. I have eight surgeons working with me, all of whom I have trained, but I still like to be in the O.R. on either side of the table. In surgery there are two components, the hands and the brain; but the brain is the most important part. If your hand is shaking a little, that is not the important part; the problems come when your brain is "shaking." I believe my hands and my brain are still in good shape.

Although I had a bout of hepatitis about six years ago, I recovered well. Last Friday I did a very complicated case and was in the O.R. for a number of hours. I still enjoy it, but I know it's time for me to slow down a little. I would like to devote myself more to writing.

What surgical areas other than coronary bypass surgery have you been involved in since your return to Argentina?

Many areas. We have done work on the artificial heart. You know Poland is very advanced in this field, and we have a combined program with our colleagues there. We have modified the artificial heart to avoid thrombosis, and we are moving ahead on this in patients next year. We have been doing cardiac transplantations. Our institute is a center for all kinds of organ transplantations, one of the largest in Latin America. At present we are doing heart, lung, double lung, liver, kidney, et cetera.

In 1976 we set up a basic science department. We also established the Favaloro Foundation. Here *[showing records]* are some of our statistics for the last seven years since we set up the new heart institute. . . .

> Let's see: 278,000 outpatient consultations, 15,841 catheterizations, almost 200,000 noninvasive studies, 337 transplants, 17,499 surgeries. . . . That's quite an operation. How big is your staff at the institute?

We have over two hundred full-time members on our staff at the institute, including all positions. We have published over one hundred peer-reviewed papers in international journals. Our people are working in cardiac mechanics with the University of Essen in Germany; coronary flow and angiogenesis with the group in Rome, Italy; arterial dynamics with French investigators; circulatory assist devices with Poland; electrophysiology with Laval University in Canada; thrombosis and hemostasis with Leuven University in Belgium; lipids with Milan University; biomathematics with the University of Arizona; and so on.

Latin America was once far behind the rest of the world in cardiovascular research. I don't think that anyone could say that this is true today.

12

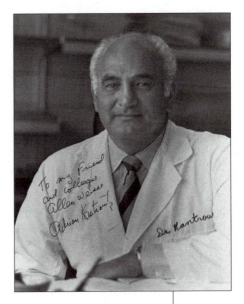

ADRIAN KANTROWITZ, M.D.
(1918–   )

One evening in the fall of 1967, I was seated at a table with the sur-geon Adrian Kantrowitz in the Oak Bar of New York's Plaza Hotel. Kantrowitz leaned toward me and told me some exciting news. He had been practicing heart transplantations in puppies to perfect the technique, and was about to take the heart of an anencephalic infant (one born without a brain and with a survival of only a few days at most) and transplant it into another infant with a severe congenital heart defect. Kantrowitz and his colleagues were sure that they could do this successfully. Would I be interested in join-ing their group at Maimonides Hospital in Brooklyn as a team cardiologist?

Although the offer was tempting, I had other, far less spectacu-lar but nonetheless personally compelling projects for cardiovas-cular research that I was keen to pursue. A few weeks later, on December 3, the news from Cape Town, South Africa, was received: CHRISTIAAN BARNARD had performed the first human cardiac trans-plantation in his patient Louis Washkansky.

In the public mind, Kantrowitz will probably always be remem-bered, along with NORMAN E. SHUMWAY, as one of the early research-ers in cardiac transplantation who had the rug pulled out from under them with the announcement of Barnard's coup. However, whereas Barnard, as he later admitted, squandered the sudden celebrity he enjoyed, Shumway meticulously continued his research into the rejection phenomenon, something that was immediately recognized to be the major problem with cardiac transplantation and the bane of all its practitioners in the early years of the procedure. Unlike Shumway, Kantrowitz turned his attention to other aspects of the surgical treatment of the failing heart. In these and other pursuits of his remarkably fecund mind, this most underrated surgical researcher of his time has managed to make his mark and win the appreciation of his peers.

Any investigator is lucky to hit upon one major accomplishment to contribute to our body of knowledge. While Adrian Kantrowitz produced many novel ideas, the one that is the most original, longest lasting, and with the most impact on the welfare of cardiac patients is the concept of "diastolic augmentation," later termed "counterpulsation."

Kantrowitz knew that the major part of coronary flow to the heart muscle occurs when the heart relaxes in diastole and the aortic valve closes. His idea was to deliver into the root of the aorta at this time a pressure pulse that might enhance coronary flow through any partially narrowed arteries as the result of coronary atherosclerosis or thrombotic occlusion. This diastolic pressure augmentation, it was found by Willem Kolff and Kantrowitz separately, could be delivered by the sudden inflation of a balloon mounted on a catheter introduced via a femoral artery and advanced to the arch of the aorta. As soon as the left ventricle contracted in systole, the balloon could be deflated, lowering the pressure in the aorta during this phase. It soon was realized that by lowering the aortic pressure during systole from its precounterpulsation level of pressure, the amount of work and thus oxygen demand of the heart muscle could be reduced, benefiting the other side of the supply-demand equation of the coronary circulation.

Although used initially in patients with cardiogenic shock, where it has only modest beneficial effects, the intraaortic balloon was later found to be of invaluable use as an adjunct to open-heart surgery, enabling many patients to be weaned successfully from the heart-lung machine who might otherwise be lost during this critical period. More recently Dr. Kantrowitz has attempted to use this concept in a permanently implanted device in patients with severe, intractable heart failure.

It is the gift of the innovator to see farther and sooner than the rest of us. In the case of Adrian Kantrowitz, it was his sad lot, for a time, to have seen too far and too soon for those with whom he was surrounded in Brooklyn. No doubt it has been this aspect of his career that, for a time, tarnished his image among the less-informed members of the medical community. What struck me about him, however, was the equanimity, even cheerfulness, with which he has accepted his lot, and the determination he has demonstrated to move ahead despite such considerations. Another important aspect of his personality, I believe, is his complete lack of artifice. Most of us—consciously or not—tend to underplay our shortcomings and emphasize our successes as we recall the past. Kantrowitz is as brutally honest about his failures as he is ebullient about the success he has enjoyed in a life dedicated to surgical research. At eighty-two years of age, this longtime pilot of his own airplane continues to fly high in all other aspects of his life as well.

Ryebrook, New York
December 1, 2000

Surgery, especially academic surgery, tends to be classified into a number of dynastic lines. People are described as having come out of the department of ALFRED BLALOCK or OWEN H. WANGENSTEEN, for example. Your beginnings were quite different, I believe, and I'm very interested in learning about how you got started in surgical research.

I think that very early in my career I was interested in surgery as opposed to internal medicine because I had a talent for doing things with my hands rather than "thinking." I graduated from medical school in Brooklyn in December 1943. At that time it was called the Long Island College of Medicine [now SUNY Downstate Medical Center]. This was in the middle of World War II and, actually, all the medical students were either in the army or the navy, and we were permitted a nine-month internship before going on active duty. A nine-month internship, which I took at the Brooklyn Jewish Hospital, doesn't give you an opportunity to learn much more than the words that are used in medicine. After I completed this, I had my basic training and eventually wound up serving some time in Europe with an infantry battalion that was then sent to Japan. I spent about six months in Japan and was then discharged.

Now, I went into the service in the middle of the war, and I did not have any significant combat experiences, which meant that I did not accumulate many points for discharge. The way it worked was that you accumulated a certain number of points for discharge, obviously more for combat, additional points for being wounded and so on, and when you reached a certain number, you were discharged. Because I had accumulated an insignificant number of points, I was in the army for six or eight months longer than most of the other young doctors who were in the war. And, in all honesty, that was fair enough because they had spent two or three more years in the service before I had entered the army. The point is that when I came back to civilian life and began looking for a residency in surgery, there were none.

The nearest I got was with Leo Davidoff, a prominent neurosurgeon who was actually trained by HARVEY CUSHING and was at Brooklyn Jewish. During my internship there, I had been assigned to his service at one point and had designed an instrument for him. One day, as I was assisting him at surgery, I observed that, as part of the routine of opening up the cranium, you had to put a bunch of hemostats on the galea* and then wrap a four-by-four around them to make a bundle and let it just hang outside the surgical site. This is what he learned from Cushing. Well, this gave me an idea, and I invented an instrument for him. I took a Carmalt clamp and placed one end of an eight-inch length of rubber tubing over each blade, thus making an adjustable elastic rubber band. And then with one maneuver you could clamp all the ties from the galea. It was more convenient; it was neater; it looked nice. Before this, I don't believe that Davidoff had ever spoken to me or even knew my name. But after I showed what I had devised to the

---

* Galea aponeurotica: a fibrous layer of connective tissue superficial to the skull but deep to the scalp running from the frontal to the occipital areas of the skull.

surgical resident, he thought it was a good idea and showed it to Dr. Davidoff. Davidoff looked at it and, while I was there as second or third assistant, used it a few times. He called it a "Kantrowitz clamp" and would say in the operating room, "Give me a Kantrowitz." Boy!

I remember standing at the far end of the operating room table and hearing Davidoff say—not to me but to the resident—"This is a good instrument. Tell him to write it up." I wrote a one-page article with a photograph of this thing, and I put Davidoff's name on it because it was my understanding that this is what was done; you put your chief's name on the paper. I gave the paper to the resident; he gave it to David-off, who approved it and said, "This is very good. We will have it published," and two or three days later it was returned to me after he had taken off his name. He certainly didn't need his name on another publication; he had plenty of his own. This was my first of some 350 publications, and I'm very proud of it.[1] It is still used by some neurosurgeons and is still called a "Kantrowitz clamp."

More than ever now, I wanted to be a surgeon, and, more than that, I wanted to be a neurosurgeon. That would certainly make my mother happy! Before I left to begin my army service, I spoke to Dr. Davidoff about this. I told him I was very much interested in neurosurgery and that when I came back from the army I wanted very much to take a residency with him. He said, "Sure," and I figured that was it. When I did come back three or four years later, I made an appointment to see Davidoff, who had moved from Brooklyn Jewish to Montefiore Hospital in the Bronx.

He greeted me, "Oh, Dr. Kantrowitz." He remembered my name from having said it so many times in the O.R. "How are you? How was the war?" He was very pleasant, and I reminded him about our earlier conversation, which he remembered. He then called in his secretary and told her to bring in her book. "When is the next opening?" he asked her. She looked it up and told him that there was not an opening for three years. My heart sank, but Davidoff consoled me. "You don't have to have a Jesus Christ complex. You don't have to be a neurosurgeon. You will be a surgeon." Then I managed to get a year in surgery at Mount Sinai and then at Montefiore to complete my training in general surgery. So I never did become a neurosurgeon, and Davidoff was quite right; I lived without it.

As a matter of fact, though, I have a son who *is* a neurosurgeon. He uses a clamp, but I don't know if he calls if a "Kantrowitz."

Well, the gene was finally expressed.

That's true. My father was a doctor, my three children are physicians, all married to physicians, and I have a grandson who is thinking of becoming premed.

How did you get seriously involved with surgical research?

During my surgical residency at Montefiore, there was a six-month period during which there was no assignment for me, so I said that I would like to do a research project. There were no pump-oxygenators (for open-heart surgery) at the time, and I had thought of a scheme to bypass the left side of the heart and thereby expose the interior of the left atrium and the mitral valve without a heart-lung machine. If you cannulate the two pulmonary veins from the left lung that lead to the left atrium, and put a tourniquet around the right pulmonary artery so that, temporarily, there will be no blood flow to the right lung (and thus no pulmonary venous flow from the right), you can collect all the blood ordinarily coming to the left atrium and then return it with a pump to the femoral artery. Then you can open up the left atrium and expose the mitral valve in a blood-free field without the use of a pump-oxygenator. I wanted to work this out for a six-month period when I was actually assigned to the Department of Medicine.

My chief was Louis Leiter, a very nice man. I explained to him what I wanted to do, and he told me that it sounded crazy, but he was very tolerant. (This young man wants to do this, and, after all, he does have a publication.) They wound up giving me a research grant for three hundred dollars, as I recall, for the six-month period.

There was another problem. At Montefiore Hospital, they would not permit you to operate on dogs, but only on cats. The reason they allowed cats was because, for some reason, the neurosurgeons used cats as experimental animals, and perhaps the barking of dogs, which might disturb the patients, was another consideration. This didn't bother me; I had done some dissections in cats and was familiar with their anatomy. I made my own cannulae and designed the experiment cat after cat after cat; but it didn't work, at least not in the beginning. The interesting thing was that I was not disturbed by this because, with each failure, I saw why it didn't work and I was able to fix it. However, I did run out of money very quickly; three hundred dollars was not a lot to do this project.

So I set out on a program of getting my own cats. Montefiore Hospital is located in the Bronx, which has many tough neighborhoods. Now if you look in the back of these apartment houses, there are lots of cats; and these are very rough and tough customers. You can't fool around with them, but I bought a trap for about two or three dollars. It was made by a company called Havahart, and it was a cage about two feet long with doors at either end so that when the cat entered the cage the doors closed and trapped it. Because I could not capture all my cats, I made deals with the janitors in this area to pay them a quarter for each cat they caught. All they had to do was call me on the phone, and I would come with a burlap bag to pick it up.

It was during this period that I met my wife, Jeanie, and we would go off together to try and capture cats.

That reminds me of how JOHN GIBBON used to prowl around Boston at night in the early days, picking up cats for him and his wife to work on.

Absolutely. We started by going into these backyards with a burlap bag to try to entice these cats with food or milk. Jeanie tried to help me, but they were much smarter than we were, so we came to rely on the traps.

Eventually I had operated on about fifty cats, and despite the failures, if you were an optimist you could see how this could eventually work. We finally got to a point of a week or two to the end of my research time, and with the sixtieth cat we operated on, we finally achieved success. We opened up the atrium; we were able to observe the mitral valve under direct vision for a thirty-minute period as planned. We actually filmed this, the first motion picture of a mitral valve in action.[2] This beautiful black cat survived, living with us for a year or two until one day when he just disappeared on us.

This was your first foray into cardiac surgical research. What prompted you to conduct this particular research project?

I had thought about this for some time before I actually began the project. I published my results on this in 1950, just about the time that Charlie Bailey, [DWIGHT] HARKEN, and [RUSSELL] BROCK were doing their work on blind mitral commissurotomy. I went to observe Bailey doing one of these procedures, and I said to myself, "That's ridiculous. Why try to open the mitral valve blindly when you could open the left atrium and look at what you were doing." So I felt that the closed mitral commissurotomy was no competition and that my way would be the best way to do it. As it turned out, the closed mitral commissurotomy was a very successful operation for its time, and thousands of them were done. The interesting thing was that it was done first in England in 1925 by a surgeon by the name of [HENRY] SOUTTAR.

I'm aware of that story and that they just didn't send him any more patients. But I think your idea for exposing the mitral valve was great. Was it ever attempted in humans?

No. The work on the cats was done while I was still a resident. By the time I might have been able to try this in humans a few years later, they were beginning to have some success with the heart-lung machine and total cardiopulmonary bypass. So although I think it was a good idea to be applied before the pump-oxygenator became available, progress in that effort made my own innovation no longer practical for attempts in humans.

How did you establish yourself as a cardiac surgeon?

Back in 1945 or 1946 there really was no such thing as a cardiac surgeon; there were thoracic surgeons, and what little cardiac work that there was—mainly ligating patent ductuses and repairing coarctations—was done by these thoracic surgeons. Still, I wanted to be a cardiac surgeon and went to see one of the most prominent thoracic surgeons in the field, a man by the name of Max Chamberlain, who worked primarily at Mount Sinai in New York. This was even before I had completed my general surgical residency. I told him of my ambition, and he told me in a very polite way that in New York City each year there were two patent ductuses to be repaired, and he did both of them; there was no such thing as "cardiac surgery."

I completed my surgical residency and went out into practice for about a year. However, during this time I was actually thinking about this whole idea of "counterpulsation." I went to Louis Leiter, who had become my mentor, even though he was an internist and not a surgeon. I told him I wanted to do a year of research on heart surgery. Leiter, as well as Harold Rifkin, another internist who had befriended me, suggested that I take a year to go to a cardiac physiology laboratory to learn techniques and learn something about the physiology of the heart. I thought this was a good idea. At the time CARL WIGGERS at Western Reserve in Cleveland was the dean of cardiac physiology, and he had an NIH grant for a half-dozen fellows in the research laboratory. He accepted me for a position there, and during my time with Wiggers I learned an enormous amount. He was a very warm person and had some great people working with him, including three or four senior associates. Bob Berne was there at the time as well as Matthew Levy and Bob Alexander. They were all terrific and later went on to head their own departments; Berne at the Medical College of Virginia; Bob Alexander at the Medical College of the University of Georgia; and Matt Levy, who now is chief of the Department of Investigative Medicine at Mount Sinai in Cleveland.

At first, the idea was not really "counterpulsation" but "diastolic augmentation." What I wanted to do was devise a way to increase coronary blood flow, and since this was best accomplished during diastole—during systole the coronary arteries were squeezed by the surrounding heart and were relatively resistant to filling—I wanted to enhance flow during diastole. Later on, it was pointed out to me by STANLEY SARNOFF at one of my presentations that by introducing a pulse during diastole and reducing the pressure head during systole, we were also decreasing the work and oxygen demands upon the heart.

Well, this was fine with me and further emphasized the benefits to be obtained. I think it was Dwight Harken who introduced the term "counterpulsation." After that first paper, I later called it "phase shift balloon pumping."

Did you actually have the idea of diastolic augmentation before you came to Wiggers's laboratory?

We are talking about events of about fifty years ago, but I did have the idea that somehow you might be able to improve coronary blood flow. When I got to Wiggers's lab, I discussed this openly with all of these people. DONALD GREGG was there at the time, and they knew all about coronary blood flow. They thought it was a good idea and emphasized that raising pressure during diastole, when the coronaries could best receive the blood, was the thing to do.

We worked with dogs, and I designed an experiment in which we put a cannula in the femoral artery so that we could route the blood through a delay line. We then perfused the left coronary artery either from the aorta or with a delayed pressure pulse from the femoral artery and showed that introducing the delayed pulse during diastole could increase the coronary blood flow by 10 to 15 percent.[3]

After the time in Cleveland, I went back into practice as a general surgeon at Montefiore for a few years and began repairing hernias and even doing a couple of mitral commissurotomies. I was even able to do a little research during this period. Then, in 1955, an opportunity came up at Maimonides Hospital in Brooklyn. They had a cardiac surgeon who was leaving and were looking for someone to replace him. There weren't that many cardiac surgeons around at that time, and most of them were in private practice. By this time I had done enough research to establish something of a reputation. The job was a full-time position, which was fine with me, and I was hired as chief of cardiac surgery. I applied for an NIH grant to support some of my research, and they gave it to me right away. The name of that grant was " Experimental Construction of an Auxiliary Ventricle," and it was for about fifteen thousand dollars, and that was back in 1956. Following this, I got another couple of grants for research projects, and then a couple of years after all this had begun, I got a call from a friend at the NIH, Robert Ringler, who told me, "Adrian, if you can get an application in here in one week, you may be able to get a program project grant." I didn't even know at that time what a program project grant was, but it is a long-term grant covering many aspects of research and for several years. We did get that application in a week later, and this tremendous accomplishment was primarily due to my wife, Jeanie, who really deserves credit. She was the one who organized everything. She has worked with me for years. She has run the laboratory all along, and it was she who enabled us to get the grant application in on time. It was for three or four million dollars, a tremendous amount at that time, and it enabled us to hire people, purchase and construct research equipment, and pursue many aspects of the research in which we were interested.

To get back to counterpulsation: how did you finally apply it to humans?

This is skipping ahead a bit. Before we ever got to the intraaortic balloon in humans, we had the idea of implanting a *permanent* left ventricular assist device (LVAD), although we called it "an auxiliary ventricle." We devised one that could be implanted in the arch of the aorta and got it to work in dogs. It seemed very feasible to use this for intractable heart failure in humans, and our first patient was a thirty-three-year-old man with a dilated cardiomyopathy and in intractable failure. In retrospect, it was a poor choice of patient, although the pump, which worked on the counterpulsation principle, seemed to work well. However, on the first postoperative day he died from pulmonary complications and bleeding secondary to thrombocytopenia, probably related to liver disease.

Our second patient was Mrs. Cerasso, a sixty-three-year-old lady who was bedridden with congestive heart failure for years. We implanted the pump, and she did beautifully at first. Hemodynamically and clinically, she responded well for the first week, and we had every intention of sending her home with the first successful permanently implanted left ventricular assist device. However, on the seventh or eighth postoperative day she began to have little strokes, which culminated in a fatal massive stroke on the thirteenth postoperative day. At autopsy she had large clots in both arms of the assist device.[4] We had used it acutely in dogs with no problem, but after several days in a patient, thrombosis became a real problem. A few months after this, [Michael] DeBakey used a different type of device in a patient, but he was smarter than I was; he realized that it could only be used as a temporary device and not a permanent one because of the clotting problem.

We agonized over this for a year or two before we decided to focus on a temporary device along with our attempt for a permanent device, something we continue to this day.

Your brother Arthur was involved with this work in the beginning and then you separated. Could you tell me about this?

My brother Arthur is five years older than I. He is a physicist whose area of expertise is in aerodynamics. However, aerodynamics is not that different from hemodynamics. He helped me on that very first study out of Wiggers's laboratory and also was in the operating room with Mrs. Cerasso and coauthored the paper in which we reported this early attempt at a permanent LVAD.

He had left Cornell and joined the Avco Company in Boston as director of their laboratory. In the final analysis it just wasn't practical for him to attempt working with me at a small Jewish hospital in Brooklyn when, as emphasized by his board of directors, he could be working at the MGH (Massachusetts General Hospital) with Harvard in Boston. We've always remained on good terms.

What happened with the development of the balloon pump? In 1962 Moulopoulos, Topaz, and Kolff reported on the use of an intraaortic balloon in dogs.[5]

In all honesty, I was unaware of what Kolff and his associates were up to, and was working on my own balloon at Maimonides. This happens. Later on, I learned that he had used an intraaortic balloon in dogs before we had, and, in our publication on this, we credit him with that although he never used such a device in humans. However, what the engineer Topaz developed for Kolff was a condom balloon, which filled the aorta, occluding it, and therefore did not prove workable. We learned this early in our own lab, where we developed a polyurethane balloon which, when expanded, filled up to a desired size and did not obstruct the aorta, allowing for a more successful passage of blood in the aorta, forward and back as the balloon was deflated and inflated, making practical application possible. What we also did differently applied to the gas used for inflating and deflating the balloon. Kolff used carbon dioxide because he felt that if any of the gas leaked into the circulation, it would do no harm. We used helium, which, if it entered the circulation, could be expelled by the lungs without doing harm. The advantage of helium was that its density was only one-twentieth of that of carbon dioxide. Therefore, with the narrow catheter bores being used at the time, the helium offered much less resistance to inflation and deflation of the balloon. Subsequent to our use of helium, all the manufacturers of balloon catheters adopted it as well. In the permanent device we are now using, we can use room air because of the larger size tubing involved.

After we had success with this in dogs, we wanted to try this in humans, and CLARENCE DENNIS lent us his support in this with our administration. He said, "Absolutely!" After all, he had come out of Wangensteen's department, where, if something seemed logical, they went ahead with it.

How much contact did you have with Dennis?

Actually a good deal. He was chairman of the Department of Surgery at Downstate when I was in Brooklyn, and we thought the same way. When he attempted the first use of a heart-lung machine in a human, I scrubbed with him and it was a patient I had referred to him. It was an excellent choice, we thought: an eighteen-year-old girl with an atrial septal defect. We placed the patient on cardiopulmonary bypass, and the pump worked perfectly. However, when we opened the heart, we found that, instead of a simple atrial septal defect, it was much more complicated, an A-V communis* with a cleft valve as well. We only had a few minutes to decide what to do. Dennis closed the atrial

---

* A defect involving both the atrial and ventricular septae, with free communication between all four chambers of the heart.

septal defect, hoping that this would help the situation, but the patient died. Some time later when John Gibbon was about to perform the first successful closure of an atrial septal defect on his heart-lung machine, he called Dennis to ask if he had any advice. Dennis told him just to be sure it was only a simple atrial septal defect and not an A-V communis.

Dennis was a very lovely man, I thought, when I was a medical student at Downstate and he was chairman of surgery.

He was a very lovely man and a great supporter of mine. But as a surgeon he was, perhaps, too meticulous, too careful in handling every detail. [WALTON] LILLEHEI and other surgeons who were his contemporaries at the University of Minnesota just got in and *did it*. Perhaps, if his approach were more like theirs, he would have had more success.

So how did you finally get to use the temporary device, the aortic balloon, in patients?

I had approached the administration at Maimonides, and they were not too enthusiastic about it. However, by this time I was not only chief of cardiac surgery but also general surgery and had a number of residents under my control. Being not very old myself, I had a very good relationship with them, and we alerted the emergency room physicians to be on the lookout for a patient in cardiogenic shock, near death, in whom we could attempt this when all else had failed. Every time there was a patient with cardiogenic shock who was brought into the emergency room, we would be there with our equipment ready to go.

The first patient we did was unconscious with a systolic blood pressure of 30 or 40, no urinary output, and unresponsive to all the drugs that were being given. We got the balloon pump in and working. The blood pressure immediately came back, the urine began to flow, and she became conscious. God Almighty, this was great! But I was very nervous; where would we go from there? I didn't want to screw it up. We stopped the pump and the blood pressure fell again, so we restarted it. And we kept this up for four or five hours, and I believe we published the chart on this patient, showing how every time we pumped her she improved, and every time we stopped she deteriorated. Finally, we were able to stop the pump and the blood pressure did not drop, and she went on to make a complete recovery. That was just pure luck because she did have sufficient viable myocardium left to allow for this to happen. The next two patients died.[6]

You then organized a cooperative study of intraaortic balloon counterpulsation in cardiogenic shock. Could you tell me about this?

Initially, we had made balloons and modified an oscilloscope to act as a balloon pump drive unit—the electronics were all there. Of those first three patients, as I said, we had one survivor and two deaths. However, we had clear hemodynamic data to show that the balloon increased cardiac output and took over part of the work of the damaged left ventricle. What we had to demonstrate was that others could reproduce this, and we also needed a significant number of patients in whom this was done to produce statistically significant results.

So we went to the NIH, accompanied by a few rather prominent medical people, among them ED SONNENBLICK, HENRY MCINTOSH, and TOM KILLIP of Cornell–New York Hospital, and proposed a cooperative study of cardiogenic shock, with eight, ten, perhaps fifteen centers where such a study could be conducted. The NIH said it was a good idea; that they would support it; but that, in order to produce statistically significant results, the study would have to be randomized between treated and untreated patients with this technique.

Why would you have to randomize a study like this in cardiogenic shock where over 90 percent of the patients die and where, even with medical therapy, the results are not much better?

Perhaps the figure then was closer to a 99 percent mortality, and none of those who accompanied us were willing to participate in such a randomized study. So we went to the John A. Hartford Foundation for support, and they said, "Sure. How much money do you want?" There was no commercial source for any of this equipment, so I set up a separate shop from Maimonides where we built and supplied catheters and pumps to study about a hundred or two hundred such patients at these cooperating institutions. We finally managed to study about eighty-seven of these patients at ten cooperating institutions where some benefit was demonstrated.

As it turned out, this wasn't the case for most cases of cardiogenic shock, as shown by your subsequent experience and that of others.

The reason for this is that in massive myocardial infarction and cardiogenic shock at least 30 percent or more of the left ventricle is destroyed and it won't come back after you turn off the pump. However, in about 20 percent of patients with cardiogenic shock there is enough viable myocardium left to permit recovery, as that multicenter study we conducted showed.

What was the role of Maimonides in all this?

By this time, I was a brand-new chief of surgery there. I had done the first heart transplant in the United States in this little hospital; I had done the first balloon pumps insertions in there; I had done the first implant of a permanent left ventricular assist device in Brooklyn; I had done some early work on cardiac pacemakers—and my colleagues there thought I was crazy.

When I read the paper on the use of the intraaortic balloon in cardiogenic shock,[7] I saw that a number of first-rate hospitals—affiliated with Harvard, Cornell, Duke, and so on—were involved, while no patients were done at Maimonides.

What happened at Maimonides was that all these people who thought I was off the wall convinced the research committee not to approve the protocol being performed among patients there. So what we ultimately became was the coordinating center for the study.

The irony is that while intraaortic balloon pumping didn't help much in cardiogenic shock due to acute myocardial infarction, it has come to be a Godsend in a number of other situations, mainly in supporting high-risk patients and getting them off cardiopulmonary bypass in open-heart surgery.

It's amazing. At a meeting in Athens last summer on intraaortic balloon pumping, one speaker got up and addressed the audience, saying, "Dr. Moulopoulos and Kantrowitz and their associates have saved more patients than all of you doctors combined."

While you were working on the balloon, there was something else you worked on, the use of noncardiac muscle to support the heart.

Using it around the heart didn't work, but using it around the aorta was introduced in the laboratory, again intending it as a permanent counterpulsating modality. We used a hemidiaphragm and stimulated it through the phrenic nerve with a generator. It did work in dogs, but the effect on increasing cardiac output was minimal.

Over the years, however, there has been a resurgence of interest in this approach, using the latissimus dorsi now, I believe; and the skeletal muscle gradually seems to become like cardiac muscle.

It tends to develop a resistance to fatigue; that is correct. In our experiments we didn't know about that because they were acute studies, and you have to stimulate this muscle four or five weeks before you develop this resistance to fatigue. Even then you can only apply a stimulus for every other beat. When we used the hemidiaphragm and wrapped it around the heart to apply systolic augmentation, we simply could not get it to work.

But you did have some interesting spin-offs on nerve stimulation.

Yes, we did. We stimulated the bladder; we successfully stimulated the intestine in adynamic ileus, and this is still used. We also made a paraplegic stand up. We put electrodes on the extensor muscle. I had hopes that, if you were clever enough, you could work out the muscle stimulation in such a way as to get them to walk, which, incidentally, is what they are now doing. But those were the very first experiments using this approach.[8]

As for using muscle around the heart to alleviate heart failure, enthusiasm for it is waning. There are several places that have tried it and published on it, but now when you talk to them, they do not believe that it really works and no one is doing that anymore. The same is true for the Batista operation.*

Tell me about your experiences with cardiac transplantation.

While I was at Maimonides, we also did a series of experiments in puppies with heart transplants, over four hundred of them eventually. We learned a great deal about how to do the operation; we recognized what rejection was and how some drugs would help in this event; and, interestingly enough, there were some dogs that would survive heart transplantation without any need of immunosuppression. We did these transplants in puppies and with hypothermia because we anticipated doing the operation in small infants with the same technique. This was before [CHRISTIAAN] BARNARD [had his success with a human heart transplant], and no one knew whether cardiac transplantation would work in humans or not.

I recall that, at one time, it was thought that the heart might be less susceptible to rejection than the kidney, and that in younger animals or infants rejection might not be as likely as in adults.

That didn't turn out to be the case, but it was reasonable to try this in humans. To do this, we had to have the cooperation of many people. We discussed this with Clarence [Dennis], and he encouraged us to go ahead. We approached the research committee at Maimonides Hospital, suggesting that the best pairing would be an infant with an inoperable congenital heart defect with an anencephalic infant as donor since these babies, born without a brain, never survived beyond two or three days after birth and most of them had normal hearts. They approved it grudgingly, and only with the understanding that the chief of pediatrics would be in charge of the donor. And it wasn't until the chief of pediatrics said, "This child is dead; you may remove the heart," that we could proceed.

---

* A procedure involving excision of a portion of a diseased left ventricle in order to reduce the volume of that chamber, thus the tension developed upon contraction of that chamber, and thereby improve the efficiency of the heart with increases in stroke volume and cardiac output.

The way he would decide that the donor infant was dead was when he could no longer hear heart sounds on listening to the chest with his stethoscope. This ruling caused such a delay in performing the transplant, that the heart we transplanted had been damaged by anoxia due to this delay, and that was why the heart stopped after we transplanted it. The recipient child, who had an Ebstein's anomaly, lived only six or seven hours after we closed the chest.

Now, this was done two or three days after Barnard had operated on [Louis] Washkansky, and there was a tremendous hullabaloo. Now we were not aware of what Barnard was up to, and, beyond that, you cannot set up this sort of operation in three days. This was not a copy of Barnard, and, as a matter of fact, we had tried to do this back in May of 1966, a year and a half before Barnard's operation on Washkansky, but at that time we felt that the donor heart was too anoxic and unsuitable for use, and didn't go through with it.[9]

> Of course Barnard was something of a Johnny-come-lately as far as the concept of cardiac transplantation was concerned, but you touched on something when you mentioned having to transplant a heart damaged by anoxia that recalls something he was really on to. In his biography he mentioned that when he once discussed transplantation with NORMAN SHUMWAY and RICHARD LOWER, they said that the only time they could do a transplant was in a patient who was on the table for open-heart surgery and they couldn't get the patient's heart started again. Then they could put some donor's heart in. Barnard realized that, logistically, this would be impossible to do. And when he transplanted the heart of that young woman, brain dead following an automobile accident, he arranged the transfer in as short a time as possible with Washkansky in one operating room and the girl in an adjoining one.

That's the only way you could do it, but at that time in the United States you could not do the operation on the basis of brain death of the donor, but only when the heart was stopped.

What led to your deciding to leave Maimonides?

I didn't decide to leave Maimonides; I was fired, and I would very much like to tell you how this came about. It was directly as a result of the kind of innovative research and surgery we were attempting to do. In retrospect, a hospital like Maimonides was not the place to attempt such work.

First off, there were those first three patients in whom we inserted the aortic balloon. We lost two of them, and in one case there was a rupture of the left ventricle. When the research committee reviewed this, some of my "friends" said, "Look, you killed this patient. You blew out his left ventricle by distending it with your pump."

How could you do that when you were blowing up the balloon during diastole?

That's right; the aortic valve was closed when the balloon was distended; you cannot blow out the left ventricle this way. This made no difference. I had operated on three patients, and two out of three had died.

Then we had done two heart transplants, one in an infant and the second, a week or so later, in an adult who also died. Then, although we were not the first, we introduced the use of cardiac pacemakers, devices that we made ourselves because you couldn't buy them. And people who could not go along with these new ideas began to reach the opinion that "this guy is out of his mind!" He had to be stopped, and [WILLIAM] DRESSLER was one of those people. I had a great deal of respect for Dressler; he was a terrific clinical cardiologist, but he was an older man and not receptive to these new ideas. For example, he had a patient with Stokes-Adams attacks,* and I said that we ought to put in a pacemaker that we had built in the lab. Dressler went to the director of the hospital and said, "That man is too much; he wants to put a battery in my patient!" The director called me in and told me to stop pursuing Dressler, although we later did put a pacemaker in this patient and she did very well.

So it was not one event but a whole series of things that led to this. I was supposed to be a "nice Jewish boy" from the Bronx, and if I wanted to be heart surgeon, okay, be a heart surgeon. But to transplant a human heart, this was too radical, and you cannot appreciate how

---

* Loss of consciousness due to inadequate blood flow to the brain, resulting from excessively slow heart rates occurring with complete heart block. These attacks are ultimately fatal.

radical that was in the minds of these people I had to work with at that time. It was unthinkable. Then the balloon pump: a "wild" idea, not good for anything. "Look how the patients with cardiogenic shock died." And it would be years before the value of the intraaortic balloon in other conditions would be recognized and so widely used. It also took a long time before people recognized the value of pacemakers.

All of this was too much for them. A good politician could have survived all that, but I am not a good politician. They went to the president of the hospital and convinced him of how unconventional I was. Finally, I was called in to see the president of the hospital, who said, "Adrian, don't you think you'd be happier someplace else?" This had nothing to do with my results; my results were not better than those of anybody else, but they were as good as anybody else's. I was not the greatest surgeon in the world, but I was a perfectly competent cardiac surgeon and, in some respects, even better than some others.

A small Jewish community hospital was not the kind of place I should have been doing this work. This kind of work should have been coming out of a university. But that's not so horrible. For a long time my wife was ashamed of the fact that I was fired, but Galileo was fired; they really gave him hell when he said that *maybe* the earth is not the center of the universe; maybe it was the sun. After twenty years he went to the Church and said, "You're right. The earth is the center of the universe, not the sun. I was wrong." But he knew that the idea, once introduced, would eventually succeed.

How did you get to Sinai in Detroit?

When it became public that I was leaving Maimonides, I was offered several opportunities, but the reason I chose Sinai was that they had a beautiful dog lab all set up in a research building they had just built. One of the reasons they were attracted to me was because of my interest in research. Another was that they wanted me to start an open-heart program there in a brand-new surgical suite they had constructed. The NIH approved a transfer of my program project grant to Sinai, an unusual action, especially at that time when such transfers of sites were not looked upon favorably. As a result of this, when it became known I was about to leave Brooklyn, literally all of the surgical house staff, research people, ICU nurses—all of them wanted to come with me, and we took a whole batch, twenty-five of them, along with us. Before this, Sinai had been unable to attract any staff for an open-heart program. Within a month of my move we had a complete staff and were performing open-heart surgery there.

Although it was not broadcast, before they hired me, they knew why I was really leaving Maimonides, and wanted to know what really had been going on. They called Clarence Dennis, and he told them, "If you could get Adrian, it would be the greatest thing in the world for you." I would not have gotten the job without his recommendation.

How long did you work at Sinai in Detroit?

About fifteen years.

Why didn't you continue the transplantation work with anencephalic babies when you arrived there?

By the time I got to Sinai, there were about ten or fifteen surgeons in the United States and some in Europe who had done heart transplants, and they all quit because the patients were all dying. The only one who continued was Shumway, and I was on the NIH site review committee that reviewed Shumway's program and I fought very hard to give him the support he needed. And I really didn't have to fight that hard because everyone agreed that Shumway should certainly continue the work. We gave him enough money to do one patient a month; that's twelve a year. That's what was needed for him to work out the problems, essentially rejection.

When I got to Sinai, the chief of medicine there told me, "Look, Adrian, it would be better if you did not do transplants here *now*. It's too tough now, just when we're trying to get the program started. Wait until you do some open-heart procedures and things go well. Then you can think about it." I agreed; I had already not done any more transplants at Maimonides and decided to put it off for a year or so in Detroit, and then reevaluate the situation. In the meantime we did some nice work in dogs. For example, we took a whole patch of the right ventricle with the right coronary artery and replaced a portion of the left ventricle with it. We replaced the right ventricle with a piece of the diaphragm because we felt the right ventricle was not that important.

> That's fascinating, because years ago I recall someone even burning most of the right ventricle in situ in dogs to demonstrate that, functionally, you didn't need a right ventricle.[10]

In this way we demonstrated that you could use right ventricle to replace damaged parts of the left ventricle. We were also deeply involved in getting the intraaortic balloon pump accepted. Then there were other projects that came up, and we just never resumed the transplantation work. You must remember that the status of cardiac transplantation at that time, thirty years ago, was not what it is today. We didn't understand immunosuppression well then; we didn't have the drugs to use that we have today. It was not a surgical problem; it was an immunological problem, and I'm not an immunologist.

> Given the shortage of hearts, even today, there seems to be two ways that one can go: one way is the left ventricular assist device (LVAD), and the other is the total artificial heart. You are still using counterpulsation.

We actually just discharged a patient from the hospital with one.* We do a thoracotomy and put this balloon in as part of the wall of the aorta. This is what we did thirty years ago in dogs and then lost those three patients, but nothing goes easily; we are finally doing it in humans after we kept improving it. And that is only because I am really interested in doing research. People who are not interested in research would not keep doing it for thirty years.

> This is a counterpulsating device, while all the other LVADs being introduced are continuous-flow assist devices.

The others are all axial flow pumps, which DeBakey and [ROBERT]

----

* This procedure was done successfully on October 30, 2000, on a seventy-four-year-old terminally ill man who postoperatively survived fifteen months, carrying on well with normal activities with only one hospital admission to observe the functioning of the equipment.

JARVIK, for example, have. There are four or five almost identical versions of this. They are small, which is great, and they rotate at about 25,000 rpm, and they go from the apex of the left ventricle to the aorta. But the patients have to be anticoagulated, and if the device stops—for whatever reason—then there is a wide-open connection from the aorta to the ventricle, and blood goes from the aorta into the left ventricle, dilating it and stopping the heart. So you can never stop pumping because the heart will dilate and fail.

But, if this happens, won't the heart start again on its own in some patients after having the LVAD in for a while?

Yes, absolutely, but you don't know which patients these are, and when you can stop the thing. The proponents of these pumps suggest that you can put these pumps in and they will work forever. Now, I know of nothing that will work forever. They are using them as a bridge to transplantation, and for that it is a reasonable approach, but it is an awful lot of surgery for a bridge.

Now, our device may be used as a bridge, even though we devised it for long-term use. It can be also turned off and on as the patient requires it symptomatically, and that's the way this patient is currently using it.

How many are you going to put in? Is this the first?

We are going to put in ten; this is the fourth; the first three died. That's not a fair impression to give you. You'll think that everybody I operate on dies! What happened was that in the first case I made an error. I am not saying that I do nothing but make errors; but I make enough of them. Our technique of isolating the aorta and letting the left ventricle pump blood to the head worked perfectly in calves, in whom we perfused the distal aorta from below. We didn't stop the heart. In this first patient, when we clamped the aorta, the left ventricle suddenly looked at such a high resistance that it dilated and failed, and we couldn't take the clamp off the aorta because we had already opened it. We learned from this that we could not depend on the patient's left ventricle to supply blood to the head, so in the second patient we supplied blood from external pumps to the head and below the area of the aorta in which the pump was to be implanted. This patient, after being terminal and bedridden following two cardiac arrests, and unconscious before we did him, lived almost six months and did beautifully postimplantation. He developed a leak in the balloon, and we lost him. We did not have a good relationship with the medical team at that hospital, and we were not given the opportunity to examine the specimen at the autopsy. They told us that their pathologist would send us a report.

That's crazy!

I know it's crazy, and their pathologist didn't know anything about these devices. He was a very sincere man, however, and tried to cooperate. We were able to look at the body but not examine the operative site and so on to determine why the balloon ruptured. We had tested twenty pumps in an accelerated life test, and all of them had gone 250 million cycles without a single failure. That is the equivalent of eighteen years.

The third patient was another very sick patient, and we did him at a different hospital where we had a better relationship with the staff, and we knew we could not make any progress if we could not understand what went wrong whenever it did. You don't learn anything if everything is fine; you have to learn from your failures. This patient was in even worse shape than the preceding one, with pulmonary disease and bilateral pneumonia in addition to his heart disease. It was stupid to do it, but he lived five weeks, dying a pulmonary death with the pump still working. During this time we saw these black particles in the air line and finally realized that what was happening was that when the pressure in the tubing became negative to deflate the balloon, it was drawing in surrounding edema fluid from that abdominal wall, and the protein in this fluid, due to the desiccating effect of the air flowing through the tubing, was precipitating it into hard particles. These were present throughout the system from the drive pump to the balloon, concentrated at the point where the balloon had ruptured in the second patient. The gnawing through of these particles, we surmised, was what had caused the puncture of the balloon in the second patient, even though we had not the opportunity to conduct a proper post-mortem examination of the surgery. This was corrected for the next patient, who went home and is doing well after two months.

You never got involved with the total artificial heart.

No; that is purely Kolff, who is the father of that idea. I just felt that that was just too tough a problem to solve. Does it have a future? Not in your lifetime; not in my lifetime; not in Kolff's lifetime. Twenty years from now? How about forty? Maybe.

But by that time, LVADs will be so good that they will be competitive with heart transplants.

All these devices have tubes coming out of the chest. Doesn't that present the constant problem of infection?

Not with us, because we worked it out. Twenty years ago, in the seventies at Sinai Hospital, we implanted essentially the same device we are using now in three patients. One died from bleeding complications about a week postoperatively. Of the other two, one survived three months, but both developed an infection involving the whole tubing of the device. And when you have an infection of a foreign body, you have to remove it. In these cases we couldn't do it. We knew that this device could never be practical unless you solved the problem of infection of the device with part inside and part outside. Having part outside was an advantage; you could have all the complicated parts external so they could be accessible for repair or adjustment, but you had to prevent the infection that arose as the tubing went through the skin into the patient. We got support from the NIH, and, first in pigs and then in humans, we were able to devise a way to culture fibroblasts from the skin of the recipient and coat the neck of the skin access device with these prior to insertion; a firm fibroblast-to-fibroblast seal would be formed that would prevent infection. That is what we have done with the CardioVad system.

Throughout the course of the work on artificial cardiac devices, you see a number of Japanese names popping up as coauthors in papers from your lab and Kolff's: Tetsuzo Akutsu, Yukihito Nosé, Yoshio Kondo.

Kondo is a magnificent surgeon, and we did the puppy heart transplants together, and then he did it on his own, staying with the dogs until the middle of the night. He later went back to Japan, but we had many fellows from Japan—twenty or thirty—who stayed with us for training, and whenever I visit Japan, they have a reunion for me.

Regarding Tet Akutsu, another surgeon, I have been accused of being persistent, even stubborn; but, like Kolff, he believes in the total artificial heart and has devoted his life to it. He was first with Kolff and then came to me, and the way this happened was that when Yukihiko Nosé, who had been working with me for four or five years, wanted to spend some time with Kolff, they arranged to trade places. Kolff was finally pushed out of the Cleveland Clinic, just as I was pushed out of Maimonides, because they thought *he* was too radical. So when Kolff went to Utah, Nosé kept up the lab in Cleveland until some medical people got together and said that *he* was too radical and drove him out. Nosé went to DeBakey in Houston and has done a marvelous job there.

Do you have any regrets about anything?

Regrets? I suppose I could have been nicer to my wife, my poor wife, who has suffered through all this. I suppose she deserved better. She used to go with a baseball player; she would have done better with him!

Especially with what they are earning today!

Seriously, though, it bothers me that I did not foresee the problems that lay ahead of me in the kind of things I tried to accomplish. It was devastating to lose these patients after all the work that had gone into these various devices. But in my business you have to be in it for the long haul. Look at Kolff and Akutsu; they've been working on the total artificial heart for twenty-five to thirty years. I have kept up with my own research because it's what I am interested in, and it's something I think I do well. I love to do it. It takes a long time for these devices to succeed—the intraaortic balloon, for example—but if you keep working at a good idea, you hope, you believe, that one day you will succeed.

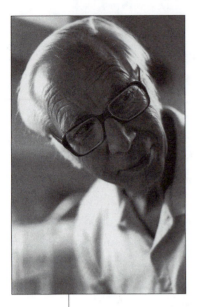

13

WILLEM J. KOLFF, M.D., PH.D.
(1911–   )

If Nobel Prizes in medicine were awarded to those whose work had led to the saving or prolonging of lives, or making life more bearable for those with serious illnesses, Dr. Willem Kolff would have received such recognition many years ago. His invention of the first practical and widely used artificial kidney, alone, has allowed for the recovery of countless individuals who have suffered acute renal failure. For those with advanced chronic renal disease, his device and its successors have maintained patients over prolonged periods either with or without subsequent kidney transplantations.[1]

The development of the artificial kidney represents but one of a number of artificial organs to which which Dr. Kolff has devoted his boundless energy and inventiveness over a long and fruitful career. Other advances in artificial organs that have emanated from his laboratory include those for sight, hearing, the lungs, and his other major contribution to the field, devices for the treatment of heart disease, especially the total artificial heart.

Early on, with the introduction of the rotating-drum artificial kidney in Holland, he noted that the darkish venous blood that had been withdrawn from the patient for removal of waste products was becoming bright red following exposure to the artificial kidney, indicating that oxygen was being added to the blood in the process. It was this recognition that led Kolff to the development of the earliest membrane oxygenator type of heart-lung machine for use in open-heart surgery. This machine was initially used at the Cleveland Clinic, his first base of operations in the United States, and later elsewhere. He also devised an intraaortic balloon for cardiac support, utilizing the counterpulsation principle to increase coronary flow, reduce myocardial oxygen demands, and improve cardiac performance.

His major efforts in the cardiovascular field, however, have been directed toward the development of the total artificial heart (TAH), an enterprise in which he has been engaged for many years. It was this work that made possible the initial efforts to this end at the University of Utah in Salt Lake City, where Dr. Kolff had transferred after leaving the Cleveland Clinic in 1967. The first patient to receive this device was the dentist Barney Clark, in December 1982. Clark survived 112 days, and although several other TAH implantations were performed after this, the program ended a few years later due to continuing problems. Undeterred by such setbacks, Kolff has continued to work on improving designs and stressing the future role of such devices. Now that the Food and Drug Administration (FDA) has approved the TAH as a bridge to cardiac transplantation, such patients can be brought to surgery when donor hearts do become available in much better shape than heretofore, although many transplantation centers have yet to avail themselves of this approach, leading to another of Dr. Kolff's personal crusades at present.

The next step, due to the limited availability of donor hearts given the great demand for them, will be the permanent insertion of a TAH to provide patients with productive and meaningful lives over a prolonged period of time.

My first interview with Dr. Kolff, en route from Washington, D.C., to Philadelphia on May 19, 1983, emphasized his work on the kidney. My second interview with him took place in Newtown Square, Pennsylvania, seventeen years later, on December 7, 2000. For this book, I decided to reproduce those portions of the first interview related to his cardiac work and then provide an update on Dr. Kolff's work in, and ideas about, this field to which he has devoted so much effort.[2]

Things seemed to be going pretty well for you in Holland. Why did you leave?

In the first place, I thought the Russians would be coming in. Second, I thought Holland was overcrowded; it had lost its colonies, and there would not be enough space for our four children—five by the time we immigrated. Last, I had been working on a heart-lung machine in Kampen at a hospital with only one surgeon and one internist. A ninety-bed city hospital was too small to start an open-heart program. So I felt I had to give up my independence and join a large team, where they could use and develop both the artificial kidney and an improved model of the heart-lung machine.

When I came to the United States, though, none of the surgeons were interested in using the heart-lung machine because Charles Bailey had just started doing his mitral commissurotomies. This was a blind procedure done without bypass, which the surgeons loved because they hated complicated apparatuses anyway. It was only four or five years later, when the limitations of closed-heart surgery became evident for valve problems other than mitral stenosis and also for complicated congenital heart disease, that interest in open-heart surgery with bypass was revived. In 1955, five years after arriving in Cleveland, I took out of the closet all of my heart-lung equipment that I had brought with me from the Netherlands and began to work with it again.

Were you aware of the work by JOHN GIBBON on the heart-lung machine?

Yes. Gibbon was professor of cardiac and thoracic surgery at Jefferson, and I stayed at his home in Philadelphia during my first visit. We became very good friends and he invited me to join him at Jefferson, but I felt it would be unwise to be working in his institution on exactly the same project. I also sensed that his relations with the chief of surgery were not the best, so I decided in favor of the Cleveland Clinic, where there was more space and at least some guarantee of a salary on which I could support my wife and five children.

> Despite all your problems in Cleveland,[3] you certainly accomplished a great deal while you were there: you made further advances with the artificial kidney and construction of the twin-coil disposable kidney; you devised an intraaortic balloon pump with Moulopoulos and Topaz;[4] and you developed the membrane oxygenator. Tell me about how you and DONALD EFFLER introduced elective cardiac arrest in open-heart surgery.

Experimental elective cardiac arrest in dogs using potassium citrate was introduced by [DENNIS] MELROSE and his group at Hammersmith Hospital in London. They showed that reperfusing the heart with normal blood could then easily restart it. This was desirable in correcting cardiac defects in open-heart surgery, since the surgeons were not used to suturing moving targets. Donald Effler and LAWRENCE GROVES, the cardiac surgeons at the Cleveland Clinic, came into my laboratory and worked together with me, doing this in dogs. We did many of these, and the ten last consecutive puppies went without a hitch.

Then in the operating room this was tried on three children with congenital heart defects. Yet the first baby died, although the second and third lived. You see, no matter how many successful animal experiments you have, you can still lose your first patient when you attempt something new clinically. You must have some leeway for some failures when you are beginning something new and worthwhile.

> Did you experience the same pressures in the Netherlands when you lost fourteen of your first fifteen patients placed on the artificial kidney?

No. There was never any pressure on me there to stop, and if there had been I wouldn't have paid any attention. But if I had been doing that work at the Cleveland Clinic, they would have stopped me.

You have to find ways of evading that sort of obstruction. For example, at the Cleveland Clinic, the urologist DR. EUGENE POUTASSE and I decided to attempt some renal transplants, maintaining the patients on the artificial kidney until they were ready. We reasoned, however, that if their natural kidneys remained in place, this might, in some way, affect the survival of the transplants adversely. We planned bilateral nephrectomy in these patients prior to the transplants.

Knowing that there was little room for trial and error, we elected to do a number of these cases at once before any prohibitions could be set up against this should there be an initial failure or two. Six bilateral nephrectomies were scheduled by the surgeon in just a few days, and the transplants rapidly followed before any potential opposition to this could develop at the clinic. Fortunately, they all turned out well, and at the Saturday morning clinic conference, we were able to present six patients with transplants, all in excellent health. IRVINE PAGE, who was very negative about the work we were doing, was called upon to make a comment. He had no choice but to congratulate us.

I knew Charlie Bailey, and he had to do the same thing in regard to the mitral commissurotomy operation.* Now it's worse than ever with the IRB [Institutional Review Board for Research on Human Subjects] and the FDA breathing down your neck. It took our surgeon, WILLIAM DeVRIES, twenty-two months to get permission to implant the first artificial heart. Twenty-two months!

I would like to start at the beginning of the total artificial heart and follow through on its history. You actually began work on this in Cleveland . . .

In 1957 Peter Salisbury gave his presidential address to the American Society for Artificial Internal Organs (ASAIO). He spoke of the possibility of an artificial heart inside of the chest, and when I came home to Cleveland, I said to DR. TETSUZO AKUTSU, "Let's do it." We had also heard about a genius from New Zealand, Selwin McCabe, who was working on artificial hearts at the NIH. He made them by cavity molding of plastisol, a polyvinyl chloride. He could make valves, too. Although we had different ideas about shape, we basically copied his technique and gave him credit for it.

McCabe got into some political trouble and had to leave the NIH. I wanted to get him for the Cleveland Clinic, but when they heard

---

* For details, see the introduction to the interview with Dr. Bailey in this volume.

about the kind of difficulty he was in, this didn't get approved. So Tet Akutsu and I began this work. He presented it at the ASAIO meeting in the spring of 1958.[5] That was the beginning.

I was then put in touch with S. Harry Norton, a retired engineer from Thompson Products, and he made for us the first electrohydraulic heart using solenoids which, when activated, compressed hydraulic fluid in which the right and left "ventricles" were suspended. We took a dog with this electrohydraulic heart to the X-ray laboratory and made angiograms, where you could see beautifully how the contrast material was pumped from the right side of the artificial heart into the lungs of the dog and then back to the left side. When my associates and I were presenting this at a later ASAIO meeting, although we had planned our time carefully, it seemed I might run overtime due to the showing of the movie. As it was running, I asked the chairman of the meeting, "Do you want me to stop now?" He said, "No," and, according to what some people in the audience later told me, they would have killed him if he had answered, "Yes."

This was a beautiful presentation of the feasibility of the artificial heart, and Harry Norton continued to work with us for some time. Later, another engineer, Kirby Hiller, from NASA Lewis Research Center, helped our group and asked, "Why do you use all this mechanical hardware and electrohydraulic systems? Why not just use air, which is light and easily controllable?" I agreed to this, and we built what we called NASA Towers. This was a very beautiful kind of machine where you could program the air pressure wave you wished to use and the amount of pressure you wished to employ and experiment with various combinations to give the best results. And it was easy to get grant money for this kind of machine because when something is complicated and looks like very clever engineering, people respect it. When you come in with a simple device, you can never get any money to support it.

The problem with NASA Towers was that you needed a pilot's license to drive the damn thing. It was always broken down when we needed it the most. Then and there, I decided that if we were going to build an artificial heart, it would have to be very simple, and this is what has guided us ever since. We have also come to concentrate on air-driven hearts as the most practical.

You were at the Cleveland Clinic from 1950 to 1967. Why did you leave?

The Cleveland Clinic had broken its promises to me so often that it became quite clear that I could never accomplish there what I had set out to do. I was very friendly with the people there, but they just thought differently from the way I did. I managed to circumvent a lot of the obstruction by having appointments in two departments: surgery and research. Then the day came when I was told that I could only be a member of one. I realized then that I would be losing whatever leverage I had and decided to leave.

The same evening I learned that I would be given a choice of either one department or the other by the clinic, I called up C. William Hall in San Antonio. He had been an associate of Michael DeBakey in Houston and had been running the artificial heart program for him. I figured the best place for me would be one with a strong regional medical program because that was where an artificial organs program would have the best chance of succeeding. I asked Hall who had the best regional medical program, and, without hesitation, he said, "Salt Lake City." Keith Reemtsma was head of surgery there at the time. I knew him and had a good relationship with him. Although there were other opportunities offered me, I decided to go to Utah to set up a biomedical engineering institute. What especially impressed me was the promise of the associate dean at the medical school, Dr. Tom King, that at the University of Utah there would be a very short chain of command. No red tape would be allowed to stand in my way, and I would report directly to the vice president of research for action on my grant and contract applications.

I have been in Utah for sixteen years now, and it has worked out very well.

One of the major accomplishments, if not *the* major accomplishment, in Utah has been the artificial heart program. Although you actually began this work in Cleveland and a number of people have been involved behind the scenes, I think most people are interested in how you brought ROBERT K. JARVIK and DeVries into the picture.

Robert Jarvik came to me as a premedical student after having been unable to get into any American medical school. He had been going to the medical school in Bologna for two years, but there were Socialist strikes at the time and he did not wish to go back. A Ph.D. from Ethicon first told me about him in 1971 and described him to me as a very ingenious fellow. He assured me that if I took Jarvik on as an assistant, he could probably get funds from Ethicon to pay for him. I spoke to Jarvik, who was on the East Coast, over the telephone and asked him to come out to Salt Lake City. While awaiting word from Ethicon, he needed something to live on, and I asked him how little he needed to manage. This was not because I begrudged him the money, but only because I didn't have it in my budget. He asked for two hundred dollars a month. Three months later, Ethicon called and told me that funding for his support by their research committee was turned down. So until he got his own research grants many years later, I supported Jarvik and we had a very good relationship. It could be described as a father-son sort of thing, but sometimes the son revolts against the father.

DeVries came to Cleveland while I was still there in 1967, I believe, and was assigned to work with us on the artificial heart. He was still a medical student in Utah at the time, but he wrote a paper on "Consumption Coagulation Shock and the Heart," a problem we found in animals with artificial hearts. This became a classic after publication in 1970.

He completed medical school in 1970 and went to Duke University for one of those terribly long ten-year residencies in thoracic and cardiovascular surgery. He returned to Utah intending to get involved with the artificial heart program, even though another man had just been appointed head of cardiothoracic surgery at the University of Utah and there really wasn't room for two. The other fellow, however, decided to go into private practice, and DeVries was appointed to the position.

I don't believe that there is anyone alive with his head on straight who does not know about Barney Clark, the first human recipient of the total artificial heart in Utah.[6] I think you should know, however, that in some quarters, the University of Utah has been criticized for the way this achievement was publicized. The sometimes circuslike atmosphere there

has been contrasted, for example, with the low profile of the transplantation team under NORMAN SHUMWAY at Stanford.

It is very unfair for others to criticize the Utah people for the way they handled the publicity. To begin with, there is no comparison with Stanford; heart transplantation is no longer newsworthy, having been around since 1967. As for the situation in Utah, you must understand that all these reporters were not invited. They came, probably about a hundred of them, with TV cameras, radios, photographers, et cetera, and we had to accommodate them. You have no idea of what we had to contend with. Finally, it was a choice between dealing with the press in an organized way, as Chase Petersen [vice president for Health Sciences] did very well, or letting them write whatever crazy things they might pick up from all sorts of odd and uninformed people who happened to be in the vicinity. The reporting of Dr. Petersen was factual, accurate, honest, and complete. I made a statement to the assembled press conference only on the day before the surgery to warn them against overoptimism, and spoke only a minute on the following day in response to a question.

The only thing we were not prepared for was that the newspapers would put such a monetary value on any extra little thing they could get. Photographs of Barney Clark as a young man were obtained from the family and sold in Europe for hundreds of dollars. I have also seen a letter from a reporter to a medical resident whom he mistook for one of the surgical residents in the intensive care unit where Barney Clark was located. It was an invitation to dinner, but also an ill-disguised bribe to get some inside information about the patient. This sort of thing went on for the entire period of his hospitalization. Even at the funeral there were more than twenty reporters about and two helicopters flying overhead.

While you're answering these charges, you might address another: that the publicity regarding Barney Clark was welcomed by Utah to use as a wedge to pry money loose from the federal government in support of your program.

This is a loaded question, and it is incorrect. I just said that we had no

other choice but to give the proper information. Yet it did have a beneficial effect in that the NHLBI [National Heart, Lung, and Blood Insti-
tute], following Barney Clark's implantation on December 2, 1982,
increased its allocation with many more millions of dollars.

We have not been very lucky in getting money from the NIH. We
have support for an electrohydraulic heart and also for an air-driven
heart. On the other hand, I have submitted the same proposal in four
different versions for left and right ventricular assist devices. So far it
has not been approved. For a feasibility study we were awarded fifty
thousand dollars, an amount with which we could do very little. Then
one reviewer said that our projected study of blood coagulation was
unnecessary. In the last study section, another reviewer said that the
coagulation study was not sophisticated enough; and so I got nowhere.
We have not had much luck with the NHLBI either. Another manufac-
turer, using Jarvik's motor with Jarvik's pump, got funded for the elec-
trodynamic heart. We did not.

The NIH was against our putting a total heart in any patient. Fortunately, Schweiker, the secretary of health at the time, ruled that the
FDA and not the NIH was the agency to rule on the use of new drugs
and new medical devices. If we had to go through the NIH human
experimentation committee, do you know with whom we would have
had to deal? It is said, but probably only half in jest: two priests, a clean-
ing woman, a banker, and a union leader. This is the kind of committee that frustrated all the studies of Jack Norman, who was trying to
develop a left ventricular assist device for DENTON COOLEY. The protocol they had to adopt was so impossible that every patient was three-
quarters dead before he could be admitted to the study. All twenty-three
of the patients they tried it on died—not a single one left the hospital
alive. That's even worse than the first fifteen patients I treated with my
artificial kidney. So you can see why I wanted to avoid the NIH review
committee. We got funded from independent sources for Barney
Clark's surgery, and they couldn't stop DeVries from operating because,
not being subsidized by the government, he was free to act.

**The public is often unaware of how such advances come about, and
many of those involved are overlooked or forgotten by posterity. To drive**

home this point, I would like to quote a memo you sent to your staff before Clark's surgery. "When the artificial heart will be implanted into a human recipient, the principal surgeon in charge is the one who takes the greatest risk to his career, the greatest part of the blame when things go wrong, but also the greatest publicity. It is this last part I want you to ponder long before the time of the actual implantation. It may be very difficult for those of us who have worked so very long on the total artificial heart to accept that the total publicity will be handled by a surgeon. His name will be flashed on the TV screen and over the news media. If some of us are mentioned, it will be due to the surgeon's generosity in thinking of us at that moment. You must also assume that although he will probably think of us during the first, second or third news release, he cannot continue to do so. Also, when the artificial heart's successful transplantation in man is described, this will be done by the surgeon, most likely at a surgical meeting of a society to which we do not even belong. . . .

"What I want to warn you about is that you may not like the way the publicity is going to be handled. Some of this may be inevitable, some of this may be unjust; none of it is done with a particular design towards hurting you. Our main reward must be to know that we have done our best, and that, in time, patients will be saved who are now doomed and that they will be saved through our efforts."

I wanted them to know what was coming and have them be thankful for whatever credit they got and not be bitter because, after all, if anything went wrong, it would be the surgeon who went to jail and not them!

What is the future of the artificial kidney and the artificial heart?

I am convinced that, with the introduction of cyclosporin A and other effective immunosuppressive agents to prevent rejection, kidney transplantation from almost any individual to another will be possible in the future and eliminate the need for the artificial kidney. After all, we have two kidneys and need only one to live.

As for the heart, you will never get enough good hearts that you can use for transplantation. Not by any stretch of the imagination. And there are perhaps fifty thousand patients dying each year in the United States who might be good candidates for the artificial heart.

How far do you think we are from a totally implantable artificial heart?

With an outside source of power delivered transcutaneously with the use of coils, at least five years. I had a contract for years for a better approach, a nuclear-driven heart where the amount of radiation exposure would be minimal. But the nuclear-driven heart is without prospect with the current hysteria over nuclear energy, a hysteria quite unrelated to the validity of the concept. Before it dies down, you and I will long be buried.

With all the projects you have going and all that you have accomplished, you must have been very well organized. Your former associate at the Cleveland Clinic, Donald Effler, calls you the most ambitious man he has ever known.

I don't think "ambitious" is the right word. It has an unpleasant connotation, meaning ambition for oneself. But I can develop a very strong driving force, and I will persevere. I very rarely give up, and if I have to relent temporarily, I usually come back to the project later.

I have certain goals I wanted to reach, usually in terms of an artificial organ that could create happiness for people. Not simply through the simple prolongation of life, but only *happy* life.

These are honest and good goals, and deserve to be pushed. It is true that I cannot stand it if something blocks me from reaching these goals. I may get a little difficult when people try to block me, and if one way is occluded, I'll find another.

Financially, I have always walked a tightrope but have managed to keep my balance. Calamities and disasters have turned out to my advantage in the long run. For example, when my wife and I were in The Hague for a funeral, the Germans invaded the Netherlands. For us, that was the beginning of World War II. I went to the largest hospital in the city and was given the opportunity to set up a blood bank. It was a wonderful experience because, through necessity, everybody helped. It was the first blood bank in Europe, and it is still in existence.

In Utah once, a large number of our sheep were stolen. I first thought this was a disaster. They were stolen in a year that I had grants and enough money; the insurance paid us back in a year when we were nearly totally broke, and it saved us.

When our laboratory at the university burned down in 1973, it was a disaster. However, twenty days later we moved to the old St. Mark's Hospital. Dr. Don Olsen has remodeled its surgical wing into the most advanced experimental laboratory for artificial organs in the world. We could never have afforded such a facility on the university campus.

You're seventy-two years old now and have been going full blast all your life. Are you thinking of retiring soon?

I'm having a good time. Why should I?

———

Newtown Square, Pennsylvania
December 7, 2000

———

The last time I spoke with you, we only touched on this topic: when you were in Kampen, Holland, before coming to the United States, apparently you already had an interest in heart devices. Could you tell me how you first became interested in them?

The best way to start this [story] is from an observation I made using the artificial kidney. When we were using this rotating-drum device, we could clearly see that when the blood withdrawn from the patient was "blue" (unoxygenated), it became "red" (oxygenated) after passing through the artificial kidney. That meant that we had an oxygenator, and I followed through on that observation. In 1955, at the Cleveland Clinic, I took the twin-coil artificial kidney, and I replaced the cellophane with a polyethylene membrane; and that was the first membrane oxygenator that was successfully used in people. I also realized even back in Kampen that in the near future membrane oxygenators could be used for small children, as indeed they would, but that they would be too cumbersome with the then-available technology. Therefore, we began to work on various types of heart-lung machines while I was still in Holland. In the early days in Cleveland when we did a ten-year-old boy with the early model, which consisted of a membrane wrapped around a fruit juice can, we needed ten of these oxygenators to perform the operation. Presently, with the capillary hollow fiber oxygenators, which are basically the same as the hollow fiber kidneys, you have such a large surface area that you could now oxygenate a very small volume of blood within them very efficiently.

One of the reasons why I moved from Kampen, where I had a wonderful life, was that the hospital there was too small for open-heart surgery. I needed to work in a large place like the Cleveland Clinic where open-heart surgery could be performed. That was in 1950, shortly after Bailey began to do those closed mitral commissurotomies. And surgeons loved it; so why use complicated machines when they could do the operation simply with their fingers? So I had to wait five years before I could use the machines that I had brought with me from Kampen and Zwolle in Holland.

You might be interested to know that, as far back as 1948, in Holland, I was able to get an extra cow in Kampen, which was not easy to do since the Germans had eaten almost all of them. Our quota for the city of Kampen was five cows per week, but I managed to get an additional one, and in that extra cow we were able to demonstrate that the heart-lung machine that we had at that time could pump and oxygenate five liters of blood per minute. The cow didn't seem to like the machine, so we put her to sleep and distributed her for consumption.

I'm trying to get this straight in my mind, because there were a number of different heart-lung machines early on: the Gibbon model, the bubble oxygenator of RICHARD DeWALL, the disc oxygenator of BJÖRK. . . . Was yours the initial one used at the Cleveland Clinic?

Yes, and it was made in Kampen. Five years later, when I came to the Cleveland Clinic, the surgeons were just beginning to realize that for congenital heart disease they couldn't do much blindly; they needed a pump-oxygenator. MASON SONES joined the clinic about two years later than I. He was interested in congenital heart disease, but the surgeons couldn't do anything for most of these patients. So Sones began to push for open-heart surgery. Knowing about this, I put a dog on our juice-can oxygenator and called Sones to come and see what could be done. As a result of this, we began to do open-heart surgery in the Cleveland Clinic in 1955, and the results were published in the *Cleveland Clinic Quarterly.*[7]

As the patients got older and larger, such as with that ten-year-old boy, we realized that the juice-can models were too cumbersome, as I just described to you. So I brought up from the basement the machines I had made in Kampen and that were gathering dust there. We cleaned them up, and we eventually were able to use these in adults. A Björk oxygenator, in which I had made a small modification, was one of them. He had used stainless steel discs, but I had very little money, so I used Dictaphone discs of the same size.

Effler and Groves were the surgeons at the clinic. Also in Cleveland at the time there was a competing heart surgeon at another hospital who had a non-M.D. assistant by the name of Jones. Jones had modified the Björk oxygenator in such a way that you could add more blood and spin the disc much faster, enabling open-heart surgery on larger patients. I used this knowledge in our own modification. Another type of oxygenator that we used clinically in adult patients was a revolving coiled-tube type, five of which I had brought with me from Holland, and this had a large surface area for a small amount of blood. This also proved to be a good oxygenator. Very soon the Cleveland Clinic had a very large and successful open-heart program, and all the new buildings you see there were built with the money made from the open-heart program.

Let me ask you about the intraaortic balloon. Were you aware of Adrian Kantrowitz's efforts when you started work on it?

No. We had started on that way before Kantrowitz. Kantrowitz has been very good about acknowledging our work, and we have been very good friends. I am very grateful to him because he introduced it in Maimonides Hospital in Brooklyn and the reaction was, "Eh! Maimonides is not a very good hospital, and we don't need this kind of assistance in *our* hospital." But Kantrowitz stuck with it, and after the first fifteen patients, people began to listen to him. We just had the first International Conference on the Intraaortic Balloon Counterpulsation in Athens, Greece, at the end of last August and into September.

When did you first begin using this balloon in patients?

That's another example of how we had to wait. It was five years before we could start this because the Cleveland Clinic did not want to do anything with it.

Let's now talk about your real "baby," the total artificial heart. The last time we spoke, it was in the aftermath of the Barney Clark experience with the Jarvik 7 and all the problems with thromboembolism. Will you bring me up to date on all the developments since then?

During the period following the Barney Clark experience, there were two large hospital corporations. One was Humana and the other was the Hospital Corporation of America (HCA). Humana saw that the total artificial heart had a great future, and they wanted to be ready for it. They wanted to have the administrative experience to manage this, so they offered the University of Utah an agreement in which Humana would assume all financial responsibility for one hundred consecutive patients. They would not interfere with medical management; they would not interfere with personnel; all they wanted was the administrative experience.

I thought that was wonderful, and I arranged a meeting with the president of the university and a whole team of representatives from Humana.They were very serious about this and sent their representatives for a second meeting after that first one.

Dr. Lee, the dean of the medical school, was not very much in favor of pursuing this agreement. He didn't actively obstruct this project, but he certainly didn't help. The superintendent of the University Hospital in Salt Lake City was afraid he would lose his job. He felt that getting involved with Humana would be like getting the head of the camel in your tent. The rest would soon follow, and you would never get him out. So he was definitely opposed to it. The man who should have followed through—and why he did not I have never understood—was the vice president of Health Sciences, Chase Peterson. You recall that when Barney Clark was treated, it was he who met every day with the press to give the status of Barney Clark. For my part, I was very busy with the Institute for Biomedical Engineering. We had about seventy-five people and a budget of five million dollars, and I had to continually work at getting grant money for the institute.

One day, suddenly I saw that somebody was moving out all the technical recording equipment that had been used on Barney Clark. I said, "What are you doing?" He answered, "Oh this is going to Louisville, Kentucky" (Humana headquarters). Five or maybe even ten years later, I learned from a perfusionist in Louisville what had happened. This perfusionist had gone to Humana and said, "Why give all that money to the University of Utah in Salt Lake City? Why don't we do it here in Louisville? In this way we will get all the glory and save all that money. Why not ask Dr. DeVries to come to Louisville?"

I had known nothing of this. All I knew was that the equipment we had used for Barney Clark was being removed. DeVries, the surgeon, had decided to go to Kentucky and told his technician to move all the equipment there. That's how I learned about DeVries's departure. I immediately blocked the export of that equipment which belonged to the University of Utah. But when DeVries left the University of Utah, the artificial heart program went with him.

When DeVries went to Louisville, Humana had every intention of doing one hundred consecutive cases, but the hospital there was a community hospital and did not have the sophisticated backup that you need to support that kind of work, especially as regards blood clotting et cetera. For that reason his patients continued to have strokes, and it was the strokes in Louisville that destroyed the artificial heart program.

How many patients did he operate on in Louisville before they stopped the program?

Five.[8]

I'm sure that didn't deter you from pursuing this research. How did you proceed from the Jarvik 7 to subsequent models?

First, nobody cared about the name of the artificial heart until it was put in a patient. Then all kinds of people began to turn up claiming to have it named for them.

There was Clifford Kwan-Gett, an excellent surgeon who worked for me a long time, and he made one of the most important contributions to the artificial heart, commonly called the "Jarvik heart." It was the development of the seamless continuity between the pumping membrane and the walls of the artificial ventricle. This greatly reduced the possibility of clotting. Kwan-Gett had come with me from Cleveland and later became a very successful heart surgeon in Salt Lake City. But the strange thing was that Kwan-Gett was on the board of the company that manufactured the Jarvik heart and at first never raised a voice against his own company calling it the Jarvik heart. However, when the Barney Clark story hit the newspapers, he came to me and demanded to know why it had not been called the "Kwan-Gett heart" rather than the "Jarvik heart." I asked him why he had never mentioned this before, but he persisted in this and I had to appear before an ethics committee at the University of Utah and then before an ethics committee of the American Medical Association, I believe, to explain why I had allowed it to be called the Jarvik heart and not the Kwan-Gett heart. It was very disagreeable. My defense was that we have artificial hearts under a variety of names—the Zwart heart, the Wertheimer heart, and so on—but we've never had a Kolff heart. We could have had a Kolff-1, -2, -3, -4, but that was not the way I operated. If an assistant, under my guidance, worked on an artificial heart model, we would name it for him, and no one ever protested about it. I suggested to the Society for Artificial Organs to let Dr. Kwan-Gett appear and state his case, but they refused. We then reviewed all the papers that had been published concerning the total artificial heart and totaled all the names of people who had their names on these papers. There were 147, and Jarvik was one of the 147, with his name on perhaps twenty papers. Kwan-Gett had his name as first author on about seventeen papers, so he had had every opportunity to put his name on it.

Were there any other developments with the artificial heart in Utah after DeVries left?

The University of Utah never followed through on the artificial heart because they never had a heart surgeon who was interested. Fortunately, a very good surgeon at the Latter Day Saints Hospital in Salt Lake, James Long, took over, and he has managed to keep the artificial heart program alive in Salt Lake City.

As for Jarvik, I arranged for him to become president of a company that was first called Kolff Associates to make artificial hearts; later it became Symbion. Jarvik had some problems with the FDA, which shut him down. By that time, I was out.

Don Olsen was the head of the Artificial Heart Laboratory in Utah and a very good veterinary surgeon. He had trained all the people who had visited Utah to learn how to put the artificial heart in calves before they attempted this in humans. Olsen has managed to keep this laboratory going and with Dr. Jack Copeland at the University of Arizona in Tucson set up CardioWest. When Symbion was disbanded, the brokers that put that company together in the first place gave its assets and material to CardioWest.

What technical modifications to the Jarvik 7 produced improvements in more recent versions?

The technical improvements are so minimal that I can hardly mention them. The reason why DeVries was not successful in Louisville was that he did not have the clinical support that he needed. I refer you to an article by Jack Copeland about the more recent experience with the artificial heart.[9]

What is the main difference between the CardioWest heart and the electrohydraulic heart, which has now come along?

The CardioWest is air driven and has tubes coming out of the chest. The electrohydraulic heart is produced by a company called Abiomed and is called the AbioCor and is now in preclinical testing. It is completely implantable and powered by transcutaneous energy.

The idea of having an electrohydraulic mechanical heart was mine. It was developed when Jarvik was still a student working with me. The original idea was to have a reversible motor so that you have only one moving part, and that is the impeller. When it pumps one way, it pumps hydraulic fluid to the "left ventricle," and when it turns the other way, it pumps the same hydraulic fluid to the "right ventricle." It is the utmost in terms of simplicity, with only one moving part. As you know, complications go up with the square of the number of parts, and you can't get any lower than this. I sent Jarvik to Dayton, Ohio, to a company, NuTech, that made a reversible electric motor. It is reversed by back electromotive force so you don't need any sensors—sensors always cause trouble. All that is required is three wires inside the chest. The electromotive force is deducted from the current going inside the chest. This gives you enough information to let you know the filling pressures of the heart and the cardiac output. Also novel was the use of saline as the lubricant; the other models use some form of silicon oil. If you have a leak of silicon oil, you're in trouble, while saline causes no such problems.

When we competed for a contract from the NIH, they didn't believe that we could reverse the motor, so we had a "reverse site visit" to Washington, where we showed them that we could reverse the motor by back electromotive force five hundred times per minute. This brought our approval score up to that of Abiomed, but the NIH gave the grant to them anyway, so I never got any funding for this project.

Have you done any work on left ventricular assist devices?

Yes, but we did not get funding, and so we couldn't do much. The NIH mistakenly viewed the left ventricular assist devices to be simpler than the artificial heart. This is not so. The insertion of the artificial heart is easy compared to the left ventricular assist devices. The LVADs do have the advantage that, if something goes wrong, the natural heart may be good enough to sustain the patient. It is also known that, after a time, the sick heart may recover and not need the device.

The advantage of the total artificial heart over the LVAD is that it is simple and not dependent upon the right ventricle working properly as the LVAD is. If you wish to have both left *and* right ventricular assist devices, then the total artificial heart is much simpler. Space is also a consideration: when you take out the natural heart, you can easily install the total artificial heart. The currently approved LVADs are very heavy and cumbersome.

What about the newer devices that may be as small as a double-A battery?

Both DeBakey and Jarvik are working on smaller units that can be implanted in the left ventricular wall and may help, especially if part of the left ventricle is functional.

> You recently made a proposal to Mount Sinai Hospital in New York to set up a total artificial heart implantation center. What impelled you to do this?

I think that it is an international scandal that wherever there are transplantation centers, people die like flies while waiting on the transplant list. I want these patients, before they're almost dead, to be able to receive an air-driven artificial heart, which is FDA approved as a bridge to transplantation, relatively inexpensive, and easy to put in. It has been well substantiated that if you take the kind of patients that Copeland has described and who get the CardioWest artificial heart, these patients, who may be in advanced heart failure, with poorly functioning kidneys, liver, and lungs as a result, after insertion of the artificial heart will be asking for breakfast two mornings later and walking around within a week. By insertion of the artificial heart, these patients can be put in excellent shape so that when they finally do receive a transplant, the success rate is 95 percent or better. Whereas if you transplant a patient who is not in good condition, the results of the transplantation are poor.

> Given the shortage of hearts for transplantation, do you ever foresee a time when the total artificial heart implantation will be accepted as a permanent device?

Inevitably this will come; it has to come; but it requires a different way of thinking by the medical profession. I have heard from all those medical advisers involved with putting in artificial kidneys, hearts, heart-lung machines, "I would rather be dead!" You never hear that from a patient!

> Of your five children, three have become doctors, but Jack seems to have been most closely connected to you professionally as a cardiac surgeon.

Jack has been very important to me. He did the implantation of the total artificial heart—the Jarvik heart that later became the Symbion heart and still later the CardioWest heart—in brain-dead patients with the permission of their families. He did this when he was at Temple in Philadelphia. The most important thing he did was to determine the correct way to implant the artificial heart. If you do not put it in the correct way, you are in trouble. When the artificial heart was put in Barney Clark, the surgeon could not close the chest. Now Robert Jarvik, who had visited Jack in Philadelphia to observe his technique, said to DeVries, "Why not take it out and put it in the way Jack Kolff does at Temple?" So they did this and were able to close the chest. If that had not happened, the artificial heart program would have been dead in its tracks.

What is your son Jack doing now?

It had been agreed upon that, after Barney Clark, since Jack had helped so enormously with the implantation of the artificial heart in the brain-dead patients, and before that, had come at his own expense to Salt Lake City to teach Don Olsen how to do it in calves, the second artificial heart to be implanted would be by Jack at Temple University, where he had a good team ready at that time. Jarvik broke his word on this and refused to contribute an artificial heart for this from the company he now headed. He wanted to charge $120,000, which Jack did not have. So Jack started a transplantation program at Temple, now one of the largest in the country.

How old were you when you retired from the University of Utah and why?

I was eighty-seven when I retired, and the reasons were personal family reasons.

Do you have any current projects?

I have two: one involves the hospital at Kampen; the other is the desire to create artificial heart/transplantation centers, which I believe to be inevitable. In Kampen they were planning to tear down the old hospital to build a nursing home, so at first it was a campaign just to save the hospital. Later the idea came to create a museum there; and still later the idea for setting up an annual artificial organ festival. This is now being planned, and I am getting a great deal of help. We formed a committee to stop the demolishing of the hospital, and finally the city council of Kampen voted unanimously to save the hospital and make it a national monument.

> **What ever happened to the four rotating-drum artificial kidneys that you brought with you to the United States? It would be great to have one on display in the new museum.**

They have all disappeared. We have made a replica for Kampen.

Anything else you wish to get on the record?

Wherever they have cardiac transplantation centers, people are dying while they are on the waiting list. It is more expensive to die slowly in an intensive care unit (with perhaps two or three admissions) than it is to receive an FDA-approved, reasonably priced, air-driven artificial heart. I believe that once you have a number of patients in good health, maintained with air-driven artificial hearts, you have ideal candidates for receiving the more sophisticated, as yet experimental, electro-hydraulic and other hearts. The artificial heart is coming; there is absolutely no doubt about it!*

In 1984, a man in Stockholm walked around with an artificial air-driven heart in his chest and a portable Heimes heart driver over his shoulder. He served himself four times at a smorgasbord, and no one in the restaurant knew he had an artificial heart. He sent a telegram to the United States to say, "I am the happiest man in Europe." But the FDA has not yet approved the use of a portable driver.

---

* On July 2, 2001, at the Jewish Hospital in Louisville, Kentucky, Drs. Laman A. Gray and Robert D. Dowling inserted a total artificial heart (AbioCor) in a man in terminal heart failure. Of the five patients who received this device, by February 2002 four had subsequently died primarily from thromboembolic complications.

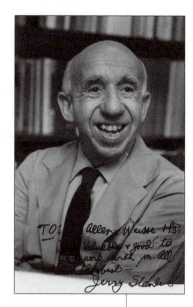

14

JEREMIAH STAMLER, M.D.
(1919–   )

It is unlikely that when they named their son, the parents of Jeremiah Stamler were aware of what the future held for him. But how prophetic it would have been had they known that years later, when he grew into manhood, like that Jeremiah of the Old Testament, he would be preaching to the masses—and to society's policymakers—about their shortcomings, not in relation to the error of their ways regarding Jehovah, but in their personal health practices that had made them so susceptible to heart disease.

As one of the founding fathers of preventive cardiology, Dr. Stamler has carried on a relentless campaign for over half a century to determine the underlying causes of certain common types of heart disease and what could be done by individuals themselves, as well as their doctors, to prevent these problems. After all, despite the great advances in treating heart diseases both medically and surgically, preventing them from occurring in the first place turns out to be the most effective approach to longer and healthier lives.

Beginning his research career in 1948 as a protégé of the great LOUIS N. KATZ, at the Michael Reese Hospital in Chicago, Dr. Stamler became an "established investigator" of the American Heart Association and assistant director of the Cardiovascular Research Institute there under Dr. Katz. Although he continues to travel widely, Chicago has remained his home base ever since. After leaving Michael Reese in 1958, he assumed a groundbreaking role in several areas for the Chicago Health Department. In 1972 he became the first chairman of the newly established Department of Community Health and Preventive Medicine at Northwestern University Medical School, also holding the Dingman Professorship in Cardiology. He remains there, active full-time in research, as professor emeritus.

His efforts in the epidemiology and prevention of heart disease are so numerous and widespread that it would be impossible to enumerate them all. Suffice it to mention as representative his role in studies such as the Hypertension Detection and Follow-up Program (HDFP), the Coronary Drug Project (CDP), the Multiple Risk Factor Intervention Trial (MRFIT), and the Dietary Approaches to Stop Hypertension (DASH) trials on dietary factors relating to people with above optimal levels of blood pressure.

Dr. Stamler's contributions to so many national and international efforts in the epidemiology and prevention of heart disease are so well recognized that it is possible to overlook the decade of his early work in the laboratory with Dr. Katz and others, an experience that dictated the future course of his research. For this reason, I have chosen to emphasize these formative years, recognizing that, in so doing, I may have not done full justice to his more recent and ongoing efforts in his field.

New York, New York
March 28, 2000

When you mention the name Stamler, there are two things that come to mind: one is "Chicago" and the other is "coronary disease epidemiology and prevention." But the first is sort of misleading because you are really a local boy, aren't you?

I was born in New York. When I was six months old, my parents decided it would be nicer to rear a youngster in a smaller community, so my father, who was a dentist, set up a practice, which continued on Main Street in West Orange, New Jersey, for more than fifty years. So I grew up in West Orange and was always grateful for the very nice childhood I had there.

Then I went to college at Columbia, where I had a rich and wonderful experience. I was a premed, and the only adverse aspect of all that was the overt anti-Semitism of the time. Columbia and Cornell medical schools elected not to admit me even though I was Phi Beta Kappa with an A average and with a great many activities of the kind deemed appropriate by higher-ups. Cornell didn't even interview me, and the dean at Columbia's P & S (College of Physicians and Surgeons) did so with transparent reluctance. At that time, P & S accepted from its own undergraduate school, Columbia College, only two or three Jewish students a year, and Cornell none or one. I finally was accepted by the Long Island College of Medicine.

Fortunately, things are different now. At the fiftieth anniversary of our Columbia class's graduation in 1990, the John Jay award, the highest award the college gives, was granted to five Chicagoans in a ceremony in Chicago, and I was one of them. At this time there was a Jewish dean of the college and a Jewish president of Columbia University present, and I thought to myself, "What am I going to say?" In my brief thank you, I was pleased to note that "obviously things are different and better."

> I also graduated from the Long Island College of Medicine, but this was in 1958, by which time it had been taken over by the state and renamed SUNY–Downstate (Brooklyn). It was always considered the kind of school that just produced general practitioners for the community, but I would like to get something into the record here. About fifteen or twenty years ago someone actually checked into the number of medical school graduates nationwide who went into academic medicine and research, and it turned out that Downstate was in the top ten or fifteen in the country, right up there with Hopkins, Harvard, and Yale.

It was never a rich school, and when I was there during the war it was particularly depleted of clinical faculty because many had gone into the armed services. Older clinicians had been mobilized to fill in, but I was very lucky to be profoundly influenced by one person who is very relevant to our discussion. That was JEAN OLIVER, the professor of pathology, who was a brilliant researcher as well as an extraordinary human being. He teased nephrons out of the kidney and worked with the physiologist Thomas Addis in California to study the pathophysiology of the kidney with particular reference to Bright's disease. Jean Oliver first got me interested in "hardening of the arteries." All the other pre-clinical people were rather *comme ci, comme ça.*

Then, in the clinical years, I had an extraordinary resident named Joe DiPalma, who had had tuberculosis and therefore was not taken into the armed forces. He later became professor of medicine and then dean of Hahnemann Medical College in Philadelphia. I spent a tremendous amount of time with him on the wards at Kings County Hospital in Brooklyn, and he was interested in cardiovascular diseases.

Later on, during my nine-month internship at Kings County, Bill Dock came to the Long Island College of Medicine as professor of medicine, and he was a remarkable person. He had a scintillating mind, constantly generating fruitful ideas. We used to have lunch with him, and he would stand on the cafeteria line, watching the medical students getting ham and cheese sandwiches, milk shakes, pie à la mode, and he would say, "They're digging their graves with their forks." At that time it was already clear to him that the main general etiological exposure factor for adult cardiovascular disease was diet.

After I finished my internship in the fall of 1944, I went into the army for two years; most of us wanted to serve in the army during the war. I went to Carlisle Barracks, Pennsylvania, for six weeks for medical basic training, where, on the last day, I noticed a posting notifying us that there was a shortage of psychiatrists and radiologists, and inviting anyone interested to apply for one of the army schools in these areas. I figured I would be an internist and that any training in radiology would be very helpful, so I signed up for this.

So I went to the army X-ray school in Memphis, Tennessee. I believe I was in the last class that went through this training under an extraordinary guy, a career army officer named Al DeLorimer, a fine person, a good doc, and an excellent organizer. The staff consisted of about nine persons for only eleven students, a tremendously good ratio of teachers to students, and they gave an intense course on one subject, beginning with up-front sessions on safety, then, mainly, diagnostic radiology, with a little therapeutic radiology at the end. I learned there a lesson that became very important to me for the rest of my life, relating to international teaching activities: when my wife, Rose, and I organized ten-day teaching seminars on cardiovascular epidemiology and prevention for the International Society and Federation of Cardiology (now the World Heart Federation), we applied what I had learned in Memphis about the merit of having a good faculty that knows the subject, knows how to teach, likes people, with a good faculty-to-student ratio to create an intense learning community to study a single subject in depth within a short period of time.

After we finished this training, all eleven of us were classified as grade D radiologists. I never quite knew what this meant: A, B, and C are passing, F is failing, and D?! Then I got assigned overseas, which turned out to be the island of Bermuda, with the Army Transport Command. That was a paradise, and it was late in the war so my wife was able to join me. I was in charge of the laboratory and the X-ray department.

What did you do when you got out of the army in 1946?

I got out in October 1946, and, by that time, I had decided with my wife that I would try my hand for a year in research on experimental atherosclerosis. We had saved some money, and Rose agreed to work so that we would be able to manage even if there would be no income for me. It's almost unbelievable to comment on it today, but, thanks to the army photostatting system of reprints, I had almost every relevant article on experimental atherosclerosis in animals that had ever been written—all in a couple of foot lockers. I actually became interested in this overtly while I was still a second-year medical student and began reading about it.

I considered getting a Ph.D. in biochemistry, but this would take three years and I just wanted a year of training in some basics. The G.I. Bill was in effect, so while I was looking for the proper position in which I might work on experimental atherosclerosis, I spent a year at the Long Island College of Medicine as a fellow in pathology with Jean Oliver and his colleagues. I did very little experimental work while I was there; mainly library reading while I observed what the senior people were doing. My reading had led me to discover that there was a laboratory in Chicago at Michael Reese Hospital under a guy named LOUIS KATZ, an outstanding cardiovascular researcher, that had the only animal experimental laboratory that I could identify at the time doing work in this area. So my wife and I took a trip to Chicago and stayed with some friends of friends to save on expenses and got to meet SI [SIMON] RODBARD, a friend of theirs who was the assistant director of that department. They picked up the phone and called Si, and I went to meet him, which eased the way into a meeting with "the great man," Katz, who wound up offering me a fellowship with a salary of two hundred dollars a month. I had been ready to work for nothing, so I left there walking on air.

I knew Louis Katz from afar, but tell me about Dr. Katz up close during the ten years you worked under him.

Dr. Katz was a remarkable person in many ways. First of all, he was probably one of the last "encyclopedists" in the cardiovascular world. He knew the whole field. He had been intensely trained as a physiologist with CARL WIGGERS in Cleveland. In addition to being a physiologist, he was an electrocardiographer, less so a clinician but interested in many aspects of cardiovascular disease, including hardening of the arteries. He was very bright and very energetic. He told the story that when he had hyperthyroidism and needed surgery, just before they administered the anesthetic he told them, "Do everything you have to do, but don't change my personality."

He was very good to—and for—young people. People would see him on the platform at meetings, and he would seem tough and mean. And once or twice a year he would get a severe migraine headache and be literally irrational; I learned that. But for young people he was very good—for one thing—because he *listened.* You could go into him and say, "You know, Boss" (we used to call him the Boss), "that comment you made yesterday doesn't seem to make sense to me." And he would look at you and say, "All right, you sonovabitch, why doesn't it make sense?" And you would explain, and he would listen, and he would act on it. He would goad you to do an experiment to assess something one way or another. He would encourage you to do a concrete project and see it through, whatever it was: in electrocardiography, on hypertension or a circulatory problem in the dog lab, or with atherosclerosis in the chicken. He would not only press you to complete the project and then prepare an abstract for a meeting; he would say over and over again, "The final product in scientific research is a paper submitted to a journal for peer review. After the peer review what must happen is publication. If you don't do that, the rest is nothing."

He would meet with us at least biweekly on Saturday mornings, reviewing the work of our atherosclerosis research group, including Ruth Pick, Si Rodbard, and myself, and then he would meet with each fellow separately at least every two weeks and the story would always go as follows: "Okay, you're working on this; when will it be finished?" "When are we going to do an abstract?" "When are we going to get a draft of the paper?"

I remember the first paper I authored. It was a "magnificent" piece of writing (I thought) with a discussion a yard long. He and Si took it and sliced it up so that my first reaction was "My God! What have they done to my wonderful paper?"

To give you an idea of what it was like, there were two experiences that occurred when I arrived in January of 1948 that influenced my entire future research career. I arrived on January 2 and went around meeting all the fellows. And, mind you, I was a guy who had read the entire world literature on experimental atherosclerosis, a tremendous expert on a narrow question. I meet a young woman named Dr. Lenel and ask her what she is working on. She tells me that she is finishing her year's fellowship and is about to leave. She says, "I fed salt to chickens."

I look at her, amazed. I knew all about feeding cholesterol to chickens, but what the hell was going on with feeding them salt? She looked at me almost pityingly and told me, "It raises their blood pressure." I asked to see the data, realizing it might be important, and she showed them to me. This was long before the concept of multiple risk factors was recognized, and this was one of the earliest studies published on diet and blood pressure. Before that I used to put lots of salt on everything. But, from that day forward, I stopped adding all that salt to my food.

What was the second experience that influenced you so strongly?

The second experience occurred when Katz called me in for an interview and I was anxious to get started on experimental atherosclerosis. He told me, "We have a little problem. We have working with us for another six months of an eighteen-month fellowship a very capable, very intense Jewish boy from Canada who wants to have a career in research." For a Jew in Canada at the time, this was tough. It turned out that he was doing animal work in atherosclerosis involving the whole chicken lab, and, until he left at the end of June, it would probably be very difficult for me to do any work in that field.

"But," Katz said, "we have another problem for you to work on. Before the war we implanted kidneys in the necks of Goldblatt hypertensive dogs [made so by constriction of the renal arteries]." Rejection occurred, of course, but in the course of the rejection, with the inflammatory reaction, the dogs became normotensive. Katz now had a grant to study renal clearances, other circulatory functions, sequential blood pressure changes, et cetera, in that dog model and wanted me to work on it.

I was flabbergasted. I told him, "Dr. Katz, the only thing I know about Goldblatt hypertension is my brief exposure early in medical school." And about inflammatory reactions, I knew zilch at that time. As for renal clearances and so on, all I knew was what I had read in the physiology textbook. "You're throwing me into a field I don't know anything about. What can I do?" And he looked at me as only a great man like Louis Katz could and said, "How the hell do I know? Go find out!"

So he threw me into the water, as if to say, "You want to be a researcher? So swim."

Well, I began to come in every day in a T-shirt and cotton trousers—working clothes—to learn from the ground up. In dogs we produced Goldblatt hypertension by severely restricting blood flow to the kidneys through the renal arteries. We would do twenty to thirty dogs on an afternoon once a month. I became an expert surgeon in the production of Goldblatt hypertension in dogs. Back where we worked with the dogs was a group of young black men from the neighborhood ghetto around Michael Reese Hospital. Most of them had never finished high school, but they were intelligent, capable, and mature. They were top-level technicians at a time when there were very limited supplies of commercially available laboratory equipment, and they made their own manometers and other instruments for the experiments.

We didn't implant kidneys in the necks of the hypertensive dogs but injected turpentine intramuscularly, as I recall, to produce sterile abscesses, and, sure enough, they did become normotensive. And after about eight months, I had a massive amount of data showing that glomerular filtration and renal blood flow increased despite the arterial ties remaining in place. The results were reported in some of the first papers I published from that laboratory.

Why did they become normotensive?

Improved kidney function? Suppression of the renal ischemia, renin output and release? That all happened decades ago, before the availability of antihypertensive drugs, and there was a short period during which typhoid vaccine was given to lower blood pressure of patients with severe hypertension, presumably the same way, but to this day the mechanism hasn't been worked out, as far as I know. Perhaps cytokines or other substances were released by the inflammatory reaction and influenced blood pressure.

There is an amusing aspect to this story. There was one guy in Chicago at the time who was doing renal clearances in dogs. I learned about him and called him to say that I was new on the scene in Chicago and had been assigned to do renal clearances for a research project at Michael Reese. I told him that I knew nothing about doing renal clearances, and would he mind if I came to observe how he did these in dogs. He told me he was very busy, and, in brief, he gave me the brush-off. Not very nice.

To learn how to do this by myself, I got the great HOMER SMITH's textbook and read about how to do it, including the chemical analyses: para-amino hippurate for renal blood flow, creatinine and other determinations for glomerular filtration rate, all on my own. I would do the experiments during the day and the chemical determinations at night. I worked hard; there were no technicians available for the chemical analytical work on the urines and the bloods; and the grant was small. Well, after a period of eight months when I had accumulated a lot of data and prepared an abstract, I wrote a letter and sent the data to Homer Smith in New York. I get a telephone call from him: "Dr. Stamler—very interesting data. It would be useful to me to be able to sit down and talk with you." He invited me to New York, took me to lunch, and spent four hours with me discussing the work.

I thought about the character in Chicago who didn't have the time to show me anything or even let me watch him doing a procedure, and here was this great scientist, Homer Smith, very busy, with commitments up to his eyeballs, who showed me all this interest and consideration. It taught me a lesson that I never forgot about the role of senior scientists in relation to young people.

> **Richard Bing told me that Homer Smith was the most impressive man he had ever met.**

He was also interesting among medical investigators in that he was a conscious philosopher; and not only a conscious philosopher, but he wrote a book on philosophy expressing that he was an avowed, unabashed materialist. A remarkable guy!

> **There were some remarkable people in Katz's laboratory while you were there. I knew of Simon Rodbard when he was at the City of Hope in Duarte, California, when I was in training. He did some very interesting work that still appears in the medical textbooks: his theory on why the vegetations in bacterial endocarditis appear where they do in the heart. What was he like up close?**

Si, first of all, was very bright. He was a little bit on the sardonic and bitter side, probably because of his early life. He and his brothers had been reared in Memphis, Tennessee, in abject poverty. He came up to Chicago in the depths of the depression to work for Katz as a "diener" in the laboratory. At that time the pay to the "dog boys" was room and board, essentially just enough to live on with practically no money at all. While working, he earned a Ph.D. in physiology and then an M.D. By the time I got there, about ten years after he did, he had become assistant director. These early difficult experiences seem to have scarred him, and he therefore had a tendency to be a little acerbic or sarcastic, but otherwise he was a very bright and pleasant guy.

> **One always reads about how women's contributions to medicine have been overlooked, and Helen Taussig is always brought up in such discussions, but there were also some outstanding women at Michael Reese, I believe.**

One of them was Deborah Dauber. Six weeks before I got out of the army in 1946, Deborah Dauber stepped off a curb on Hyde Park Boulevard in Chicago and was killed by a car. She was in charge of the atherosclerosis research under Katz and planned the course of this research with him and carried it all out. Her tragedy proved to be my opportunity. A few people who knew the literature well in the old days would ask, "What ever happened to Deborah Dauber?" She was the first author on all those early papers on atherosclerosis.

Then there was Ruth Pick. Ruth and ALFRED PICK were one of the few Jewish couples from Czechoslovakia who survived the war and the Nazi Holocaust. It had been a very rough go, as you can imagine, and they were not happy with the Communist regime that came to be in the postwar period. With the help of RICHARD LANGENDORF, the cardiologist and electrocardiographer who had emigrated from Prague earlier, they were able to come to the United States. Ruth had been trained in pathology, but when she first arrived she was shaken up psychologically, withdrawn and uncertain of herself. Katz, wisely, put her to work in the pathology laboratory as a high-level technician, and she was included in our weekly meetings from the beginning. Gradually she opened up and became comfortable psychologically, and, at this time, she became an important contributor to some of the work I was pursuing on atherosclerosis.

I had noticed in our work with chickens that when fed cholesterol in more than minimal amounts, they developed not just hypercholesterolemia but an imbalance among the serum lipids: the phospholipids went up much less than the total cholesterol. What this observation was really reaching for was the lipoprotein story; and this was before [JOHN] GOFMAN and [DONALD] FREDERICKSON separated out and identified the important lipoproteins in the blood and related them to atherogenesis. What we recognize now as HDL (high-density lipoproteins), which are regarded as having an antiatherogenic function, are loaded with phospholipid.

So in 1948 or 1949 I postulated that if instead of having a high ratio of total cholesterol to phospholipids, this dysbalance could be overcome and a normal ratio produced, there might not be atherogenesis despite cholesterol feeding and hypercholesterolemia. Somewhere I had learned that estrogen secretion by hens caused a mobilization in the plasma of cholesterol and calcium for making eggs. But in this case the hyperlipidemia was predominantly due to elevation of phospholipids rather than total cholesterol. So I figured that if we gave cholesterol-fed chickens estrogens, we could get a hyperlipidemia but without imbalance between phospholipids and cholesterol.

Up to that time all the atherosclerosis experiments at Michael Reese involved a very simple approach to evaluating the extent of atherosclerosis: we sacrificed the animals; we opened up the aorta; we laid out the aorta and graded the severity of gross atherosclerosis, blinded as to experimental group. This was cheap and easy but questionable since it was based on the assumption that what was happening in the aorta was representative of what was going on in the whole arterial tree.

A few days after I proposed this study, Ruth Pick, who by this time had become quite settled psychologically, came to me with a request. "I would like on this experiment to cut sections of the coronaries as part of the study." I agreed, and we performed the experiment with controls (only cholesterol feeding) versus chickens given the same cholesterol-supplemented diet but estrogens as well. What happened—in one respect—was just what I had expected: in the estrogen-fed chickens we obtained an elevation of both phospholipids and cholesterol with a normal ratio. But when we opened up the aortas there was severe atherosclerosis in *both* groups. Another great idea down the tubes, and I wrote an abstract reporting our negative findings, that is, no benefit of estrogens in preventing aortic atherosclerosis. Getting the findings on the coronary sections Ruth had to prepare took a good deal more time.

But what did the coronaries show?

No atherosclerosis at all in the coronaries of the estrogen-treated cockerels but extensive coronary lesions in the birds fed cholesterol without estrogen supplements. And we didn't need any statistical analysis to determine this difference: it was severe atherosclerosis in the aorta and none in the coronaries in any of the estrogen-fed chickens. When Ruth first brought me the results of the coronary sections, I tended to ignore them as due to a sampling problem and just told her to get more sections, but they finally sat me down, Katz along with Rodbard and Ruth, and said, "You've got to listen to what this lady is saying: no atherosclerosis in the estrogen-treated group coronaries even though the aortas were full of lesions." To this day we still do not know the cause of this disparity of cholesterol deposition. But we became convinced that a key reason women have less coronary disease than men is physiologic endogenous estrogen secretion, protective, possibly, via high-density lipoprotein (as at least one mechanism).

Incidentally, why did you use chickens for all your experiments?

That began there before I got to Michael Reese. Previously most atherosclerosis research in animals had been done using rabbits, but this was criticized because rabbits are herbivores. Chickens, like humans, are omnivores; they will eat anything. Louis Katz put it this way: "We work with chickens for three reasons: number one, like humans they're omnivorous and not herbivorous; number two, they stand on two legs like human beings; and number three, they have a brain that's small, not all that different from a lot of human beings." He had a great sense of humor.

There was another woman who had a lot to do with your work, your wife, Rose.

Rose and I were married in June 1942. At the end of World War II, as I mentioned, we agreed to use our limited savings to help start my career in research. After a year as a fellow at the Long Island College of Medicine, we relocated to Michael Reese in Chicago in December 1947. Our son, Paul, was born in 1950, and, for a few years, Rose dedicated herself to family life. When Paul was a little older, Rose, who had discontinued her education at Brooklyn College following the sudden and unexpected death of her father, applied for and won a place in a bachelor's-master's program in sociology at the University of Chicago. She worked in the Population Center at the University of Chicago for a few years, where her training and work in demography provided an invaluable background to her future collaboration with our epidemiological studies and clinical trials involving heart disease and high blood pressure. She also worked, for a time, as an administrative assistant to Louis Katz at Michael Reese.

When I moved from Michael Reese to the Chicago Health Department, Rose accompanied me to work on various projects for which we had obtained grant funding from a variety of agencies. Over the next decade, Rose assumed a leadership responsibility for several important undertakings on health problems we addressed in Chicago. In the early seventies, when the NHLBI (National Heart, Lung, and Blood Institute of the NIH) undertook the national cooperative Hypertension Detection and Follow-up Program (HDFP) trial, Rose became the coordinator of that program in Chicago and a coinvestigator on the grant, with me as the principal investigator. She also served on the national steering committee for this study, which became the basis for a whole series of studies on pharmacological and lifestyle (particularly nutritional) interventions for the treatment of hypertension as well as its primary prevention. She was first author or coauthor on a number of publications that derived from this work.

Later on, she was a key force in the organization and conducting of the international teaching seminars on cardiovascular disease epidemiology and prevention, and was often called the mother of these seminars by the fellows who attended them. If I were to enumerate all her contributions, it would take an additional chapter in your book. These are just some examples.

Until the end of her life, even when weakened by heart failure, she continued actively working on the INTERMAP Study. In summary, she was a lifetime companion, friend, wife, collaborator—and a source of inspiration throughout the course of my career.

What is the INTERMAP Study?

INTERMAP stands for International Study on Macronutrients and Blood Pressure, and it is our current major population observational study on dietary factors and blood pressure. Its data, collected in the late 1990s, are from seventeen diverse population samples in China, Japan, the U.K., and the U.S.A. It involves 4,680 men and women ages forty to fifty-nine. Rose was involved in every phase—concept, hypotheses, design, organization, training, and fieldwork to get the data—until her final days in the hospital in February 1998.

> **I want to get this into the record because people don't generally realize this: that for the first ten years of your research career, 1948 to 1958, you were doing basic work in the animal lab even though you later became recognized for your work in epidemiology.**

Before I respond to that question, I would like to mention two other important findings that came out of our animal work. The first was a finding in chicks (cockerels) made hypertensive by administration of salt and DOCA (desoxycorticosterone acetate). When estrogen was administered concomitantly, there was significant suppression of hypertension development. As you know, worldwide prior to the menopause women have lower blood pressures than men. This is probably related to circulating endogenous estrogens, concordant with the findings in that experiment.

The other item I would like to mention is related to hyperglycemia (diabetes) and atherogenesis. We made chicks hyperglycemic by pancreatectomy plus the administration of glucocorticoids. Since humans with diabetes have increased atherosclerosis, we expected to find this in our hyperglycemic chicks when fed cholesterol or cholesterol plus neutral fat. It came as a surprise to us when increased atherosclerosis was *not* found in these chicks. In Canada, Lyman Duff and Gardner

MacMillan, who used rabbits, found the same results when they performed similar experiments in that animal model. However, when both the chicks and the rabbits were "treated" with insulin to control the hyperglycemia, atherosclerosis became severe in both animal models. This apparently was an early demonstration, experimentally, of the phenomenon of hyperinsulinemia leading to increased atherosclerosis. This is a current "rage" among investigators, if I may use that word, which was anticipated by this early animal work.

Now, in response to your question about basic work in the laboratory and clinical work, I would like to qualify it in two ways. First of all, I find imprecise the idea that animal work is basic and other research is not. I've thought and read a lot about what should be considered basic work, and I've come to the conclusion that *basic research is that research whose application is presently not clear.* You can do basic clinical research, basic epidemiological research, and basic animal research. The place where it is done and the methods used do not contribute to and are irrelevant to the definition.

Secondly, my branching out into other areas actually began fairly early. The first such extension was into a clinical trial with estrogen because of the findings in chickens. Not only did estrogen prevent the development of coronary atherosclerosis in cholesterol-fed cockerels, but in later experiments we showed that coronary atherosclerosis that had been induced by cholesterol feeding could be completely *reversed* by subsequent estrogen administration, even though the chickens continued to be fed a high-cholesterol diet. To make a long story short, we organized a randomized controlled trial in men under age fifty who had had one proved myocardial infarction to evaluate the effect of estrogen treatment on subsequent events and survival. We started out with patients at Michael Reese and quickly came to the realization that to get any numbers, we would also have to go elsewhere. I made contact with the cardiologists at the Veterans Administration hospitals in Chicago, and they agreed to participate in the trial. Later, other VA hospitals throughout the Midwest agreed to participate. We eventually recruited about three hundred patients, which was still an inadequate sample. This was early in the game for me and for most researchers concerned with atherosclerotic diseases. I was really not clear on many considerations regarding adequate sample sizes, statistical power, and other aspects of doing this kind of research. We started with lower doses of Premarin (mixed conjugated equine estrogens), and soon realized that the patients were not getting obvious estrogenic effects (such as gynecomastia), so we gave larger doses as starting doses to subsequent patients without building up the doses as we should have. We also erred in simply focusing on the possibility of favorable results; none of us at the time—except for concern about estrogens and breast cancer—considered the other aspect of an investigation like this: what were the possible harmful side effects of the intervention?

I had a very bright research assistant, Dolores Friedman, who came to me after we were well into the study, with the patients then getting a high dose of 10 mg per day. We had a chart on the wall listing the ID numbers of all these patients. She came to me and said, "Jerry, we better review the latest data. There is something going on with the men receiving 10 mg of estrogen as the starting dose." And although it was not statistically significant, we had had a number of thrombosis-related deaths. I nearly fell off my chair and realized that we might have been having the same experience that they also had with the first trial of the "[birth-control] pill" in Puerto Rico, where a few women had major thrombotic complications, coronary or cerebrovascular, which the investigators, even though sincere in their efforts, did not attribute to the medication. That apparently adverse outcome colored all the results in our trial, all reported in the *JAMA* and elsewhere.

That trial was my first departure from animal work while I was at Michael Reese. The second departure was partly due to my initiative and partly due to the second director of the National Heart Institute, James Watt, a career public health officer. Jim Watt was a very bright guy, very astute. He sought to expand epidemiology in the cardio-vascular field. He specifically sought out bright young people who had been well trained by outstanding people in the field. So he sought out Oglesby Paul at Presbyterian–St. Luke's in Chicago, who had been trained by Paul Dudley White, and me, trained by Louis Katz. What I had learned about experimental atherosclerosis induced in chickens by cholesterol feeding plus the interdigitating effects of salt—the beginning of the multiple-risk-factor concept—seemed meaningful for human population studies and lifestyle trials of the kind Watt wanted to bring into being. Watt and his associate, Frank Yeager, another wonderful guy, got together with Katz and me and suggested that I get involved with epidemiological work. It was agreed that I would begin to spend about 20 percent of my time on this. In these discussions Watt and Yeager laid out the rest of my professional life with the main thrusts of epidemiologic work set down: start out with mortality data; then collect cross-sectional and prospective data among living populations; and then study the effects of interventions (i.e., do trials). And that's what I have been doing ever since!

Frank was also instrumental in how I became a principal investigator. Watt and Yeager asked Katz to write a new type of grant proposal for our animal work on atherosclerosis, a *program* grant application, not just a project one—the sole type up until then. Ruth Pick and I put in a great amount of time writing up a draft of a grant for the great man as principal investigator. Katz and Rodbard reviewed and approved it. Then Frank Yeager came out to visit us and go over it all. He was very diplomatic, knowledgeable, and astute. He read the grant through, made a few small suggestions, and then sweetly asked who had prepared this—Louis Katz was listed as the principal investigator with the rest of us in a list below. Katz told him that Ruth and I had done most of the work with some input from him and Rodbard. Then Yeager said, "Well, if you're agreeable, it might be good to have them down as coprincipal investigators." This had never even occurred to Katz, but he immediately agreed.

What finally led to your leaving Michael Reese?

It was a matter of politics. My wife and I had been politically active for years. For instance, when a committee was established in the city of Chicago to protest discrimination in Chicago medical institutions, we participated. At that time Chicago was highly segregated medically. For example, the day my wife and I arrived there in December 1947, there was a strike at the University of Chicago protesting that the Lying-in

Hospital excluded blacks—ironic, because now about 90 percent of the patients there are black. The mortgage on our house, as we discovered when it was all paid, had a clause that it could not be sold to black people in the same Hyde Park neighborhood. We were amazed!

Later on, a distinguished professor of anatomy at Howard University in Washington, D.C., [WILLIAM] MONTAGUE COBB, organized a national Imhotep* conference on discrimination in medicine. People from Chicago were invited; I joined them and took a formal leave of absence from Michael Reese for two days to attend this meeting in Washington at Howard Medical School. When I got back, I was called in by Katz, who pointed out that, at this conference, I was the only white academic research physician who was a registered delegate, as distinguished from observers from certain academic organizations.

He said, "This is very embarrassing for us. The FBI has been here talking to us about you and your leftist activity, and we have decided that when you complete your final year and a half as American Heart Association established investigator, you will have to find yourself another place."

None of that has ever been discussed before by me as part of the public record for a variety of reasons, but perhaps it can be usefully made known now about how things were during the dominance of the McCarthy era and the House Un-American Activities Committee.

> Well, I guess Katz, for all his apparent fiery nature, was a man of his time. Thanks to Wiggers, he had been allowed into the academic cardiology "club," and despite all his accomplishments, he was still insecure and fearful of losing not only his own position but the ability to advance the careers of others that might not have been possible without him.

The behavior, not only of Dr. Katz but the whole administration at Michael Reese, reflected a fundamental sense of insecurity and a "bending of the knee" before the hysteria of the times. Given that Michael Reese was a Jewish institution, they felt that, in the public eye, they had to be—like Caesar's wife—above suspicion. That meant that they had to be in step with the most conservative elements in hewing to the line

---

* Imhotep was the ancient Egyptian equivalent of Aesculapius.

as promoted by McCarthy and the House Un-American Activities Committee. The Michael Reese people didn't realize that such an attitude in response to the powers that be—like that of some Jewish leaders in prewar Europe—was a worse-than-useless tactic in the face of the rising fascistic ideology and policies. It was lost on them.

I discussed all this only once with Dr. Katz, indicating how such a stance was not only irrational and nonscientific, but also dangerous, worse than futile. He wound up by saying, "and they shouldn't discriminate against Jews in medical schools," another way of saying that that was the way of the world and the reality to which I had to accommodate.

I do not in any way condone his behavior toward me, but, in a way, he and the Michael Reese hierarchy were victims of the times. It was a sad story. Now, rather than dwell on this, I like to consider all the positive aspects of my association with Dr. Katz, who taught me so much.

> **When you were having your set-to with the House Un-American Activities Committee, I received a letter from Paul Dudley White, who headed a committee for your defense at the time.[1] I've always felt that Dr. White was to you what Dwight Eisenhower should have been to George C. Marshall, who was also attacked by this element. Whereas Eisenhower, one of the few people in the country who was immune from such attacks, let Marshall down, White, the Boston Brahmin who had a similar position within the medical community, came to your aid. And when Paul Dudley White went to bat for you, although I didn't have much money at the time, I am proud to say that I contributed to that campaign.**

Thousands did.

> **How did you come to work for the city of Chicago after you left Michael Reese?**

When I learned I would be leaving Michael Reese, I began to look around for other opportunities. It turned out that the U.S. Public Health Service and the Chicago Heart Association were very interested in getting the Chicago Health Department involved in cardiovascular disease epidemiology and prevention. They worked together to convince Mayor Richard J. Daley and the czar of the Chicago Health

Department for forty years, old Herman N. Bundesen, to support this with a line item in the city budget for a "heart disease control officer." This would be the first such position in the country and the world. The idea arose that since Jerry was leaving Michael Reese (nobody made public the reasons I was leaving) and going on "to greater glory," maybe, with his interest in epidemiology and public health, Jerry could do this. So, on April 1, 1958, I became the first heart disease control officer in Chicago.

> **And eventually, this led to the Chicago People's Gas Company Study[2] and all the other important studies that followed it.**
>
> **Let's get back to White: He was sort of a paternal figure for you in all this effort. He was one of the earliest people interested in the prevention of coronary disease, wasn't he? I remember at the meetings in Atlantic City, he would exercise on the boardwalk, and people would even poke a little fun at him!**

He was very important early on and for years. He emphasized bicycling, the importance of improving eating habits, and of nonsmoking. He also worked with ANCEL KEYS when Ancel first went to Italy after the war on sabbatical to study diet and coronary heart disease.

> **Tell me about Keys.**

He was originally a physiologist, highly trained (in the U.S., the U.K., and Denmark), who went to the University of Minnesota, where MAURICE VISSCHER was head of the physiology department. Visscher was an excellent physiologist and also a distinguished civil libertarian, another one of the people who helped us in our battle with the House Un-American Activities Committee. Well, Keys and Visscher didn't get along well, perhaps because they were both very strong characters, so Keys wanted out of there.

The University of Minnesota skillfully solved the problem by establishing a Laboratory of Physiological Hygiene with Keys as director, with the facility located under the University of Minnesota football stadium stands. So Gate 27, the entrance, became world-renowned in cardiovascular research, especially epidemiology.

During World War II Keys did studies on human starvation with conscientious objectors who volunteered for this kind of study; and this heightened his interest in nutrition. For reasons I have never learned, Keys understood that, after the war, the "hardening of the arteries" problem, coronary disease in particular, would emerge as a major concern. He also understood the fundamental epidemiological truism that the incidence of this disease would be different in different countries because the exposures to risk factors would be different, including nutritional exposures, especially to dietary lipids. This led to his trip to Italy early in the postwar period, where he thought that, due to differences in lifestyle, particularly diet, the coronary rates would be lower than in the United States.

Paul White joined him, and they published their observation on the rarity of Italian patients in hospital with myocardial infarction. That ultimately led to the famous Seven Countries Study.[3]

I got closely involved with Ancel and Paul in an unusual way. My first World Cardiological Congress was in Mexico City in 1962, where we presented data from our early epidemiological work in living populations in Chicago: on serum cholesterol levels in men and women, black and white. When I walked into the congress hall to register, Paul White and Ancel Keys were standing there and greeted me. "Come with us." "Where?" "The Research Committee of the International Society." (At that time Paul was chairman of this, as I recall.) "I'm not a member of the Research Committee." "Now you are a member." So I was co-opted as a member of the Research Committee and got into international cardiology. Four years later, in New Delhi, Ancel and I were charged to create a council on epidemiology and prevention, and that's how I got up to my eyeballs in the international field.

I first heard about you when, as a young physician, I read your book *Your Heart Has Nine Lives*.[4] Who was your coauthor, Al Blakeslee?

Al Blakeslee was the science writer for the Associated Press for many, many years.

Well, after reading your book, I became a convert and began using Mazola margarine instead of butter. It was a good thing I started young

> because both my parents died later from coronary disease. In those
> days—the early sixties—you couldn't even buy a corn oil margarine like
> Mazola in the supermarket; I had to obtain it from pharmacies.

That's right. And they couldn't say on the label "high in polyunsaturates, low in saturates, and free of cholesterol" because the Food and Drug Administration ruled that, even if this is factually absolutely correct, you cannot say it because it sets in motion a train of ideas that this is good for lowering blood cholesterol and this, in turn, is good for preventing clinical coronary disease, something that—according to the FDA in the sixties—had never been proved! Therefore you could not say this, and that FDA position prevailed for years, although we protested repeatedly. All this is hard to believe nowadays, when just about everyone—finally—is convinced about all this.

> Here is an interesting postscript: Recently, when I had difficulty finding
> Mazola, diet or otherwise, on the shelves, I learned on telephoning the
> company that made it, Best Foods in New Jersey, that it had discontin-
> ued producing this product. I guess that the competition got to be too
> much.

Well, there are other substitutes now that are equivalent, and nowadays we are also concerned to have margarines without trans-fatty acids, a more recent story about an adverse dietary component.

> Your book, which was published over thirty-five years ago, included all of
> the risk factors we now recognize: high blood pressure, high cholesterol
> (dietary and blood), cigarette smoking, obesity, adverse family history,
> diabetes . . . they're all there. But what also struck me about that period
> was that we had what was called an epidemic of coronary heart disease,
> with relatively young men dropping left and right. I recall a number of
> them among my parents' contemporaries. The first question I would put
> to you is: "What made coronary disease so prominent at that time?" The
> second question is: "With all the things we are doing today, are we just
> delaying the inevitable?"

Paul White introduced that term, "an epidemic of coronary disease." You ask two seminal questions. The first one concerns the question of whether there really has been an epidemic. The answer to this is "Yes."

At its worst, in those years, from multiple prospective population studies, we found there was about one chance in five before age sixty or sixty-five of a first major coronary event for American men. These were local studies, because, for the country as a whole, there have been no national data on nonfatal plus fatal events, or for any other total population anywhere. In terms of mortality, we have meaningful trend data with a limitation. The limitation concerns comparability with evolving rubrics (i.e., definitions) in the *International Classification of Diseases and Causes of Death* in its successive editions. (I think we're now up to number eleven.) Modern terminology that clearly identifies a fatal coronary event dates back only to the sixth revision.

Let me give you an example of how such classifications or misclassifications can influence our perceptions. After I was, for a few years, the first heart disease control officer of a city anywhere in the world (Chicago), I liked to point out that I "ended" one "epidemic" and "produced" another. Ridiculous, of course. I "produced an epidemic" of rheumatic fever because we were concerned with the prevention and control of rheumatic fever and got approval of a state program to supply penicillin prophylaxis to every case of known rheumatic fever to prevent recurrences. To do that, we had to identify cases and worked with the medical community to get doctors to report cases that had not been routinely reported before. Up until our program got under way, they were reporting about seven cases per year. In two or three years this went up to three or four hundred. We were just revealing what was there in order to get these kids into this free prophylaxis program.

What epidemic did I "prevent"? If you looked at the Chicago Health Department records from the early and middle part of the twentieth century—and this was true of many health departments—a significant percent of the cardiac death certificates were signed out by coroners. These were unattended sudden deaths at work, or in the street, or at home of people who had died too quickly to be seen by a physician. These were the responsibility of the coroner system we had; there was no medical examiner system in Chicago at that time. And we had two older coroners who, without bothering to spend much time on these cases, would sign them out as "chronic myocarditis."

Now, I recalled the fourth edition of Paul Dudley White's monograph on cardiology—a great book—in which he had a polemic against that term "chronic myocarditis." He said that true chronic myocarditis is almost a nonexistent entity, a very rare condition, and that these cases being signed out as "chronic myocarditis" were actually cases of coronary heart disease with fibrosis of the myocardium resulting from severe atherosclerosis and consequent ischemia, infarction, et cetera.

That's what LEW KULLER showed about sudden unexpected deaths in his population studies.

Exactly, my good friend and colleague, Lew Kuller. So when these two older coroners retired in Chicago, hundreds of death certificates that would have been signed "chronic myocarditis" ceased to be so signed; hence, in this way we "ended" the "epidemic" of chronic myocarditis.

So it was these inadequate kinds of classification that, for a long time, distorted the picture of the coronary problem and made it hard to put together reasonably valid long-term trend patterns. Still, with all these qualifications, the data indicate that from the twenties on it was on the rise.

This reminds me of the one little foray I, myself, had in coronary epidemiology. When my medical school moved to Newark and I was to head the coronary care unit, I expected to see a lot of coronary patients with the large numbers of blacks in Newark, especially with their high blood pressures and heavy cigarette smoking. However, when I got to what was then Martland Hospital, we just weren't seeing them, and, to make a long story short, we found that they were not free of coronary disease; they were not going to other hospitals; they were simply dying outside of the hospital.[5]

Can I tell you my own story in this regard? Working with the help of a young, fine Ph.D. statistician just graduated from Tulane, Marcus Kjelsberg, I gave my first epidemiological paper on the mortality data in Chicago by gender, age, and *race*. We found a high rate of coronary disease in black and white men, possibly a little lower in the black; and a much higher rate in black women than white women. That's when I got into the business of analyzing the coroners' reports because the majority of the deaths among black women were signed out by the coroners. I reviewed every one of their records for a year, and they were a disaster—each just a few words, almost without exception. I even found one coroner's report with a description: "Found dead in bed, needle in vein. Diagnosis: coronary heart disease."

Up until that point I had two piles of published papers; one said coronary disease was higher in whites than blacks, and the other indicated no substantial difference. I gave a paper on this at a pre-lunch-break session at an American Heart Association meeting in Cincinnati. And just as I was going out the door, a young man approached me. With an obvious thick southern accent he said, "That was a very interesting paper; very valuable to me." He was Curtis Hames from Claxton, Evans County, Georgia. He said, "Where I live we don't see coronaries in blacks."

"What about high blood pressure?" I asked, to find out what he really knew about blacks. Promptly he told me that there was a terrible problem of hypertension among the blacks, so it was obvious he knew what was going on in the black population. I said, "Lets go and have lunch."

And over lunch I learned that he was born and bred in Claxton—never left except to go to medical school—and he knew every family in town and provided them with medical care, blacks as well as whites. I told him that he might be right about a low coronary incidence among blacks in rural Georgia; things might be different there than in Chicago. I told him, "What you've got to do is get a grant to study the problem." To make a long story short, I became the "godfather" of the Evans County Study. I introduced him to Frank Yeager, chief of the extramural program at the Heart Institute; Frank helped him prepare a grant proposal the way he once helped me, and that's the origin of the Evans County Study, which has contributed much and is still going on. Although a relatively small study, it is one of the few prospective studies that have been carried out including blacks as well as whites, and with representation of women as well as men among that population.

To turn to something else: do you think personality type—Type A or Type B—has a bearing on the development of coronary heart disease?[6]

My first comment is that it was always a reasonable hypothesis, if formulated as one among several of the etiopathogenetic factors producing the coronary epidemic. Given the relationship of lifestyle and stress to hormonal production, adrenergic stimulation, et cetera, it is possible that, over a long period of time, certain behavioral patterns may add insult to the injury produced by diet, smoking, et cetera. Two points: first, a hypothesis is a hypothesis and must be tested with data; and second, it never made a lot of sense as the key factor in coronary disease.

One problem with Ray Rosenman and MIKE (MEYER) FRIEDMAN, who, incidentally, were old Louis Katz fellows, was that they developed an interview method for diagnosing Type A—before the psychologists came up with a questionnaire—that was not testable. A scientific tool is one that anyone should be able to use and the data should be reproducible. They had a method that only Friedman and Rosenman could use. Furthermore, in promoting their own ideas on this, they tended to downgrade the other risk factors, including the major ones (adverse diet, serum cholesterol, blood pressure, and cigarette smoking) known to be at least as important as Type A, as their own data also showed.

In the MRFIT (Multiple Risk Factor Intervention Trial) Study, we forced them to teach us how to do the interview, and the study produced negative results for Type A/Type B as predictive of coronary risk.

What was the MRFIT study,[7] and what role did you play in it?

I was a member of the Steering Committee and the Design Committee, and I'm still a member of the Editorial Committee now heading ongoing MRFIT work. We wanted to identify a group of men who had not yet experienced any outward manifestations of coronary heart disease, but who had certain risk factors predisposing them to it. The plan was to randomize these individuals into two groups: one with specific interventions to prevent coronary disease from occurring and the other with ordinary care, to demonstrate whether or not our interventions were effective. Some of us deemed it important that this be not only a seven-year trial of preventive interventions but also a longer prospective study. In the course of identifying the 12,866 men who were randomized into the trial, based on the 361,662 who were initially screened, we also picked up over 5,000 men with a history of myocardial infarction, and over 5,000 with drug-treated diabetes. These became the foundation for prospective work on the largest cohorts with these two conditions that have ever been studied. We also acquired the largest number of black men followed prospectively and sizable numbers of Hispanics and Asian Americans, all part of the 361,662 screenees.

> It appears that as we attempt such large trials, the cooperation of large organizations, not only medical but involving the government as well, becomes mandatory.

Throughout my adult life, from the teens on, I have been concerned with public policy matters, initially in the political sphere, but as I became involved in heart research, I realized that public policy here was also very important. Observing and working with people like Louis Katz, Paul Dudley White, Ancel Keys, IRVINE PAGE, and MARY LASKER, all skilled and sophisticated individuals, I became convinced that only through sound national policy could our health goals be achieved.

The concept grew that coronary disease was becoming an epidemic problem in the West, population-wide, and that this was related to a *combination* of risk factors—not only one but two or more—common in our population, with its adverse lifestyles. It was only by addressing this problem in a preventive manner that the epidemic could finally be stopped.

> Well, in recent decades, thanks to such an approach, there has been an apparent decrease in coronary heart disease, but to answer my earlier question: is it disappearing or simply being pushed back in time?

There's no doubt that, as the coronary death rate has gone down and the all-causes death rate, too, as a consequence, we are extending life expectancy. In the fifties and early sixties in this country, especially for middle-aged white men, there was a period when life expectancy was decreasing, and this was of such concern to the Public Health Service that a special report was written as to why this was happening. And it was first and foremost due to the waxing coronary epidemic. That plateaued in the middle sixties, and then the mortality trend was steadily downward through the eighties and into the nineties—the decline was more than 50 percent for the coronary mortality rate and even greater for stroke, but in the nineties the decline slowed for coronaries and stopped for stroke. If the rate of coronary disease is reduced to that of low-risk people, who—regrettably—now make up less than 10 percent of younger and middle-aged adults, life expectancy could be increased by five to nine years for adults, as we reported in *JAMA* in December 1999.[8]

Now, can we conceive of a situation where we might eventually have little cardiovascular mortality, with most mortality in elderly people due to cancer? My answer is "Yes." How can I say this? First on the basis of animal work and second on the basis of findings on coronary rates in that low-risk group we reported, less than one-fifth of what it is for everybody else. Then look at other populations such as in Japan and China, where I have been working on several studies. We see strokes due to hypertension, but few coronaries! And cancer rates too will be reduced by elimination of smoking, by better eating patterns, and by other lifestyle improvements.

Well, we all have to die from *something* . . .

Let me comment on that truism with an anecdote. Many years ago I was invited to speak at a joint Canadian-American meeting of physicians in Ketchikan, Alaska. I had flown to Seattle and then took a hydroplane to get to Ketchikan to give an after-dinner talk for a group that was really on holiday. By the time I got up to speak, they had been drinking before and during dinner, and many of them were high. I showed my slides and gave my talk on the prevention of coronary disease and how this would improve life expectancy and so on, going on for about a half hour.

When the chair asked for questions, one guy got up and, with his slurred speech indicating that he had been putting it away as much as anyone, asked me, "A very fine talk; very interesting. But, tell me, if we are going to keep all these people alive, what are we going to do with them *before* they die after growing so old?"

A good question for a guy that was in the shape he was. I said, "I'll tell you something. I am now about thirty years into research, and in one lifetime, if one wants to be productive, one focuses on one set of questions and leaves other questions for the *next* generation."

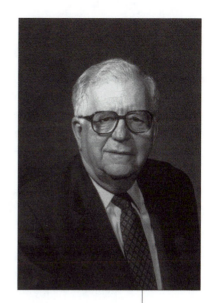

15

Eugene Braunwald, M.D.
(1929–   )

Not since the time of Paul Dudley White has one individual so dominated the field of cardiology over so long a period of time as has Eugene Braunwald. Born in Vienna, he came to the United States as a young boy, fleeing from the Nazis with his family.[1] He continued his education in New York City, where he eventually began his medical studies at New York University. Following his early training as a house officer, he began an association at the National Institutes of Health (NIH), where, over a period of years, he gathered a talented group of young investigators. Under his leadership, this team carried out a major research program on many basic aspects of cardiac function and physiology, reevaluating certain important concepts that had gone unchallenged for a half century.

Following the NIH years, he turned his talents to the creation of a department of medicine at the newly created medical school at the University of California in Davis, while continuing there some of his most important work on the limitation of infarct size in acute myocardial infarction. Recognition of his organizational and administrative ability as a chairman of medicine led to an offer from Boston to perform the same function at Harvard Medical School.

Dr. Braunwald has always demonstrated an uncanny ability to consider all existing facts, no matter how contradictory or confusing they might seem, about any particular problem and create a framework for their understanding and effective clinical application. These same skills, along with his superior ability to organize and present the latest medical knowledge, led to his becoming chief editor of one of the leading textbooks of medicine (*Harrison's Principles of Internal Medicine*) and his own textbook on cardiovascular disorders (*Heart Disease*), both of which contain important sections written by him with his usual clarity, balanced approach, and intelligence. In recent years his organizational ability has also been reflected in his heading of the TIMI (Thrombolysis in Myocardial Infarction) Trials, which have gone on for over fifteen years in evaluating different aspects of the effects of blood clot dissolution in acute myocardial infarction.

There is a line from *Twelfth Night* that seems particularly apt when reviewing the career of Dr. Braunwald: "Some are born great, some achieve greatness, and some have greatness thrust upon them." Certainly Dr. Braunwald was born with great ability. He achieved greatness by wise career choices and years of incredibly hard work. Thanks to his natural gifts and the energy and wisdom with which he has applied them, he has richly deserved the many honors that have been showered upon him as one of the great cardiologists of our time.

Boston, Massachusetts
July 26, 2000

If I were to characterize your career, I would paraphrase what Caesar said about Gaul; like Gaul, it is divided into three parts: Bethesda, San Diego, and Boston. But actually, the beginnings of your life in cardiology began much earlier, even as a medical student, and then with stops at every possible desirable place one could imagine on your way to a career in cardiology. Could you recount this for me?

I have been extremely fortunate throughout my professional life to have been at the right place, with the right people, at the right time, and I believe it is fair to say that I tried to make the most of the wonderful opportunities presented to me. In medical school there were two events that excited my interests in cardiology. The first was at Bellevue Hospital, where they had something called the Thursday night cardiac clinic.

This clinic allowed second-year medical students to interact with patients in a continuity clinic. Second-year students, after four long years of premedical studies and the first year of medical school, are so eager for this type of professional interaction without a faculty member in the room (although later the faculty member, of course, came in for supervision). This opportunity, unique to cardiology at NYU, enticed a disproportionate number of students into this specialty.

The second defining event was a three-month elective I took as a fourth-year medical student at New York University in a catheterization laboratory with LUDWIG EICHNA. Mind you, we are talking about 1951, and cardiac catheterization was not yet a routine procedure. It was a research procedure being carried out at, perhaps, ten laboratories in the country. Eichna was an extraordinary mentor and he was studying congestive heart failure, and this gave me the opportunity to get involved with serious research on the hemodynamics of heart failure patients.

Eichna was an interesting individual; my understanding is that he led sort of a monastic existence with few interests in life other than medicine.

We shouldn't say "was," because he is still alive. He is a bachelor and was very focused on medicine, although I think he also liked mountain climbing. He was in his laboratory at seven in the morning and didn't leave until ten in the evening, so he seemed to be married to medicine. He demonstrated to me that research is a serious business that can be quite demanding.

Because heart catheterization was so new at the time, I wonder where he learned it.

I believe that he picked it up from André Cournand, who was also at Bellevue Hospital. Bellevue Hospital was blessed with two catheterization labs at the time.

Your next step was Mount Sinai . . .

Yes. I took my internship and then a year of cardiology there. I was afforded great opportunities in cardiology. Cardiac surgery was just beginning, and we had a very cooperative cardiac surgeon who was also chairman of the department, Mark Ravitch. He was willing to puncture the chambers of the left side of the heart at operation, enabling us to make the first direct measurements of pressure gradients across stenotic human heart valves in 1953. We evaluated, also for the first time, the effects of mitral valvotomy. This was pretty heady stuff for a twenty-five-year-old, and I was given the privilege of being first author of the paper in *Circulation* describing these measurements.[2]

> **What contact did you have with CHARLES FRIEDBERG? You didn't do any papers with him . . .**

No, I didn't author any papers with him, but I did get to know Charles Friedberg reasonably well. He was not yet chief of cardiology; ARTHUR MASTER was the chief of cardiology, and Charles Friedberg was an internist who happened to be *interested* in cardiology. He was a spell-binding clinician. I should really go back and tell you that, during the summer of 1949 between my first and second years of medical school—this was even before those Thursday night cardiac clinics—I worked as a technician in the Department of Chemistry at Mount Sinai Hospital. On afternoons, when my work was completed, I would attend ward rounds with Charles Friedberg, and I came under the spell of this extraordinary clinician. As an intern, I saw him in the library at Mount Sinai very late at night, working on his classic textbook, *Diseases of the Heart,* from which I learned cardiology.

> **I think he was the last American to write a single-authored book on cardiology.**

That's right. So I got to know this great clinician very early in my professional life. Later on, after I had gone to the NIH [National Institutes of Health] and I started to travel and speak at meetings, I found myself on programs with him. We formed a good friendship.

Now let's fast forward to 1972. When Charles died tragically in an auto accident, he was working on the fourth edition of his textbook. Several months after he died, shortly after I had arrived in Boston, I received a call from his publisher, W. B. Saunders, Inc., asking if I would be willing to complete the fourth edition. Mrs. Friedberg had suggested this to them. It was, of course, tempting, but I had just come to Harvard and the Brigham and saw that working on this book would be an enormously time-consuming effort. I told them I just couldn't do it at that time. But I was intrigued. I said, "I'll do it, but I want to do it right. In six years I will take a sabbatical and take a full year off to prepare the text."

To make a long story short, they couldn't wait six years for the revision of the Friedberg book, but Saunders was willing to wait six years for my own textbook on heart disease, which, although multiauthored, turned out to be the successor to Friedberg's book.

I've heard a number of stories about Mount Sinai having various factions and feuds at that time. Is there any truth to them?

It is true that it was highly political, but not more political than Boston academic medicine is right now. You know, when you have competitive people with limited turf, they get to stepping on each other's toes. There were a lot of talented people at Mount Sinai in the fifties, and I don't think the situation there was very different from that at Harvard in the year 2000. I am reminded of Holly Smith's saying, "Why are academic medical politics so dirty? Because the stakes are so small."

Your next stop after Mount Sinai was Bellevue.

By the time I got back to Bellevue Hospital, I had already worked at two cardiac catheterization laboratories: under Eichna when I was a student and at Mount Sinai under Al[fred] Gordon. I had been extremely productive that year at Sinai. There were papers on vectorcardiography with Arthur Grishman; the hemodynamics of pregnancy published in the *JCI* (*Journal of Clinical Investigation*) and, of course, the first measurements of transvalvular pressure gradients in patients, which I mentioned earlier. By the end of the Mount Sinai experience, I was afforded the opportunity to take a second fellowship in cardiovascular research with "The Grand Master of Cardiovascular Science," André Cournand. It was the year before he won the Nobel Prize. By today's standards, it was a small laboratory with only three fellows, so I got to see a good deal of "The Chief." Times were different then; people weren't traveling all over the world; Cournand attended about four out-of-town meetings per year. So he was in the lab every day looking at pressure tracings with us and discussing hemodynamic-clinical correlations. That was very different from the way that labs are run now.

> I looked into a job with him at one time as I was leaving my fellowship in Utah, and in the interview he almost blew me out of my seat, he was so intense and probing about my future plans, which I admit were a bit hazy. He went on and on, like a district attorney grilling a felon. How did you find him to work with?

He was gruff, a very demanding micromanager . . . but, as I said, he was "The Grand Master." During the time I was in New York, before I even went to medical school, I attended a lot of concerts of the NBC Symphony Orchestra conducted by Arturo Toscanini, arguably the greatest conductor of the twentieth century. In order to get a first row seat, I would go up there early, getting on line outside of Studio 8, and I must have seen Toscanini at least seventy-five times close up. I thought that these two men were alike; both were prima donnas, but also at the top of their fields.

> Did you have any contact with DICKINSON RICHARDS when you were there?

He was around, but he was remote figure, a "grand old man." André Cournand was extremely respectful of him, and, of course, they shared the Nobel Prize [with Werner Forssmann]. Richards came to some of the laboratory conferences, but I never really interacted with him either personally or intellectually. He was a quiet, austere person.

> Did they have a cath lab at Columbia-Presbyterian uptown at this time, or was all the work done at Bellevue?

There was a "satellite" cath lab at Presbyterian Hospital. However, Cournand and Richards were the archdeacons of the enterprise for Columbia University.

> Aside from yourself, were there others who came out of that laboratory after a fellowship and distinguished themselves?

First of all, you have to remember that Cournand was principally a pulmonary physiologist, and at first he was interested in catheterizing the heart in order to obtain mixed venous blood. There were flocks of pulmonary physiologists in the laboratory such as Richard Riley. Others who became leaders included ALFRED P. FISHMAN, Harry Fritts, and Lars Werkö.

After Bellevue came the NIH and a fellowship with STANLEY J. SARNOFF. Tell me about him.

He was a dazzling, flamboyant figure who had an extraordinary knack for experimental design, some of which I learned from him. He knew how to develop and test a hypothesis. It was an exciting period for me to roll up my sleeves, with Sarnoff allowing me to become a full participant in experiments on the determinants of myocardial oxygen consumption. Subsequently, this became my principal interest. He was a free spirit who kept his own working hours and was also involved in commercializing his medical discoveries. He had been trained in surgery and anesthesiology and brought these disciplines to bear on cardiovascular physiology. He was the leading experimental circulatory physiologist of the fifties and sixties with a truly grand view of the circulation. He had a powerful influence on me.

Today, there is a foundation in his name that supports young researchers.

Yes. It's a very large foundation because, after leaving the NIH, Stanley developed a company called Survival Technology and most of the income from that company goes to this foundation. It is emblematic of his generosity and commitment to cardiovascular science, to which he contributed so much.

What led you to go to Johns Hopkins after the NIH?

After my two years of fellowship, I was invited to stay at the NIH, but I felt that I had to complete my residency in order to become a "complete" doctor. I chose Hopkins because I had dragged my wife, NINA (now deceased), from New York, where she had been the first woman surgical resident at Bellevue Hospital, to Washington, D.C. When I came to the NIH in Bethesda, she transferred from New York to Georgetown, located in Washington, D.C., which is not far from Bethesda. While I was training in cardiovascular research at the NIH, she was climbing the surgical residency ladder. So Johns Hopkins, conveniently located (for us) in Baltimore, was the best place in the area for me to complete my medical residency. At Hopkins there were no nights off for the house staff. (In my twenty-eight years as a chairman of medicine, I have been fighting a losing battle on this as the residents insist on more and more time off!)

Who was it at Hopkins that made you the more complete physician you wanted to be?

There were a number of great people there. The chairman of medicine, [A. McGHEE] "MAC" HARVEY, was a very hands-on chief, who tirelessly made daily ward rounds with the house staff. Phil Tumulty was a giant of clinical medicine. "Coke" Andrus was a great chief of cardiology. RICHARD ROSS, who later became chief of cardiology, taught me a great deal. I also got to know HELEN TAUSSIG, the "mother" of congenital heart disease. While I was doing a medical residency, I wasn't going to pass up the opportunity to learn from these greats.

In the two years at the NIH while I worked with Sarnoff, I did a lot of clinical cardiology, and, of course, the frontier of cardiac surgery at that time was congenital heart disease. So I became very interested in congenital heart disease when I returned to the NIH following my medical residency at Hopkins, and I published in the field. I was actually offered Helen Taussig's job when she retired as head of pediatric cardiology.

That occurred in 1959, and I was overwhelmed by this offer. By this time, Nina was working in cardiac surgery under (ANDREW) GLENN MORROW at the NIH, and I also was working in the Department of Surgery as director of the catheterization laboratory. When I was offered Helen Taussig's job, I was anxious to accept. We even began to look for a home located between Bethesda and Baltimore.

I had been very happy during my residency at Johns Hopkins. It had a great influence on my subsequent twenty-eight years as a chairman of medicine. Hopkins opened my eyes to many aspects of medical care and education that I had not appreciated in New York. And then, at the age of thirty, to be offered the opportunity to succeed Helen Taussig, a towering, almost legendary figure in world cardiology, made me feel as if I had been struck by lightning. So I went to Bob Berliner (head of intramural research at the NIH National Heart Institute) on a Friday and told him about this offer. He said, "That's terrific, but don't make any decisions until Monday."

Well, there was nothing I could do anyway over the weekend, and the following Monday he offered me the position as head of the Cardiology Branch at the (then) National Heart Institute.*

So that's how it happened!

That's how it happened.

It's not widely known that in addition to doing so much research in myocardial function, myocardial oxygen consumption, and preservation of ischemic myocardium, you did a tremendous amount of work early on in congenital heart disease.

We helped develop the use for diagnosis of indicator dilution curves, and the use of inhaled radioactive Krypton gas in the detection and measurement of shunts. But also, Morrow was starting his open-heart surgery program, and, at that time, approximately 85 percent of such operations involved correction of congenital heart defects, principally in older children. Then, around 1963 or 1964, I began to feel insecure in regard to managing infants and younger children. It was then that I recruited Bill Friedman (also from Johns Hopkins) to become the first pediatric cardiologist in the Cardiology Branch at the NIH.

In reviewing your bibliography, I noticed that you have published over eighty papers with Andrew Morrow. Tell me about him.

He was an extraordinary person. We worked very closely for nine years and had a wonderful partnership. Glenn was about six years older than

---

* A position that was obviously created to keep Braunwald at the NIH.

I and certainly was the senior partner. He was by far the most brilliant cardiac surgeon that I have ever encountered, and I have encountered the best. He had an appreciation of physiology and was a very good self-taught cardiologist. He had trained in surgery at Johns Hopkins and then at Oxford. I consider him (along with Eichna, Cournand, Sarnoff, and Berliner) to have been one of my five most important mentors.

> Let's start with your work on ventricular function, then myocardial oxygen consumption, and then the reduction of infarct size. Our generation of trainees in cardiovascular research cut our teeth on reading papers on the heart by ERNEST H. STARLING, C. L. Evans, and their associates;[3] this was a requirement. However, their work, which was conducted in the first decade or so of the twentieth century, never underwent any further scrutiny until the midcentury. I think the first to reexamine Starling's Law of the Heart were Sarnoff and Berglund at Harvard just before you joined Sarnoff's laboratory at the NIH. They found out that there was not just one curve of ventricular function with a descending limb but that an actual family of curves could be described based on sympathetic stimulation et cetera.[4] How did you get into all of this?

I got into it when I came back to the NIH from Hopkins and established my own laboratory. My colleagues and I published nine papers entitled: "Starling's Law of the Heart in Man, I to IX." This line of research, on the control of cardiac contraction, began with the great German physiologist OTTO FRANK, who worked with the isolated frog heart at the end of the nineteenth century; then Ernest Starling early in the twentieth century in the dog heart-lung preparation; then Stanley Sarnoff in the intact dog in the fifties; then we took this into man in the sixties.

> I had forgotten this, but on reading your papers, I became aware again that to study the human heart in cardiac surgery patients, you actually sewed strain gauges and other devices onto their ventricles. Do you think you could get away with this today?

Probably not, although there were absolutely no adverse effects. Actually, Glenn Morrow sewed the strain gauges on the right ventricle at operation.

What about the determinants of myocardial oxygen consumption?

That work began with Sarnoff, as I mentioned earlier, and then, about eight years later, I returned to this in my own laboratory, working with several talented colleagues—John Ross, EDMUND SONNENBLICK, and James Covell. With Sarnoff we devised the tension-time index in the fifties to predict myocardial oxygen consumption; and then in the sixties we learned that catecholamines increase oxygen consumption while reducing the tension-time index, and that's how we came to identify myocardial contractility as an independent determinant of myocardial oxygen consumption, one as important as the tension-time index.[5]

> Evans and Matsuoka, who studied oxygen consumption back at the beginning of the twentieth century in Starling's dog heart-lung preparation, actually thought external work was the major determinant of the heart's oxygen consumption,[6] but your work emphasized that this was not the whole story and that several other factors came into play as well. Is this a fair statement?

Exactly.

> Were you influenced at all by DONALD GREGG because he was the doyen of the coronary circulation at the time?[7]

Oh, yes. He was close by at Walter Reed, and I got to know him. Like Dickinson Richards, he was a towering but somewhat remote figure. I visited his laboratory on a number of occasions, and I even got to know *his* mentor, CARL WIGGERS, whom I regard as the greatest cardiac physiologist of the twentieth century, perhaps of all time.

> I was about to ask you that because Wiggers was the CARL LUDWIG of his time, producing so many outstanding circulatory physiologists.

Precisely. Wiggers was quite gruff, a person who wasted no words, of the *Geheimrat* (autocratic professor) school. He had studied with the great Otto Frank and introduced the European approach to physiology to America. You couldn't argue with him. Of course he was always right, so there was no reason to argue with him!

It became apparent that Starling's isolated dog heart preparation had problems; it was isolated, denervated, failed after a time, et cetera. You, however, used a preparation involving an intact dog that was instrumented and supported by another intact dog. I was wondering if the source of this was C. WALTON LILLEHEI's technique of cross-circulation used in operations for congenital heart defects.[8]

Yes.

Tell me now about how you got into the work on reduction of infarct size.

Three events led to this: (1) We were studying myocardial oxygen consumption in the dog in one laboratory in my department; (2) We were studying the carotid sinus control of the circulation in the laboratory next door; (3) I had visited the University of Rochester where I had met Seymour Schwartz, who was then a young instructor in surgery. He took me to his lab to show me dogs with experimentally produced hypertension in which he was reducing blood pressure by stimulating the carotid sinuses using a cardiac pacemaker. When I was flying back to Washington, it occurred to me, "Why can't we stimulate the carotid sinus in patients?" Not constantly, but on demand. So that evening I talked to Nina about it, and I asked her to consider sewing electrodes to the carotid sinuses of patients with intractable angina, and we would then stimulate these nerves using a radiofrequency pacemaker.

She had risen to be deputy chief of the Surgical Division by that time and had the authority to do it. This work is now a cul-de-sac in the history of the treatment of coronary artery disease because it was only two years later that René Favaloro developed coronary bypass surgery and blew this approach to the treatment of angina out of the water. But it did relieve intractable angina. Carotid sinus nerve stimulation reduces myocardial oxygen demands because it slows heart rate, reduces contractility, and reduces arterial pressure, the three principal determinants of myocardial oxygen consumption that we had defined.

There was one pivotal patient who brought all this home to us. This patient had had the stimulator implanted six months earlier. He came to the NIH in the throes of experiencing a myocardial infarction. We advised him to turn the stimulator off. However, against my express instructions he turned it on, that is, stimulated his carotid sinus nerves while the infarction progressed. When I turned it off, his electrocardiographic ST segments shot up; and when, on his own, he turned the stimulator back on, the ST segments came down. I realized then, "My God, we can influence myocardial infarct size!"

> But, as you say, back then the idea of carotid sinus stimulation was overshadowed by the advent of coronary bypass surgery.

That's true, but because of the demonstrated effects of carotid sinus stimulation on myocardial oxygen demands, we developed the idea that by lowering oxygen consumption in the setting of acute myocardial infarction, you could reduce infarct size.

> I recall that in his book *Clinical Heart Disease*, SAMUEL LEVINE mentions the effects of carotid sinus stimulation on angina.[9] He used the technique of massaging over the carotid sinus in the neck as a test for diagnosing angina in patients with chest pain. If it relieved the chest pain despite the physician suggesting the opposite, "Is it worse?" then that was angina. I was wondering if you were aware of this.

You're right! What a memory you have! *[Removes his copy of Levine's book from the bookcase behind him.]* But the carotid sinus nerve stimulation in the diagnosis of angina was only a way station, because it was that specific patient who was undergoing a myocardial infarction and used carotid nerve stimulation—against my instructions—to reduce his elevated ST segments who carried this an important step farther.

> Let's talk about IHSS (idiopathic hypertrophic subaortic stenosis). In the mid- to late fifties a number of people, including your own group, began to report isolated cases of this condition, but you and Morrow really put the disease on the map.

Glenn Morrow and I were there very early in the recognition of this disease. In 1959 we published a paper describing two patients with what we then called "functional aortic stenosis."[10] Later we published several larger series of such patients to define the characteristics of the disease (which was then named idiopathic hypertrophic subaortic stenosis or IHSS), its diagnosis, treatment, and natural history.[11]

> Of course we realize now that what we called IHSS then is really one
> form of a hypertrophic cardiomyopathy that can be obstructive or nonob-
> structive. But people forget that there was a good deal of controversy
> between your group and Mike Criley, who said that all the reported
> obstruction was really due to catheter entrapment.* That went on for
> years and must have caused you an awful lot of grief.

It did. Mike Criley and I had been residents together at Johns Hopkins,
and we knew each other well. In the midsixties he was a member of the
Hopkins Cardiology Division under Dick Ross, and we had this program in which every other Friday one group visited the other for a conference. On one of our visits to Hopkins he presented this notion, and
I went ballistic! I found his idea threatening because Glenn Morrow
had developed a surgical procedure for correction of the obstruction—
the myotomy/myomectomy (now called the "Morrow Operation"),
and we were referring patients with severe obstruction to him for this
procedure. If Mike was correct, then there was no purpose to the surgery (which was not without risks). It was not only a matter of intellectual pride as to whether we were right or wrong; the well-being of
patients was involved.

> Is that why John Ross developed the transseptal technique to get left
> atrial and ventricular pressures, avoiding the problem of entrapment this
> way?

No, he developed that much earlier to enable us to measure left atrial
pressures through a venous route, without requiring the assistance of
surgeons to cut down on arteries (before the popularization of the
Seldinger percutaneous technique for arterial access). By using the
transseptal approach [puncturing the atrial septum to advance a needle and then a catheter from the right atrium to the left atrium; see Fig.
3-1], we could measure left atrial pressure and then advance the tip of
the catheter just beyond the mitral valve into a part of the left ventricle

---

*A well-known phenomenon, especially in hyperdynamic hearts when, if a catheter tip
is located near the left ventricular wall, for example, on contraction, the ventricle will
squeeze the tip of the catheter and result in the recording of a falsely high pressure with
a factitious gradient created between the left ventricle and the aorta showing on the
pressure monitors.

where there was no question of catheter entrapment and that's how we proved that true obstruction does exist in what is now called hypertrophic *obstructive* cardiomyopathy or HOCM.

> And, of course, when echocardiography came in, without any catheters in the heart, this was another clincher in demonstrating the gradient and settling the matter.
>
> Now, what made you leave the NIH for San Diego? It seemed to be a very strange move for you at that time.

In retrospect, it was. I had spent twelve wonderful years at the NIH, but I was getting restless. Let me put it this way: I love eating steak, a culinary analogy to conducting research, but work at the NIH was like eating steak three times a day, seven days a week. So one part of what went into my decision was that I began to feel confined, and I wanted to try my hand at something else. But there was another piece. I was now into infarct size reduction, and I couldn't do that at the NIH because we had no emergency room to which patients with acute myocardial infarctions (AMI) were referred. As a matter of fact, in 1967 I worked very hard to develop a collaboration with the D.C. General Hospital to have our cardiology division run the coronary care unit there and thereby provide us with an entrée into clinical investigation in AMI. The leadership at D.C. General was very cooperative, but it turned out that very few patients with AMIs were actually admitted there.

> The AMIs were dying out of the hospital; we learned that in Newark.[12]

So I realized that if I was going to pursue this problem, it couldn't be in Bethesda or Washington, D.C. I was also interested in helping to develop and lead a new medical school. Looking back on it, it was pretty arrogant for me to take this job (and it was gutsy of the university to offer it to me) because I hadn't really been in a medical school since I had been a student, and now I was at the center of developing a curriculum and everything else entailed in starting a new school. I must tell you that as I look back on those four years in San Diego, from a cardiology point of view they were the best four years of my life.

Why?

We were in the desert, literally, but everything I had done before seemed to be a preparation for this work on infarct size reduction. And everything I have done since has been a continuation of the work in San Diego. We had a wonderful group. My research fellow was the late PETER MAROKO, and, of course, I brought a number of outstanding colleagues from Bethesda: John Ross, BURT SOBEL, Bill Friedman, Peter Pool, and Jim Covell. We worked together as a team, and things just fell into place.

> **Being a chairman of medicine today is such a big job. How were you able to do your cardiac work and be a chairman at the same time in San Diego?**

When I went out there, I did not expect that I would be doing much research. Obviously I had the reduction-of-infarct-size project in mind, but I really went out there to be a chairman. I felt that I was going to completely change my career after doing research for about eighty hours a week for twelve years in Bethesda. I was no longer going to be a chief of cardiology; John Ross was chief of cardiology. However, I decided that I would just do research a half-day a week and have one part-time fellow assigned to me. Back at the NIH I was involved in twenty or so research projects simultaneously; it wasn't an assembly line, but it was a *mega lab*. So now I decided that out of a possible twenty projects I would select only one—and, of course, that was infarct size reduction. As time went on, I realized that I wasn't really prepared to give up research. So even though, since leaving the NIH, now thirty-two years ago, I have always had administrative positions, research has been, at the minimum, a 30 percent effort and, at times, as much as 50 or 60 percent.

> **Things were going well in San Diego, but then you came to Harvard. I suppose the call from Boston was just too hard to resist.**

When someone asked Senator Jack Kennedy why he wanted to run for president, Kennedy said, "If you're going to be in politics, then there is only one job." So if you are going to be in academic medicine, how could you not want to be chairman of medicine at Harvard and the Brigham?

> You did something that was not only very nice but also very wise when you headed medicine at the Peter Bent Brigham Hospital. For an earlier book I interviewed Louis Weinstein, who was there at the time. When I visited him there, I learned that you had hired a number of senior people like Weinstein, who were considered by the medical establishment to be past their prime or over the hill, et cetera. You had the good sense to hire older people like Weinstein who really still had a lot to offer.

Oh, yes. There was also Dan Federman, who had been chairman of medicine at Stanford; Bud (Arnold) Relman, who had been chairman of medicine at Penn and was editor in chief at the *New England Journal of Medicine;* Lou Weinstein; and others. We had an incredible senior faculty.

> I think that allowing these outstanding people to continue to contribute irrespective of age was a great credit to you. And while you were at the Brigham you got into the whole business of myocardial stunning.* Could you tell me about that?

I have always been very interested in heart failure as well as ischemia, and the two intersect when it comes to stunning. I did not make the original observation; it was made by Steve Vatner, who had been a fellow of mine in San Diego. When I came to Boston, I brought only Steve, Peter Maroko, and Peter Libby. Steve went on and established an independent laboratory here at Harvard. Although he didn't call the phenomenon "stunning," he was the first to describe it.

But Bob Kloner and I began to realize that this phenomenon had very important implications for clinical cardiology that hadn't been appreciated. That's when we named it "stunning." So although I didn't describe it, I do think that I helped put it on the map.[13] And the most important original suggestion that we made was about the importance

---

* "Stunning" in acute myocardial infarction is a situation in which portions of the heart muscle surrounding a central area of severe ischemia do not move when viewed by radiological or ultrasonic techniques but are still viable. This jeopardized myocardium can thus go either way, being ultimately destroyed or later restored to function depending upon the management of the acute myocardial infarction.

of "chronic stunning," now called "hibernation,"* which is now recognized as the most important reversible and treatable cause of heart failure.

What made you take the chairmanship at Beth Israel Hospital at this time? You already had so much on your plate.

I look back and I wonder. In retrospect, it was probably not a good idea. But these two great hospitals, the Brigham and the BI (Beth Israel), both major Harvard teaching hospitals, were "cheek to jowl" yet operating in a very competitive mode. The search for a new chief of medicine at BI wasn't going well. Dan Tosteson, then dean of the Harvard Medical School, suggested to me, "Why don't you do this on an interim basis and maybe you can help bring the two hospitals closer together?" "Interim" was supposed to be two years, and it turned out to be nine. And I never managed to bring the two hospitals together. But maybe this will still happen. Who knows?

Let's get back to the research story: When you mentioned all the projects you carried on at the NIH, I remembered attending the FASEB (Federation of American Societies for Experimental Biology) meetings in Atlantic City, where you would show up with all your fellows en masse. You would enter a meeting room like a phalanx, and one fellow would deliver a paper, followed by applause, and on to the next, then the next, like a cheering squad.

Well, we had an extraordinarily talented team!

A tremendous team. What happened to all of them after they left?

About eighty of my former trainees have gone on to become heads of cardiology, medicine, or deans. Remember, I'm not bashful and I'm not modest, but I started this interview by saying that I was in the right place at the right time, and this threw me together with the best and the brightest young scientists. The years that I was at the NIH were the hey-

---

* "Hibernating" myocardium refers to poor or abnormal heart wall motion in patients with chronic heart dysfunction or failure due to coronary disease. The subnormal motion, related to inadequate coronary blood flow, can be reversed following revascularization by surgery or angioplasty.

day of the intramural program. The division that I ran was the first integrated cardiology division (of which there are now many). We had two hemodynamic laboratories, a cardiology ward, a papillary muscle laboratory under Ed Sonnenblick, a dog laboratory, and a biochemistry laboratory. That is commonplace now, but in 1960 it was the first of its kind. The military draft was still on during this period, and service in the Public Health Service at the NIH satisfied the requirement for military service. This aided in the recruitment of research fellows. When we went to San Diego, we were still extremely competitive in attracting bright young people and had our pick of the best. And here at Harvard you don't have to look very far for outstanding research fellows.

> Turning to the future of research, I want to begin with an example from the past: When Howard Florey wanted to test the therapeutic efficacy of penicillin, he took eight mice and injected them with lethal doses of streptococci. Then he gave penicillin to four of them. These four survived, and the untreated four died. Penicillin worked! Even in our own time, back in the sixties, if you wanted to test something, you went to the lab and took seven or eight dogs to try it out on, and if six of seven or seven of eight demonstrated your hypothesis to be valid, you reached a p value of less than .05 and had proved your point.
>
> Today in cardiovascular research we seem to be drowning in an alphabet soup of studies involving hundreds or even thousands of patients to show that a bit more of drug A is more effective than a little less; or that drug A given before drug B is better than the reverse or if they are given simultaneously. These marginal benefits at such great cost trouble me, and since you have been involved for years in the TIMI (Thrombolysis in Myocardial Infarction) study, now well into its twenty-fourth or -fifth reincarnation, I put it to you: do you really obtain any satisfaction from this kind of research involvement?

The questions in cardiovascular medicine have changed, and therefore the methods designed to answer them must change. You know, you can demonstrate infarct size reduction in the rat heart or the dog heart, and we did this for more than fifteen years. But there's a big step from demonstrating infarct size reduction in a controlled animal model to helping a patient. I know that what I am about to say will be shocking to you, but I believe that one of the most important medical developments of the twentieth century was the Kefauver Commission. In the sixties that commission, headed by the late Senator [Estes] Kefauver of Tennessee, was looking at the operation of the FDA [Food and Drug Administration] and concluded, logically, that for the agency to approve a drug or device, it was necessary to prove clinical efficacy and safety. A surrogate endpoint—such as what happens to the height of the V wave on an atrial pressure recording—is simply not enough. You need to demonstrate how many patients must be treated to save one life, or to prevent one hospitalization, or to prevent one MI.

> **Let's say that after studying thousands of patients, you determine that one of these interventions drops the death rate—I'm making the figures up—from 8 percent to 7.6 percent; would you find this satisfying?**

Yes, very. It may sound mundane, but I come back to being a doctor, and if you can reduce the mortality of MI by even a single percentage point, you're talking about saving more than twenty thousand lives per year, worldwide. Isn't that what it's all about? Now when we do these trials, we are asking many questions other than drug efficacy, and we use this population of thousands of patients in many ways. So my answer to your question is resoundingly positive. What is challenging when you devise a large clinical trial is to set up all of the other questions that can be answered.

> **I have no ax to grind like one of those old-time clinical cardiologists who has never gone into the dog lab, but with the advent of molecular cardiology at the leading edge of research today, I'm wondering if the people doing this kind of research are capable of fulfilling the faculty role of teaching and patient care that we usually associate with academic cardiologists.**

In our earlier days, yours and mine, we recognized the Renaissance figures, the Paul Dudley Whites and Charles Friedbergs of cardiology. You don't find those kinds of people anymore. In current cardiovascular research, the molecular aspects are so demanding of time and effort and energy. The fact is that when you are an M.D. cardiologist conducting molecular research, you are forced to compete with Ph.D.'s out of great technical universities such as MIT who are ten years younger than you. This requires you to run very, very fast. And you cannot carry a beeper and be available to the HMO and conduct meaningful basic research at the same time.

That's pretty tough on the medical student.

It's very tough, but in the present era, if people are going to do significant research, it requires a minimum of 80 percent of effort.

Then who becomes our faculty?

Scholarly clinicians in clinical departments.

Let's talk about your books *Heart Disease* and *Harrison's Textbook of Medicine*.

In Boston, from 1978 to 1979, I took a year's sabbatical to prepare the first edition of *Heart Disease.* If you think Eichna was monastic, I was *really* monastic. I started to work on July 1, 1978, and I completed the book on June 30, 1979. I stayed at home; I didn't shave; I worked day and night.

Harrison's has been a big part of my life. I like to feel that I have made a difference in education since I believe that *Harrison's* is the most widely read text in all of medicine. More than two million English-language copies have been sold, with translations into twelve languages. In the past month I have completed work on the fifteenth edition of *Harrison's* (the tenth edition on which I have served as an editor and the second on which I have been editor in chief), and I look forward to beginning on the sixteenth in one year. I am so proud of this effort, and I have enjoyed working with great colleagues.

Have you obtained more satisfaction from *Harrison's* or the textbook on cardiology?

It's like asking me which of my children I love the most! The satisfactions are different. *Heart Disease* gives me the feeling of deep scholarship and it immerses me in all aspects of cardiology, while *Harrison's* gives me the opportunity of making a real impact and brings me close to all aspects of internal medicine. I travel all over the world and see

Harrison's wherever I go. Once I went to a community hospital's emergency room for a personal medical problem, and I saw an opened copy of *Harrison's* on the emergency physician's desk. I found it to be reassuring. I receive letters, usually from India or Pakistan, in which the writer has picked up a mistake. They may write something like, "On page 1147 on the 19th line you say this. . . . Professor, with deep respect, I think you are wrong." And these letter writers are always correct! It might be a typo or even a serious error, but it means that people around the world are really reading this book, and this is a great responsibility.

Now we're putting both *Harrison's* and *Heart Disease* on the Internet.

The following question may strike you as odd, coming right after our discussion of your many accomplishments, but I put this to all the contributors toward the end of our talks. Do you have any regrets about anything?

If I had to do it all over again, I wouldn't have spent those nine years walking back and forth between the Brigham and Beth Israel. I would have used that time to build up a personal consultant cardiology practice. We have talked a lot about my efforts in research and education, but I identify most with being a doctor. At the NIH it was very easy for me to be active clinically; we had a floor of twenty-four patients, and I was a hands-on clinician. In San Diego, while I loved setting up a new Department of Medicine, helping to develop a new school, and working on my first edition of *Harrison's*, to my surprise and disappointment, I wasn't asked to see many patients as a personal consultant; that was part of the "town-gown" problem there. I have had no end of teaching patients to see as chairman of medicine, but I missed giving more personalized care. In Boston, during the first couple of years I was busy getting the department in order, and I didn't seek out private patients. Then I began to build a consultant practice. But in 1978, when I took the sabbatical to prepare *Heart Disease,* that sort of fell apart. Then in 1980, just when I began building up my consultant practice again, I took on the BI job. If, as a result of that effort, I could have brought the Brigham and BI together, I would have no regrets, but it didn't happen. On the other hand, more recently I've played a role in helping to bring the Brigham and the MGH (Massachusetts General Hospital) together in Partners HealthCare, and that has been very challenging and gratifying.

> You know, regarding your Brigham-BI experience, there were some in the cardiology community who thought you were making a power grab to take over Beth Israel in addition to the Brigham. In truth, you were never really keen on this and considered your experience to be a failure. It should make them take notice.

Look, I have been so lucky during my career, and most of the things I've been involved in have worked out better than I expected. I have no complaints about my professional life and only this one regret. You can't win them all. I'm certainly not bitter about it.

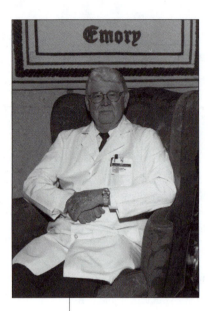

16

J. WILLIS HURST, M.D.
(1920–   )

Medicine has often been represented as a three-legged stool: patient care, teaching, and research. To extend that metaphor as we begin the twenty-first century, one might conclude that the research leg, though still sturdy, may wobble a bit from time to time, given the fluctuation of support and changing fashions in the emphasis of such work. The patient-care leg, however, with increasing costs and restrictions imposed by the managed care mentality, is showing some major cracks in the present economic climate. The teaching leg, the least apparent to the general public and relatively ignored by the media, is undergoing progressive rot, and this is of growing concern to those of us in academia.

There may be a number of reasons for this growing failure of our system to optimally train our medical students and house officers. A major blow to teaching has resulted from the decrease in hospital stays for patients. No longer can students and junior physicians observe at close hand the natural course of diseases and the effects of treatment in patients. As soon as patients are no longer at death's door, they are discharged from the hospital with a few pills and some prescriptions in hopeful anticipation that full recovery will take place. Oftentimes, they are back in the hospital with relapses within a few days as a result of such premature decisions, and they now encounter a new set of students and house staff.

Another blow to teaching has been the decline in approachable clinical investigators as part of the medical school faculty and hospital staffs. Research has become so specialized that even those trained in clinical medicine are drawn away from the bedside as they enter the more esoteric realms of modern medical research, where they must compete for funding with brilliant Ph.D.'s in the basic sciences who need have no pretensions about any interest in clinical medicine. For those faculty who would still like to keep one foot in clinical medicine and the other in patient-based research— the model of the clinical investigator—this becomes more and more difficult, for medical schools now insist that their clinical faculty obtain the bulk of their income from patient fees, especially in outpatient settings, where it is harder to demonstrate and discuss with students various aspects of the patients being evaluated and treated. The numbers must be kept up!

Finally, federal support of teaching hospitals is falling off, to the obvious detriment of the training of new specialists for the future. Not only are fewer specialty slots supported by government grants or the hospitals themselves, but many services to the indigent have been canceled at these hospitals. It is in such settings where doctors-in-training in the past obtained valuable experience.

The effects of such deterioration in medical teaching can be easily represented by another symbol, the pyramid. Constituting the base is the knowledge generated by first-rate research. The pinnacle is the expert patient care that is the ultimate goal of the medical profession. Between the two, in the middle section, is medical teaching, through which all the wonderful discoveries of our researchers can ultimately be conveyed to our patients. It is here that the crumbling of the edifice is most pronounced.

Over the past half century it has been the medical researcher who has been accorded the most prominent recognition by the rest of us, and most of those appearing in this book fall into such a favored category. Amazingly, Willis Hurst, who makes no claims about being a medical scientist, has become a major figure in American cardiology over this period, a position he has achieved through his personal character and his dedication to the highest ideals of medicine. He has also demonstrated throughout his career a keen ability to detect in others those talents for research and scientific innovation that he might not claim for himself.

One of the last fellows trained under Paul Dudley White, that great icon of American cardiology, Dr. Hurst has spent a lifetime building a superb medical service at Emory University. His extraordinary organizational and intellectual capacity has also enabled him to edit and contribute to one of the two major current textbooks in cardiology (the other being Eugene Braunwald's *Heart Disease*).

Through all the changes in the practice of medicine over the last half century, buffeted as it has been by many adverse economic and societal factors, for those of us looking ahead with growing trepidation Dr. Hurst has maintained a steady course of optimism and faith in the future that is both inspirational and reassuring.

———

Atlanta, Georgia
August 31, 2000

———

How did you come to select medicine as your field of study?

That's a commonly asked question, as you know. Medicine is the only field that involves science and a close working relationship with people. So, with an interest in science and an enjoyment in dealing with people, I decided that medicine was the profession for me. I thought about it as a child, but I really firmed up my decision on a certain day when I was in the eighth grade taking biology. As I look back, this was the most fascinating day I can remember in high school. The biology teacher was up front at his desk when a knock came at the door. It was the chemistry teacher, who barged into our classroom and began to say ugly things to the biology teacher. The two of them got into a heated argument and almost came to blows. Finally, with a huff, the chemistry teacher left. At this point the biology teacher asked the students to write down the color of the tie the chemistry teacher was wearing and to state the first words that were spoken in their argument. Well, we students were so disturbed about the affair that the two of them had staged that we couldn't answer the questions.

The biology teacher defined psychology as the *study of why people do what they do.* He pointed out that we had just experienced our first lesson: *emotional turmoil interferes with one's ability to observe.*

I have always believed that in medicine, where we deal with people, that an important part of our work is to understand the individuals we are involved with. We don't need long years of training in psychiatry to develop that interest.

The staged argument between the two teachers intrigued me, as did the dissection of the frog. I simply enjoyed all of that. It definitely enhanced my interest in the profession of medicine.

> I would like to skip forward now, past your college and medical school training in the South, to ask you about how you finally came to Boston to work under PAUL DUDLEY WHITE. Such positions were obviously highly treasured, and you must have been competing with many people from places like Harvard and Yale for such a position.

It came about this way: I went to medical school at the Medical College of Georgia and was an intern and resident at the University Hospital there. Several faculty members impressed me enormously. One was V. P. Sydenstricker, the chairman of the department of medicine, who I think was the smartest doctor I ever knew. The famous WILLIAM HAMILTON was our physiologist, and Harvey Cleckley was our psychiatrist. Dr. Harry Harper was our highly respected cardiologist. He was a perfect gentleman and role model for me at that time! His knowledge was great; he was a superb teacher. So I began to warm up to the idea of becoming a cardiologist.

It just so happened that Dr. Harper had spent some time with Dr. White. So he invited Dr. White to come to visit our school. Well, when the visit ended, Dr. Harper came to me and said, "How would you like to work with Dr. White?" I said, "I'd love to do that." Before Dr. White left, Dr. Harper spoke to him about me and, I'm sure, put in some good words for me. So, shortly after Dr. White got back to Boston, he wrote me saying he had saved a fellowship position for me at a certain time. I had to go into the service, but I had the fellowship lined up a couple of years in advance. I am sure I would never had been able to do that if Dr. Harper hadn't intervened and if Dr. White had not visited Augusta just at the right time.

Paul Dudley White, I believe, was the most dominant figure in cardiology of his time both here and, I suspect, abroad as well. You were close to him, and I would like you to tell me about your recollections of him—and don't "spare the horses."

His impact was enormous both in this country and internationally. He made this statement, which I agree with: "I take care of people with heart disease." That implies to me that he cared about the *people* who were sick. He was a gentle, extraordinarily intelligent, humanistic type of person. He wanted the world at large to go well; he hated war; he hated the destruction of the environment. He almost became a forester in his early life. His role model was Theodore Roosevelt, who was a strong environmentalist. He liked people, and because of that, got to know a lot of people, but he never attempted to influence people through anger or a domineering approach. He became so respected he could "calm the troubled water" of a group of arguing people by simply being there. He kept up with his patients; he kept up with his trainees; he produced the first major textbook of cardiology in this country, although there had been others along the way.

He was a superb writer. During the period of his early schooling, even in high school, he had studied several different languages, including, I believe, Greek, Latin, and French. His first textbook is an absolute testament to his personality.[1] Look at the references. Many of them are in foreign languages. He makes the statement in the book that he personally translated all of them. That is unheard of today. People don't or can't do that today.

His ability in teaching medicine, of course, was well known everywhere. But he also taught the lay public; he even had children's crusades in which he tried to influence them to adopt the proper diet and so forth.

Addison Messer, who later moved to Florida, and I were his last trainees.

Why were you two the last ones?

During my last few months with Dr. White, he had to make a decision. He was going to Washington more and more, where he was the major mover in developing the National Heart Institute. This activity was taking most of his time. DUCKETT JONES and others advised him that his effort to develop the institute would be one of the greatest things he could do. Accordingly, he became more and more involved in planning the activities of the National Heart Institute. So, because he was spending more and more time in Washington, Ed Bland replaced him as chief of cardiology at the Massachusetts General Hospital. Dr. White was a major mover at the National Heart Institute for many years before they recruited permanent people to shoulder the responsibilities.[2]

Did you have any involvement with cardiac catheterization in these early years? This, of course, was a major development in the forties, fifties, and beyond.

First of all, [André] Cournand visited our school when I was a senior student in 1944. I was fascinated with his slides showing a catheter in the pulmonary artery. Prior to 1948–49, there had been some experience with establishing a cardiac catheterization laboratory at Mass. General before my time, but the laboratory had never been sustained. Dr. Gordon Myers preceded me as a cardiology fellow and then stayed on the staff with Dr. White. He was an extremely capable individual and spearheaded the development of the cardiac cath lab. I was a minor member of that team. The team consisted of Myers from cardiology, Gordon Scannel from surgery, Stan Wyman from radiology, Grey Dimond, and me. Myers did all of the catheterizations. We published one paper that I am proud to have had a small part in producing. We discussed in that paper how an elevation of pulmonary artery pressure could alter the murmur of patent ductus or any other shunt from the aorta to the pulmonary artery. This allowed us to understand some of the clinical features of the Eisenmenger syndrome.*

Let me insert this story, which occurred before I joined the Emory faculty. EUGENE STEAD was chairman of the department of medicine at Emory University in 1942. He and JIM WARREN became interested in

---

* A reduction and then reversal of shunting of blood from the systemic to the pulmonary circulation through a septal defect or a patent ductus arteriosus as a result of increasing pulmonary vascular resistance and pulmonary artery pressure (see Fig. 3-1).

what Cournand was doing with cardiac catheterization. The reason they became interested is that ALFRED BLALOCK came for a visit. This was during World War II, and Blalock was involved with the armed forces and needed more scientific information about shock. Blalock pointed out that there was money available for the study of shock, and Stead and Warren decided that cardiac catheterization would make it possible to obtain the information that was needed. The clinical services at Grady [Memorial] Hospital, where they worked, were run by Emory. The emergency clinic was filled with patients who had gunshot wounds and stabbings. Accordingly, they had access to patients with shock. So they wrote a grant for the support of a shock study.

Well, in those days no one was familiar with writing grants, and so, when the secretary typed up the grant she misplaced a decimal point to the right, resulting in their asking for ten times as much money as they intended—and they got it! And it turned out that the larger sum was about right; the original sum they thought they were asking for wouldn't have done it.

At that time there were only about three cardiac catheterization laboratories in the world, and Emory's laboratory at Grady was one of them. In addition to the shock work, Stead's team revolutionized the understanding of heart failure. The first *diagnostic* cardiac catheterization was performed in that laboratory. Prior to that time the various laboratories had used the catheter to unravel the mysteries of cardiovascular physiology. Jim Warren reasoned that in a patient in whom they clinically suspected an atrial septal defect, there should be an increase in oxygen content of the blood of the right atrium. They proved that such was the case by using the cardiac catheter to sample blood from the right atrium. This work was published in 1945.[3]

While assigned to the U.S. Naval Hospital in Bethesda in 1956, I started a cardiac catheterization laboratory and performed a study on a patient with patent ductus who had pulmonary hypertension. She was similar to the Boston cases I mentioned earlier. I left the navy and returned to Emory before the lab was fully developed.

In 1950, Emory Hospital did not have a cardiac catheterization laboratory, so we transported a few patients to Grady Memorial Hospital for catheterization. When I became chairman of the department of medicine in 1957, one of my first acts was to develop a cardiac catheterization laboratory at Emory University Hospital. I recruited Dr. Robert Franch to direct the laboratory and perform the catheterizations. Now, of course, there are numerous catheterization laboratories at all of our hospitals and in all of the large hospitals in Atlanta.

I never worked exclusively in a cardiac catheterization laboratory. It was too confining for me. I enjoyed learning which patients should have the procedure and what to do with the data after it was obtained. I was more interested in correlating the data found in the lab with my clinical observations.

> Let's go back, for a moment, to your time in Boston with Dr. White. What was the relationship between Dr. White at Mass. General and that other major figure, SAMUEL LEVINE, at the Peter Bent Brigham Hospital, and what were your impressions of Dr. Levine?

I did know Dr. Levine. He, too, was a giant. Dr. Levine was a great teacher. He was a dogmatic teacher, but his dogma was usually correct! The relationship between Dr. White and Dr. Levine was one of enormous respect, but you would expect that of both of them.

> Before you went to work under Dr. White, you went from your medical residency to Fitzsimmons General Hospital in Denver for your military service.

Right. I was in the army at Fitzsimmons General Hospital in Denver, which was a superb hospital. I did not finish the required time there because of a terrible family tragedy. I received a call from a lady in my wife's hometown in Georgia telling me that there had been an auto accident in which my wife's mother and a child of her sister had been killed. My wife's sister and another child were seriously injured. So we had to go home immediately. My sister-in-law was unconscious for about six weeks. So I was released from the army because of family hardship.

My wife and I moved into the home of her brain-injured sister to assist in her rehabilitation. After three or four months, when my wife's sister was beginning to ambulate, I called Dr. White. He invited me to join him a few months earlier than planned.

After my fellowship with Dr. White, I went to Atlanta in 1949 to go into private practice. I learned a lot about myself that year. I spent more and more time with Emory students and residents at Grady Hospital. I realized that I enjoyed the challenge of academic medicine and felt I should devote myself to academic work. At about that time, Paul Beeson, who was chairman of the Department of Medicine at Emory, and Dr. Bruce Logue, who was the cardiologist at Emory, asked me to join the faculty at Emory University School of Medicine. Dr. Logue and I had a great time. Things were going well; I was enjoying teaching and writing. The Korean War heated up, and there was a new need for doctors. They were beginning to call back those who had not completed two years of service in World War II. I learned that the army didn't need anybody, but one day I walked down to my mailbox and there was a notice from the navy. So I went to the U.S. Naval Hospital in Bethesda, just outside Washington, D.C., where, after a year, I became chief of cardiology.

> It was there, of course, that you acquired the kind of reputation that made you familiar to the public. Although we in cardiology and medicine recognize you for your academic achievements, the public knows you as the physician to Lyndon B. Johnson, a relationship that began in Bethesda and then went on for another eighteen years to the time of his death. When Johnson was still alive, you told me that although it wasn't fitting to write about him during his lifetime, you would do so at some future time. Then, you did write a book about certain aspects regarding him, which was published in 1995. I would like you to summarize here what you learned from Johnson about him as a person and what you learned about yourself from this experience.

I wrote, along with Dr. Jim Cain, a book about his humor and humanism. The book was titled *LBJ: To Know Him Better.*[4]

On July 2, 1955, LBJ, who was then majority leader of the Senate, was admitted to the hospital with a heart attack (myocardial infarction). Once again I think my interest in people was why we hit it off well. I was involved with his medical care through the vice presidency, presidency, and afterward for eighteen years.

He was a very brilliant man with a remarkable memory. He also had a humorous side to him that most people were not aware of. He was, of course, an extraordinary politician of the old school and was majority leader of the Senate when I first met him. At that time he was the next most powerful political person in the country after President Eisenhower. They worked well together. Historians commonly say that he was the most effective majority leader the country has ever had.

What did I learn from him? There were some very specific things, conceptually at least, that helped me. For example, he emphasized that even a great idea won't work unless the timing is right. A person has to be able to sense when the timing is right. Historically, all through his political life, there were people who wanted him to do this and others who wanted him to do that, and he would say, "I'm for that, but the timing is wrong." When the timing was right, he made his move.

Did he ever discuss political matters with you?

I did not get involved with the political decision making. I never thought that was my role.

When he charged a commission to do something, he might say, "Now look, I know all the different ways that you can come back to me changing names and changing phrases and make it sound like a report of progress. I want you to know that I am aware of that kind of action, and that is not what I am asking you to do. I want new ideas, not rephrasing of old ones."

He also pointed out that if one approach to a problem did not solve it, that you should try something else. His mind was constantly searching for new solutions to problems.

Did the fact that you were known to be his physician for so many years affect your own professional standing in any way?

No, I would say not. Of course people were interested in the president and might, for that reason, remember who his cardiologist was.

When you got out of the service and returned to Atlanta, you were again in private practice a short time before you became chairman of medicine at Emory.

No, I returned to my faculty position at Emory in November 1955. When I returned, I found the school in turmoil. The dean was having trouble with several department chairmen, and he felt that changes had to be made. Many members of the faculty were leaving. I was thinking about leaving and going to the Mayo Clinic. DR. HOWARD BURCHELL had been enticing me to join him there. I have always had enormous respect for him. In fact, we still correspond with each other. As a side comment, I would like to point out that I ask him to check many of the articles I write. I don't like to send an article to any journal without it having been checked by the best expert I know.

The possibility of joining the Mayo Clinic was intriguing: John Kirklin was there; JESSE EDWARDS was there; Ray Pruitt was there; Ray Gifford was there; along with Howard Burchell. I had made one trip to the Mayo Clinic, and things were moving along, when I was asked if I would accept the chairmanship of the Department of Medicine at Emory. It was late in my thirty-fifth year when the offer was made. I accepted the offer and started work as chairman in February of 1957.

Why did they pick you? People usually have a little more gray hair by the time they become heads of departments.

[*Laughing*] You would have to *ask them* about that. I don't know, but one of my greatest honors I discovered in the correspondence that I found in the old files after I became chairman was that I had been considered for the position back in 1952, at which time I was thirty-two years old. I am sure that the people making such decisions knew that I was interested in students and how people learn; that I was contributing to the medical literature; and that Emory needed someone like that in Medicine. I didn't make it when I was thirty-two because someone pointed out that I was pretty young; so by the time I was thirty-six I was then considered "an old man." I knew the problems but had been away in the navy when the problems arose. I had a good relationship with students, house staff, and other faculty. At that time there were no more than fourteen or fifteen members in the Department of Medicine. We used Grady Memorial Hospital, Emory University Hospital, and the VA Hospital to carry out our teaching, patient care, and research mission. Later we added Crawford Long, which Emory owns.

My job then was to develop divisions—there were none when I started. I was also responsible for dermatology, neurology, and preventive medicine. In those early days we didn't have much money, so a lot of excellent practicing internists in Atlanta helped us a great deal. They were given clinical appointments without pay. We at Emory owe them much. By the time I left the chairmanship—thirty years later—we had all the divisions that you find in a modern department; we were doing more research; and there was about 140 full-time faculty. And, of course, the size of the department has continued to grow since then. I am pleased to note that out of our original Department of Medicine, we were able to establish separate departments of neurology, dermatology, and preventive medicine.[5]

> You have always had a close relationship with Bruce Logue. Was he older than you? Had he been considered for the chairmanship of the department at the time you were selected?

Bruce is the greatest friend I have ever had. He recruited me to Emory in the first place, where we worked together. He opened many doors for me and taught me a great deal. I think that had he wanted it, Dr. Logue could have been chairman of the Department of Medicine. Bruce is one of the finest clinicians ever. He is loved by everybody, but he didn't want to be chairman of the Department of Medicine. He urged that the position be offered to me. He is nine years older than me, and we still have lunch together.

> You always describe yourself as a nonscientist, but you seem to have a remarkable ability to recognize those who were. René Favaloro, for example, told me that when other cardiologists were reluctant to accept his work on coronary bypass surgery, you were an early supporter.

I am a clinician-teacher-clinical investigator-writer. I am not a scientist. I enjoy patients, and I enjoy working with trainees. Early in the development of coronary bypass surgery, we had sufficient data to support its use for the relief of angina pectoris. At that point we did not know whether or not the procedure would prolong life. In the early seventies the operation was performed only to relieve angina that was refractory to medical treatment. I delayed saying that the procedure prolonged life until the studies showing that this was true became available. At this time, about 1978, coronary arteriography was improving; the surgical technique was improving; and everything was moving in a positive direction. In 1978 I participated at the American College of Cardiology meeting at one of the Controversies in Cardiology sessions and supported the view that coronary bypass surgery not only would relieve angina pectoris but, in properly selected patients, would prolong life.

> You brought to Emory many outstanding people whom we could mention, but probably the most outstanding was ANDREAS GRUENTZIG. I counted at least four obituaries you wrote about him after his death.[6] You had a father-son relationship, I gather.

I never felt I was that much older than he was, but Andreas himself made that remark to people. His father had been killed in World War II, and I was about twenty years older than Andreas. We did hit it off well, and I suspect he did think of me in that way.

> Gruentzig was in Switzerland when he introduced the angioplasty procedure, and Spencer King at your own place told you about it. There is a story told about how Gruentzig came to work at Emory, which may or may not be apocryphal: you supposedly went to the governor to pull some strings so Gruentzig could come on board without any of the usual hurdles that foreign physicians must face. Is this story true?

Not exactly. Spencer King first told me about Andreas, and I had seen one of his poster displays at the American Heart Association meeting. Andreas was giving courses in Switzerland, and Spencer went over to see him. When he came back, Spencer told me, "You know, I think he wants to leave Zurich. Maybe we can get him here." As time passed, it became clear that Gruentzig did want to leave Zurich and that he had contacted several places in the United States. I invited him to visit us at Emory. He liked what we had to offer. He was impressed with the president of the university because, although he was not a physician, he asked probing questions about angioplasty.

It turned out that Gruentzig wanted several things. I had to find a faculty position for his first wife, who was a psychologist. He wanted a permanent resident's visa. He didn't want to take a state board licensure exam, which was ordinarily required of immigrating physicians. He wanted a full professorship. He wanted an office with a window. He wanted a decent income. I persuaded the Department of Psychiatry to support his wife, and she had a position there for some time. As for the board exam, my former trainees were in charge, and they recognized that Gruentzig should come as a national treasure. Then, I believe, Spencer King approached Mr. Griffin Bell, who lives in Atlanta, and asked him to help Gruentzig obtain a permanent resident visa. Mr. Bell was the former attorney general of the United States. So we were able to pull all this together. I kid my Emory colleagues by telling them that Gruentzig's final request after he got here was for a parking place. That was the most difficult request for me to accomplish! He actually rode back and forth to the hospital on a little mechanical scooter, and I was scared to death he would get killed on *that*.

Andreas, of course, was a charismatic, brilliant creative person. He was an honest innovator who was on a daredevil course. But, let me emphasize, he would never endanger a patient.

In his presentations I always detected a note of caution in what he did.

That's what I mean. He was obviously an intense pioneer, but he would never hurt anyone.

He started our postgraduate courses in angioplasty, and people from all over the world came to hear him. We placed television sets in the auditorium for the audience to watch while he was back in the lab performing the procedure. He was constantly working on new, improved catheters. At the same time, he was interested in other things, which people didn't realize. Angioplasty, of course, was his baby, but, at the same time, he was profoundly interested in prevention of heart disease; he was interested in catheter techniques to close an atrial septal defect; he was creative in many areas, although he spent most of his time in angioplasty of the coronary arteries.

But the daredevil streak was there. He drove his car faster than he should. My wife and I cautioned him about being the pilot of his own plane. He enjoyed living on the edge like that. When I got the message that his plane was down, it was amazing because, within hours, I was getting messages from all over the world. There simply is no way to know what he would have accomplished had he and his wife not been killed in the plane crash.

I'd like to talk with you about your textbook. How did it get started?

In the early sixties there were three textbooks: Dr. White's, and he decided he would not continue with it; Charles Friedberg's book, and Paul Wood's book. Paul Wood was a guest at Emory as a visiting professor at my invitation in 1962. He had come to the American College of Cardiology meeting in Denver and was returning to England via Atlanta. I had not known Dr. Wood before except by his reputation, which, at that point, had established him as the leader in cardiology of the world. Brilliant, caustic, sharp, quick. I was with him for two or three days, and although I had not known him before, he seemed to be extremely tense and uptight to me. I felt that something was bothering him. When I asked him about his textbook, he told me, "I don't know what I'm going to do. Now there is so much new work coming out that by the time I finish the end of the book, the first part of the book needs revising."

He could not, I think, bear the thought of producing a book that was less than perfect. He realized that he could not be expert in all aspects of cardiology and said, "I just don't know what I'll do." He left Emory and went back home and died two weeks later of a myocardial infarction. I concluded from what he was saying that one man could no longer produce a textbook of cardiology. I decided after Wood's visit, having had a little experience in writing and editing the cardiovascular section of *Meakins' Textbook of Medicine,* that I would ask a group of people to help me create a multiauthored textbook of cardiology. My idea was to select people to contribute to the book who had expressed views that I agreed with. The book was to be titled *The Heart.* Bruce Logue and I met every Thursday for about one year. We reviewed every word of every chapter; made suggestions for alterations, and sent chapters back for approval, et cetera. The first edition was published in 1966.[7]

Friedberg had been publishing his excellent single-authored book. You might be interested to know that I was with him on a teaching assignment at the University of Alabama after our book had come out, and his was the only other book available at that time. I have always thought highly of him because of his reaction to our book. He commented to me that *The Heart* was a good book and that he was pleased that it was on the market. He was a great man and very kind to me in this regard whenever we appeared on programs together. Regrettably, he was killed in an awful auto accident. Because of that, *The Heart* became the only book available. It was published in four or five foreign languages, and, as the years went by, we revised it every four years. I was pleased that the book was so popular. Then my friend Gene Braunwald's book came along. I think Friedberg's publishers were interested in him continuing the Friedberg book—

They were.

—and Gene, whom I had known since my tour of duty at the U.S. Naval Hospital in Bethesda, and I actually talked about it. Gene and I made a gentlemen's agreement that we would not come out with new editions the same year. So subsequent editions of our books came out every two years, with Hurst's *The Heart* alternating with the Braunwald book. Now, of course, there are several books on the market.

> **Something I always thought interesting is that each edition of your book on the heart has had a chapter on iatrogenic heart disease, written by you.**

I think that it is a very important subject. I'm sure my interest in it goes back to Dr. White's influence. I divide iatrogenic heart disease into two parts: one is when something is done by a physician that causes a problem that is obvious, for example, a catheter puncturing the wall of the right ventricle; that's obviously iatrogenic. The other aspect of this— and I am sure this is Dr. White's influence—is that when a doctor puts undue restrictions on a patient, limiting his enjoyment of life, this too is important and also an iatrogenic problem. Dr. White was the world's expert on *not* doing that. If a patient came to him, he always tried to strike a positive note, trying to say something good. If he could, when he listened to the heart, he would say something like "Good heart sounds!" and you could see the patient's eyes light up. If you say nothing or listen too long, patients may think you're hearing something terrible and not telling them.

> **You have always been interested in electrocardiography, and you have written monographs and books on the subject. Do you think that with all the new techniques being introduced—echocardiography and so on—that today's cardiologists are as expert in electrocardiography as they might have been twenty to thirty years ago?**

There's no question that many members of the profession are not extracting all the information they should from the electrocardiogram. What some of them don't realize is that there has been a lot of progress in electrocardiography in recent years. Another reason for poor interpretations is the *excessive* reliance on computer-read ECGs, where the error rate is about 20 percent. Also, remember the software is rarely changed, and computers don't go to school or read the literature. Accordingly, the computer readout is usually out of date. The reason an electrocardiogram is made by a clinician is to answer the question: "What heart disease could the patient have to create this tracing?" Today electrocardiograms are being recorded without physicians asking that important question. Do the abnormalities in the tracing fit the other data collected from the patient? This question must be answered because, in this day and time, patients may have more than one type of heart disease—the electrocardiogram showing one disease and the rest of the data suggesting another disease. But I would say that the wheel is beginning to turn again, and that physicians are beginning to understand that they can extract more information from the tracings than they have done during the last twenty-five years.

> **There are many good books on electrocardiography, and Bob Grant's book is among them.[8] I must tell you a little story about him. Back in**

the days when we had those great spring meetings in Atlantic City, one evening after the meetings a few of us young guys were on our way to dinner and who should be standing outside the meeting hall but MAXWELL WINTROBE, my old chief, who asked if he might join us. We were honored. Then there was another fellow standing on the curb who also asked to come along, and, of course, we welcomed him as well. When we got into the cab, I introduced myself, and then he said, "My name is Bob Grant." I was overwhelmed, having admired his work from afar. It was like supping from the Holy Grail for me, having dinner with him. You knew him, and I would like to hear your comments about him.

I heard about Bob Grant when I was a cardiology fellow with Dr. White. I wrote him to please send me some reprints of his work. He sent me a copy of the manuscript of his first book before it was published. Every sentence excited me. I arrived in Atlanta in late 1949, to enter in private practice, and found myself spending most of my time with Emory students and house staff at Grady Hospital. That's when I first met Dr. Grant. I then joined the Emory faculty and continued learning from Dr. Grant, who left Emory about a year later. My first little book on electrocardiography was based on his work. Dr. Grant was one of the most creative people I have known. He was a magnificent human being. Later in his career he became head of the National Heart Institute. A clear thinker, a beautiful writer. I couldn't do my work today without having had that exposure to Bob Grant.

The work I continue to do in electrocardiography is based on *his* work, but the advantage I have now, which he did not have, is the ability to correlate the findings in the tracing with the results of modern high technology.[9]

Let's get personal for a moment. Every time I read about you, I read that you get up about four o'clock every morning. What I want to know is, when do you go to bed?

[Laughing] Sometimes it's even earlier than four. People always ask me when I started doing that. I think I started this in medical school. I had learned as a high school student that if I could not solve an algebra problem in the evening, that it was better for me to go to bed and get up in the morning and try to work it out. The wiring in my brain is that

I am smarter in the morning. I like to say that a few hours sleep wipes my slate clean so external forces do not impede my thinking. Also, when you become a doctor, you want to spend as much time as you can with your family, and early morning work does not conflict with family time.

I read and write at four in the morning and sometimes earlier. My bedtime varies all over the place. For years I couldn't sleep more than four hours in a row, but I would catnap at will. I have learned from people who have roomed with me that I don't waste any time going to sleep. I go to sleep instantly once I close my eyes. I wake up in an instant as well. I suppose I am a very efficient sleeper. I usually get to bed at ten or eleven o'clock, but rarely do I sleep more than five hours in a row. I am still an efficient catnapper.

By the time you get to be a hundred, it may be six!

Another aspect of this is absolutely ridiculous. In the morning I sit in my *working chair* with dictionaries, pencil sharpener, et cetera, at hand where I do my writing. This chair is in the den. On the other hand, if I just want to sit and think, I move to another special chair, which is my *thinking chair.* It is located in the living room. I don't turn on the light; I just sit there and think about how to write a sentence; how to solve a patient's problem; how to solve a trainee's learning problem; and how to solve my personal problems. I look upon thinking as a conscious act, and I need to have a place where I do that intensively. I tell people—I have a place to eat, a place to sleep, and a special place to think.

One of your children is a cardiologist, and I read that he took his cardiology training with you. That seems a rather dicey decision to make. I know at least one instance of this that proved disastrous.

I recognized that it might not be wise for my son to train under me when I was chairman of the Department of Medicine at Emory. So he went to medical school at the Medical College of Georgia and completed his internship and residency at Parkland Hospital of Southwestern Medical School in Dallas. He called me one night during his third year as a medical resident and said, "I'm thinking about going into cardiology." I said, "That's fine—where do you want to go?" He replied, "How about Emory?" I said, "I think it can be arranged." During his fellowship I did arrange for him to work with Bruce Logue, Spencer King, and others so he was exposed to many people other than me.

> In historical terms relating to medicine, I think of you as one of a line of good ole southern boys who went North and then came back and did as well or better on their home turf: Gene Stead, GEORGE BURCH, TINSLEY HARRISON. . . . Do you think of yourself in this way?

First of all, let me say that I enjoyed the Massachusetts General Hospital enormously, and it would have been wonderful to stay in Boston, but the hospital and city were filled with superb people. I did feel that my roots were in the South and that I should return home.

It's interesting that you brought up the name of Eugene Stead, who was Emory's first full-time chairman of medicine. He has been my mentor in medical education for many decades, and I still visit him at his home on Kerr Lake in North Carolina. He is ninety-two years old now and is still mentally active and creative. I have always listened to Gene Stead. At the time they offered me the chairmanship at Emory, he was chairman at Duke, so I went up to see him. I also went to Yale to talk with Paul Beeson, who had also been chairman at Emory before moving to Yale; I wanted to talk with him as well. When I went to visit Stead, he made some comments about what SOMA WEISS had said to him when Emory offered him the position as chairman of medicine. Soma Weiss had urged him to go to Emory when other people did not encourage him to do so. Soma Weiss saw Emory's future financial support coming from Coca-Cola and the Woodruff Foundations. So Stead's advice to me was the same he had received from Soma Weiss: *Go where you are needed.*

He also told Stead: *"So far, you have been a man of promise; now is your chance to see if you are a man of achievement."* Stead gave me that same advice. I can't say I was more comfortable in the South than in the North because I never met finer people than those who were at the Mass. General. But I was from the South and felt that I might be needed there.

Years ago when I was interviewing Louis Weinstein, I asked him why he never had become a chairman of a department or a dean even though he had been offered such positions many times. He told me that in earlier times the chairman of medicine was usually also the best doctor, the most knowledgeable, as well as a good administrator. It seems that today the departments of medicine are so big that there's very little time for a chairman to be a doctor. What is your comment on this?

There is some truth to what you are saying; in earlier times departments of medicine were tighter organizations; they were not as diverse and far-flung as they are now. I enjoyed my own chairmanship enormously. I continued my consultative practice of cardiology; I spent much time on the wards of the hospitals with patients, house staff, and students. I felt that I always learned from my colleagues. I could solve problems with a phone call rather than having to have a big committee meeting. The most important thing was that we worked together and learned from each other. Now departments of medicine are so large that all the subspecialties seem to go their own way. Even units within divisions function as separate units. On the one hand, that is the way medicine has advanced, but, on the other hand, the separateness blunts the learning opportunities.

I wish to point out that a chairman still has the opportunity to write his or her own job description as long as he or she satisfies the dean. So even with the administrative headaches today, I believe the chairman can still be a doctor, teacher, and investigator.

If you were thirty or forty years younger, would you take a job as chairman today?

Absolutely. Recently, when Emory was searching for a chairman of medicine, some of my colleagues said that I should apply for the job. Although I am eighty years old, I responded, "I won't take it unless I get a thirty-year contract."

Yes, I would jump at the chance to be chairman again, but I would do my best to alter the current system. I would carve out those things that I believe in. I would try to have the smallest number of administrative meetings. I would continue to see patients. I would continue to teach and write.

Are there any particular disappointments or regrets you have experienced along the way?

I enjoyed being chairman. I also enjoy my work now. I teach nine or ten sessions a week and write the rest of the time. I usually have one or two books in the works most of the time. So my personal activity is very rewarding. But the profession of medicine itself has changed, and this influences everything we do in academic medicine and in practice. As a profession we have to face the fact that both the government and the private sector have failed in their efforts to deliver health care. I don't believe that continually manipulating the two approaches will solve the problem. That means that someone must come up with another view to change things. It will take patients themselves to say, "This is not good," before change can be made. They're beginning to do that.

The ethical lines of medicine that I grew up with have shifted. Many things are going on within the profession and its relationship to industry that troubles me. I think we must have a reassessment of the ethical behavior within what I would call the medical-legal-political-industrial complex.

In academic work, I believe the attending physician who has a patient, and teaches the house officer and student who are assigned to the patient, holds the future of medicine in his or her hands. As I see it, in that teaching system there should be as much time spent with the student and house officer as with the patient. The attending physician has two important functions: to take superb care of the patient, and to be sure that the people he or she is training understand everything that is going on. In many institutions now, where the HMOs are involved, the physicians are not permitted to take the amount of time needed to deal with the patient's problem, much less to teach the trainees, who will soon be practicing physicians. The HMO may even penalize the attending physician for taking time to teach.

You see, the attending physician's role in the training of house staff and fellows is the most important position in a medical school because medical schools have never delivered skilled physicians to the public. Medical schools only *introduce* students to skills. In fact, medical schools only introduce students to language; the language of physiology and biochemistry, et cetera. In medical school the student has very little opportunity to use that kind of information in a thought process as applied to the patient before him or her. The skilled attending physician must have time to lead the house staff and fellows to become good thinkers and skilled physicians. When this is not done, we run the risk of delivering to the public doctors who are not as skilled as they could be.

> Let's hope, to paraphrase your patient-mentor LBJ, that sometime in the future someone will recognize when to do the right thing at the right time. I hope it's sooner rather than later.

As you know, I have written or edited a number of scientific books and articles. Three of the books have been on teaching medicine, and one is a children's book about the heart. It was written with my ten-year-old grandson. My reason for writing is to organize my thoughts. The discipline of writing forces me to increase my knowledge base and to communicate more clearly. This, I believe, makes me a better teacher.

My most recent book, however, will come out in November 2000, and it is a work of fiction. I wrote it with one of my sons who is a psychologist. The title is *Prescription for Greed,* and, although pure fiction, it deals with the interrelationship among doctors, lawyers, politicians, and industry. It highlights some of the problems we face as a medical profession.

> Even though it is fiction, I hope we will learn something about the status of medicine today from it. I would like to say, however, that although you seem to be basically an optimistic person, the picture you have drawn of our current state seems to be filled with dark clouds. Are there any silver linings you might detect in the future?

Of course, the long-term future of medicine is bright. The disappointments I have just discussed about the delivery of health care by the government or by the private sector will gradually be solved. The solution to any problem begins when the problem itself can be stated clearly. Now it is clear—the current health-care delivery system is a disaster. Patients are unhappy. Physicians are unhappy. Hospitals are closing, and academic centers are struggling. The current system has forced us all to participate in activity that we realize is less than the best. When the chaos is recognized by a critical mass of creative people, the problem will be solved. The time for new approaches is definitely approaching.

Today, medical journals are filled with new information coming out of the research laboratories of the nation. New and important information is also available on the Internet. The scientific revolution in medicine accelerated after World War II, and the last fifty years have been filled with scientific discoveries. The discovery rate is still accelerating. The new work in molecular biology, genetics, prevention, transplantation of organs, et cetera, is magnificent.

Computer systems such as Weed's knowledge coupling will give the physician assistance in his or her problem-solving efforts.

I could go on, but the fact is clear, scientific medicine is marching on. Our problem is the delivery of medical care. This will be solved now that a mass of people recognize that we must do better.

Finally—I wish I could do it all again.

17

THE TWENTY-FIRST CENTURY

There is a certain kind of hubris that attaches itself to the turn of every century, and nowhere is this more apparent than in the fields of medicine and science. At the beginning of our own new era, should any members of a scientific gathering rise to voice expressions of doubt or caution about the future, they are likely to be shouted down by pronouncements from others that "this is, after all, the twenty-first century!" implying that we have reached some kind of a pinnacle that cannot be questioned or denied. Similar expressions of confidence were surely voiced at the turns into the twentieth, nineteenth, and eighteenth centuries, and perhaps even earlier. Realization of our limitations seeps into our collective medical consciousness only a bit later into the future.

However, it must be said that the twentieth century was a banner one for cardiovascular research and progress, as the personal histories of the contributors to this book so effectively demonstrate. Yet with each door opened, another locked one is revealed, and finding the right keys to those portals becomes our future task.

Improved diagnosis and therapy constitute the dual goals of our profession, and in both respects what lies ahead looks promising. In terms of diagnosis, electrocardiography, introduced early in the twentieth century, has, in some ways, remained the backbone of diagnostic cardiology. Adding enormously to this capability was the later introduction of cardiac catheterization and cineangiography, once seen as the ultimates in diagnostic technology. As we enter into the twenty-first century, however, we see that ultrasound (echocardiography and Doppler) and nuclear medicine have to a great extent provided useful alternatives to these other modalities. Chamber size, pressures, contractility, and flows may all now be determined without the breaking of the skin or the spilling of a drop of blood. Soon the differentiation between types of tissue and alterations in tissue response to various diagnostic maneuvers will also be determined by such methods. Although examination of the coronary circulation still routinely requires cineangiography, there are techniques being developed (using magnetic resonance imaging, for example) that will eliminate the need for catheterization to reveal coronary artery anatomy.

The rise of molecular biology has already impacted upon our understanding of certain cardiac diseases by defining their genetic basis (e.g., hypertrophic cardiomyopathy). Once we pinpoint the genetic basis of a disease, we can surely find ways to eliminate or alter the expression of such faulty chromosomes.

Atherosclerosis in the guise of coronary heart disease has been recognized as the bane of the developed countries of the West for over half a century. We have learned about the multifactorial basis of this disease (e.g., hyperlipidemia, hypertension, smoking), but perhaps we have barely scratched the etiological surface. We have recently been alerted to the possible role of other elements, nutritional and otherwise (e.g., selenium, homocysteine blood levels, various vitamins). We are now becoming aware of an inflammatory component to atherosclerotic development by the presence of elevated C-reactive protein levels in the blood of susceptible patients. An infective component (e.g., chlamydia, helicobacter, chronic periodontal disease) has also been implicated. Studies must be done to clearly evaluate the extent of such influences and how best to control them.

Open-heart surgery has been a high point in the progress of twentieth-century cardiology, but newer modalities in medical and surgical therapy have modified its use and will continue to do so. The introduction of coronary artery balloon angioplasty has eliminated or delayed the need for coronary artery bypass grafting in many patients.

The use of stents has improved the long-term patency of vessels subjected to angioplasty; and methods for improving and prolonging the usefulness of the stents, themselves, by impregnation with anticoagulants and other substances along with the use of radiation, are rapidly being developed. The recent report showing that coating stents with an immunosuppressive drug, sirolimus, caused no stent stenosis after a six-month period, whereas untreated stents had a 26 percent stenosis rate,[1] is a major step forward in this area, and we now await longer-term follow-up and confirmatory findings among larger groups of patients.

Given the recognition of risk for neurological or neuropsychiatric complications from the use of the pump-oxygenator,[2] "off pump" bypass procedures for coronary bypass surgery are now being recommended. To reduce the amount of surgical trauma and other complications involved with such major surgery as sternal-splitting incisions used routinely in the past, minimally invasive techniques using multiple small portals to permit access to the operative site are also becoming increasingly popular, not only for coronary surgery but for valvular surgery as well. Certain congenital heart defects and valve diseases such as mitral stenosis may now be approached by catheter interventions without the need for any surgery at all.

The successful use of the stent in coronary disease has been reflected in similar devices for carotid artery disease and even for the relatively noninvasive treatments of aortic aneurysms ("endovascular exclusion").

We all die eventually. For the cardiac patient, the terminal event is often severe, refractory heart failure, now becoming the major challenge to the cardiovascular medical community. Nearly five million Americans have this condition today. It is the most common reason for hospital admissions for patients over the age of sixty-five, and the numbers are growing. Surgery—that is, cardiac transplantation—has been the most dramatic response of the medical profession to this syndrome. However, the supply of donor hearts is limited and shows no signs of growing; problems in rejection and the risk for the future development of neoplasia still persist; and the ethics of transplantation for elderly patients, often with other complicating medical problems, is another major concern. The total artificial heart, in the works for almost forty years, may finally be showing signs of success, while alternatives—a permanent implantable counterpulsation device (Kantrowitz) or ventricular assist devices (DeBakey, Jarvik)—may offer more practical and reliable solutions.

In an important randomized long-term study of patients in end-stage heart failure, surgeon Eric Rose and his colleagues found a 48 percent reduction in the risk of death from any cause in patients receiving an LVAD when compared with a group receiving medical treatment alone.[3] There was also an average increase in survival of about eight months among the operated group. However, even with these benefits, the patients receiving the device had nearly an 80 percent mortality at two years and frequent problems with infections, bleeding, and device malfunction. Hopefully, with increased experience with the implantation of mechanical devices to assist or replace the failing heart, greater benefits will be derived from such surgery in the future.

The rise of molecular cardiology, besides its role in genetics, has offered avenues of hope for patients with coronary heart disease or end-stage heart failure. Genetically engineered substances can be introduced via catheter into the coronary circulation or directly into the myocardium to stimulate angiogenesis or improve cardiac function.[4] The recent demonstration by Piero Anversa and his colleagues that, unlike it was formerly believed, myocardial cells are capable of regeneration in areas bordering myocardial infarctions,[5] suggests that new ways may be found to enhance this process in the heart attempting to heal itself after such damage. Equally exciting is a recent report from the same group indicating that primitive cells from the body of a cardiac transplant recipient migrate to the transplanted heart, suggesting that these cells may have the potential of contributing to the function of the grafted heart at some time following surgery.[6] If stem cell research is allowed to progress, the results of such work might provide another source of myocardial cells to replace diseased or depleted myocardium in the patient with heart failure.

Finally, pacemaking, once used only to restore normal heart rates in patients with heart block, may help improve cardiac function in heart failure by sequencing pacing sites within the heart to orchestrate the most efficient contractions of that organ.

Such is the potential extent of newly developed technologies envisioned, and, no doubt, the summary provided here might turn out to be an underestimate of what will be accomplished in the next few decades. It is not the science, however, but the social and political aspects of medicine that give one the greatest pause. The organization of the American health-care system leaves much to be desired. As long as millions of our citizens still have little or no access to even the minimum elements of medical care, it must be considered a failure. The growing influence of managed-care organizations, government bureaucracies, and other constraining elements upon physician autonomy will continue to have a detrimental effect on our ability to deliver good health care to our patients. The extent to which these trends will discourage future generations of bright young men and women from even entering the medical field can only be guessed at.

In viewing the current status of American medicine—in which heart disease occupies such a prominent place—one can construct a triangulated paradigm, in which one side becomes inadmissible. We want our health-care system to be universal, to be excellent in quality, and to be cheap (i.e., affordable). It can be made universal and excellent, but given the high cost of technology now in operation and being developed, it would not be cheap. It could be made universal and cheap, but this would require the abandonment of high-cost high technology. As a result, it could not be excellent. As for the final pairing, "excellent" and "cheap," this constitutes a contradiction in terms.

Yet even with the high total cost of medical care, if a good portion of the funds currently devoted to administration, marketing, litigation, and other nonmedical expenses were to be transferred to direct patient care, there might be enough money to institute a single-payer system throughout the United States. But even if there had to be some increase in cost, wouldn't it be worth it? Perhaps if we spent less money on alcohol, tobacco, junk food, gambling, and gas-guzzling, environment-polluting, and accident-prone sports utility vehicles most people don't even need, we might find the wherewithal to meet the country's medical bill.

This book, by design, has been "cardiocentric," but it is necessary to place medicine in a larger, world context. Coronary atherosclerosis is not a world problem; AIDS *is*. Michael S. Gottlieb, an immunologist, points out that although we may keep the disease under control within our own borders with the multiple drug regimens established and, perhaps, a vaccine, the disease is spreading virtually unchecked throughout Africa, Asia, and the former Soviet Union.[7] According to United Nations statistics, the worldwide number of those infected will be over 150 million by 2021.

There is no doubt that in the twenty-first century there will be tasks to be performed; there will be promises to be kept; and there will be important discoveries to be made. We will all be very busy. We must also remain humble and hopeful in anticipation of the great work that lies ahead.

BIOGRAPHICAL NOTES

ABBOTT, MAUDE E. (1869–1940)

Canadian physician who became curator of McGill Medical Museum and began to collect and catalog a wide variety of congenital cardiac malformations. This eventually became the basis of understanding these diseases—critical information when surgical techniques to correct them began to emerge.

ABELMANN, WALTER H. (1921–   )

German-born cardiologist who was prominent in Boston cardiological circles, with a special interest in cardiomyopathies.

ADAMS, FORREST (1919–   )

Formerly chief of pediatric cardiology at UCLA, with important contributions to knowledge about toxoplasmosis and congenital heart disease.

AKUTSU, TETSUZO (1922–   )

Japanese surgeon with an early interest in cardiovascular devices, which he pursued in the United States at the Cleveland Clinic (Kolff), the Maimonides Medical Center (Kantrowitz), the University of Mississippi, and the Texas Heart Institute in Houston (Cooley) before his return to Japan.

AUSTRIAN, ROBERT (1916–   )

Johns Hopkins–trained physician who worked at SUNY-Downstate Medical Center in Brooklyn 1952–62. Best known for his extensive work on pneumococcal infections and pneumococcal polysaccharides, leading to the development of a polyvalent vaccine now recommended for susceptible individuals.

BAHNSON, HENRY T. (1920–   )

Contributor across a broad range of clinical investigative surgery at Johns Hopkins and the University of Pittsburgh.

BAILEY, LEONARD (1942–)

Transplant surgeon at Loma Linda, best known for his attempt at placing a baboon heart in a critically ill infant, "Baby Fay."

BALDWIN, ELEANOR (1904–51)

Member of the Department of Medicine at Columbia's College of Physicians and Surgeons (1934–51) and frequent collaborator with André Cournand.

BARNARD, CHRISTIAAN (1922–2001)

South African surgeon who, after completing his doctoral (Ph.D.) work in the surgical department at the University of Minnesota (1956–58), returned to Cape Town and Groote Schuur Hospital, where he headed a team of surgeons who performed the first human heart transplant (in Louis Washkansky). Although Washkansky soon died from complications, Barnard's attempt led the way to further operations of this type in Cape Town and elsewhere.

BARRATT-BOYES, BRIAN (1924–)

New Zealand surgeon who introduced a number of open-heart procedures to that country, especially for congenital heart disease. He was also a pioneer in using aortic valve homografts and coauthored, with John Kirklin, a highly regarded textbook on cardiac surgery.

BEAN, WILLIAM B. (1909–89)

Gifted clinician, medical researcher, and historian who spent the bulk of his medical career at the medical schools of the University of Cincinnati and the University of Iowa.

BECK, CLAUDE S. (1894–1971)

Distinguished surgeon at Western Reserve who used a variety of techniques for relief of valvular and coronary disease. He also promoted the open-chest technique for cardiac resuscitation prior to the establishment of closed-chest methods.

BERLINER, ROBERT W. (1915–2002)

Outstanding researcher in renal physiology and administrator at the National Institutes of Health, where he served as director of intramural research for twenty-three years (1954–68). He was later dean at Yale Medical School (1973–84).

BERNARD, CLAUDE (1813–78)

Major French figure in the development of nineteenth-century biological and physiological thought. In addition to developing the technique of cardiac catheterization, he pioneered in studies on gastric juice, pancreatic function, the autonomic nervous system, and neuromuscular transmission, to list only some of his contributions. Perhaps he is best remembered for his concept of the internal environment (*"milieu interieur"*), which held that the body fluids of higher animals provide a medium that makes possible the conditions for existence of the cells they surround and nourish.

BEST, CHARLES H. (1899–1978)

Canadian physiologist, most noted for his work, while still an undergraduate student at the University of Toronto, with Frederick Banting on the discovery of insulin. In 1923, he was excluded from the Nobel Prize that was awarded to Banting and the head of the laboratory, J.J.R. Macleod. Best had a distinguished career thereafter, heading the physiology department at the University of Toronto (1929–65) and coauthoring a highly popular text in physiology.

BHARATI, SAROJA (BIRTH DATE NOT AVAILABLE)

As an assistant to Dr. Maurice Lev for many years, Bharati worked on the pathology of congenital heart disease. She is now a well-recognized expert in her own right.

BIGELOW, WILFRED G. (1913–   )

Canadian surgeon who introduced the concept of hypothermia in heart surgery to reduce metabolic requirements and thus preserve myocardium; today, this is a routine aspect of open-heart surgery. (See Callaghan entry for Bigelow's role in pacemaker development.)

BILLINGS, FRANK (1854–1932)

Leader in Chicago medical circles who also performed research and developed the doctrine of focal infection.

BILLROTH, THEODOR (1829–94)

Surgeon, teacher, and scientist who worked mainly at the surgical clinic of the University of Vienna. He was one of the first to introduce antisepsis on the Continent, the first to resect the esophagus, and to perform total laryngectomy. The types of gastric resection he developed still bear his name today (Billroth-1 and Billroth-2).

BING, (SIR) RUDOLPH (1902–97)
Vienna-born impresario who, following initial successes in Europe, became general manager of New York's Metropolitan Opera (1950–72).

BJÖRK, VIKING O. (1918–   )
Swedish surgeon noted for a number of accomplishments in cardiovascular surgery, but best known for the mechanical heart valve he developed with the engineer Don Shiley.

BLACKSTONE, EUGENE (1941–   )
Surgeon with extraordinary skill in statistical evaluation of surgical techniques who was an important contributor to John Kirklin's efforts and now continues this work at the Cleveland Clinic.

BLALOCK, ALFRED (1899–1964)
Among his other accomplishments, this Johns Hopkins surgeon, at the urging of Helen Taussig, devised an operation in cyanotic infants with congenital heart disease which involved diverting unoxygenated systemic blood back into the lung to improve survival (Blalock-Taussig or "blue baby" operation). When such patients became a little older, they could have their disease corrected by open-heart surgery, once it became available.

BLOOMFIELD, ARTHUR L. (1888–1962)
Distinguished physician and teacher at Johns Hopkins (1912–26) and later Stanford, where he headed the Department of Medicine (1926–54).

BLUMBERG, BARUCH S. (1925–   )
Virologist who shared with D. Carleton Gajdusek the Nobel Prize in 1976 for "discoveries concerning new mechanisms for the origin and dissemination of diseases." Blumberg's work concerned hepatitis B and Gajdusek's the "slow virus" causing Kuru disease.

BLUMGART, HERRMAN L. (1895–1977)
Outstanding physician-cardiologist at Harvard and Boston's Beth Israel Hospital, where he headed research and clinical programs from 1928 until his retirement in 1962.

BOYD, WILLIAM (1885–1979)
Scottish-born pathologist who spent most of his professional life in Canada at the University of Manitoba and the University of Toronto. A great teacher and author of an extremely popular textbook of pathology.

BRAUNWALD, NINA S. (1928–92)

Wife of cardiologist Eugene Braunwald, but a major figure in her own right: she was a leading cardiac surgeon and performed important research at the NIH at a time when women were discouraged from entering this highly specialized field.

BROCK, (SIR) RUSSELL C. (1903–80)

Guy Hospital surgeon who performed the first pulmonary valvotomy for obstruction to the outflow tract of the right ventricle (pulmonic stenosis) as well as pioneering surgery for mitral stenosis in England.

BURCH, GEORGE (1910–86)

Influential cardiologist and chairman of the Department of Medicine at Tulane (1947–75). He published extensively on such topics as electrocardiography, the effects of hot climates on the heart, congestive heart failure, and the use of radioisotopes in the diagnosis of heart disease, as well as serving as editor in chief of the *American Heart Journal.*

BURCHELL, HOWARD (1907–   )

Among the deans of American cardiology, Burchell, who was born in Canada, spent much of his entire career at the Mayo Clinic, providing the medical arm to John Kirklin's team in advancing open-heart surgery there.

CALLAGHAN, JOHN C. (1924–   )

While working on hypothermia as a fellow under Wilfred Bigelow at the Banting Institute in Toronto, Callaghan, with Bigelow and engineer Jack Hopps, developed an early pacemaker to prevent cardiac standstill, which they had observed occurring in some of their dogs at the low body temperatures induced.

CANNON, WALTER B. (1871–1945)

Harvard physiologist (1898–1942) who was the first to use X-rays in physiological studies (of the gastrointestinal tract), among many other achievements involving the nervous system. His autobiography, *The Way of an Investigator* (1945), remains an enlightening and uplifting guide for those attempting to tread a similar path in science.

CARPENTIER, ALAIN (1933–   )

French cardiovascular surgeon who introduced major advances in valve prostheses as well as pioneering cardiomyoplasty, the use of noncardiac muscle in patients with advanced heart failure.

CARREL, ALEXIS (1873–1944)

French-born experimental surgeon who emigrated to the United States in 1904 and developed many of the cardiovascular techniques that were later incorporated into clinical surgery involving the heart and blood vessels as well as transplantation. Much of this work was done at the Rockefeller Institute. He was the first American citizen to be awarded the Nobel Prize in physiology or medicine (1912).

CASTLE, WILLIAM B. (1897–1990)

Boston hematologist and discoverer of the "intrinsic factor," leading to the elucidation of the cause of pernicious anemia.

CHARDACK, WILLIAM M. (1914–   )

Surgeon at the University of Buffalo who developed the fully implantable permanent pacemaker with engineer Wilson Greatbach.

CHESNEY, ALAN M. (1888–1964)

Early thyroid researcher who later became a faculty member and then dean at Johns Hopkins Medical School. In the latter post he served twenty-four years of a four-decade span at his alma mater.

CHINARD, FRANCIS P. (1918–   )

Chinard's research in the field of indicator-dilution studies shed light on many aspects of the normal and abnormal circulation. He was chairman of the Department of Medicine of the New Jersey Medical School from 1968 to 1975.

CHRISTIAN, HENRY A. (1876–1951)

Pathologist and internist at Harvard who authored many papers as well as textbooks of medicine but is probably remembered best as chief of medicine at Boston's Peter Bent Brigham Hospital (1910–39), during which time many future leaders of American medicine trained under him.

CHURCHILL, EDWARD D. (1895–1972)

Surgical researcher and teacher who served as chief of surgery at Massachusetts General Hospital for many years, beginning in 1933, interrupted only by distinguished World War II service. His major contributions included surgery for hyperparathyroidism, constrictive pericarditis, and bronchiectasis. Many future outstanding surgeons trained under him.

Cobb, William Montague (1904–90)

Physical anthropologist, anatomist, and physician who taught at Howard University's medical school from 1928 until 1973, mainly in the anatomy department, which he headed between 1947 and 1969.

Comroe, Julius H., Jr. (1911–84)

Outstanding pulmonary physiologist and later philosopher of research, first at the University of Pennsylvania and then at the University of California in San Francisco, where he headed the Cardiovascular Research Institute.

Cooley, Denton A. (1920–   )

Perhaps the most naturally gifted cardiac surgeon of our time. Although no great innovator, he contributed to advances in aortic surgery while working with Michael DeBakey at Baylor until 1969, when he left to head the Texas Heart Institute, also in Houston.

Crafoord, Clarence (1899–1984)

Swedish surgeon who participated in many aspects of the advance of cardiac surgery, including surgery for coarctation of the aorta, the development of a heart-lung machine, and the second successful open-heart operation involving removal of a left atrial myxoma.

Cross, Frederick (1920–   )

Cleveland surgeon who, with Earle Kay, developed a rotating-disc pump-oxygenator for use in open-heart surgery.

Cushing, Harvey (1869–1939)

Father of neurosurgery who trained under the legendary William Halsted at Johns Hopkins but was also influenced by William Osler, whose biography he wrote and for which he received a Pulitzer Prize.

Cutler, Elliott Carr (1888–1947)

Moseley Professor of Surgery at Harvard, where he succeeded Harvey Cushing, and chief surgeon at the Peter Bent Brigham Hospital. In 1923 Cutler and cardiologist Samuel Levine joined in an early attempt at surgically repairing mitral stenosis in a young girl. Although unsuccessful, this surgery probably stimulated later researchers to continue this work.

Damman, John F., Jr. (1917–   )

Former chief of pediatric cardiology at the University of Virginia School of Medicine.

DENNIS, CLARENCE (1909–   )

Protégé of Dr. Owen Wangensteen at the University of Minnesota who later became chief of surgery at the State University of New York–Downstate Medical Center in Brooklyn (1952–72), where he continued his work on open-heart surgery.

DEVRIES, WILLIAM C. (1943–   )

Cardiac surgeon who headed the team at the University of Utah that performed the total artificial heart replacement in the patient Barney Clark in 1982.

DEWALL, RICHARD A. (1926–   )

Thoracic surgeon who trained under Dr. Owen Wangensteen at the University of Minnesota and then developed the bubble oxygenator, which allowed for Lillehei's team to begin open-heart surgery with total cardiopulmonary bypass.

DEXTER, LEWIS (1910–95)

One of the early practitioners of modern cardiology at the Peter Bent Brigham Hospital in Boston, where his active cardiac catheterization laboratory produced a number of the new generation of cardiologists, the "Dexter fellows."

DOCK, GEORGE (1860–1951)

The most outstanding trainee of William Osler and the father of William Dock. George Dock was the first full-time professor of medicine in the United States at the University of Michigan when he was appointed to that position, in which he served from 1891 to 1908.

DODRILL, F. DEWEY (1902–97)

Detroit-based surgeon who was one of the pioneers in developing heart-lung machines and other methods for the performance of open-heart surgery.

DOTTER, CHARLES T. (1920–   )

Unquestionably the father of interventional radiography, at the University of Oregon, where he was chairman of radiology for thirty-two years. His angiographic catheter approach to the opening up of arterial vessels to the lower extremities provided a road map for Andreas Gruentzig to attempt the same for the coronary arteries, a debt freely acknowledged by Gruentzig.

DRESSLER, WILLIAM (1890–1969)

American cardiologist who described the syndrome bearing his name that occasionally occurs some weeks following an acute myocardial infarction (pericarditis, fever, leukocytosis) and which is probably related to an auto-immune reaction as a result of the myocardial necrosis.

DUBOST, CHARLES (1914–91)

French surgeon who, in 1951, performed the first resection of an abdominal aortic aneurysm with restoration of continuity.

DuSHANE, JAMES W. (1912–   )

Formerly chief of pediatric cardiology at the Mayo Clinic in Rochester, Minnesota, DuShane was instrumental in helping set up the subspecialty board in pediatric cardiology.

EBERT, PAUL A. (1932–   )

Professor and chairman of cardiovascular surgery at New York Hospital–Cornell (1971–75) and then at the University of California in San Francisco (1975–86).

EDWARDS, JESSE F. (1911–   )

At the Mayo Clinic in Rochester, Minnesota (1946–60) he was the pathologist specializing in cardiac diseases during the Kirklin era, contributing significantly to that program. In 1960 he moved to United Hospitals in St. Paul.

EFFLER, DONALD B. (1915–   )

Colorful and enterprising thoracic and cardiovascular surgeon who was at the Cleveland Clinic during the development of open-heart surgery and especially coronary bypass surgery, in which that institution was an early leader.

EICHNA, LUDWIG W. (1908–   )

Professor of medicine at New York University, later becoming chairman, Department of Medicine, at SUNY-Downstate in Brooklyn (1960–74).

FERRER, M. IRENÉ (1915–   )

Cardiologist at Columbia's College of Physicians and Surgeons, where she often collaborated with Réjane Harvey and André Cournand. She had a special interest in cor pulmonale and electrocardiography, and she delineated the clinical features of the "Sick Sinus (brady-tachy) syndrome."

FISHMAN, ALFRED P. (1918–   )

Physician and physiologist whose interest in the pulmonary circulation resulted in major contributions to this field of study.

FLEMING, (SIR) ALEXANDER (1881–1955)

Discoverer of penicillin, for which he shared a Nobel Prize in 1945 with Howard Florey and Ernst Chain.

FLOREY, HOWARD (1898–1968)

Australian-born investigator who, at Oxford with Ernst Chain, renewed interest in the use of penicillin as suggested by Fleming over a decade earlier. This led to the clinical introduction of penicillin as an antibiotic and a Nobel Prize in 1945.

FRANK, OTTO (1865–1944)

German scientist whose work on the frog heart led to Ernest Starling's work in the dog and the latter's concept of the Law of the Heart. This was later modified by the work of Stanley Sarnoff and Eugene Braunwald at the National Institutes of Health.

FREDERICKSON, DONALD B. (1924–2002)

Investigator whose work with lipid metabolism at the National Institutes of Health provided a helpful classification of the dyslipidemias.

FRIEDBERG, CHARLES K. (1905–72)

Author of the classic textbook *Diseases of the Heart,* the last influential single-authored work by an American on this subject. Dr. Friedberg worked for his entire career at Mount Sinai Hospital in New York, following a four-year fellowship study period in Amsterdam and Vienna.

FRIEDMAN, MEYER (1911–2001)

Cardiologist who, with Ray Rosenman, linked the effect of personality features (Type A, Type B) on the propensity for developing or not developing coronary heart disease.

FURMAN, SEYMOUR (1931–   )

Surgeon at Montefiore Hospital in the Bronx who introduced intracardiac pacing (via catheter) in heart block in 1958.

GARRETT, H. EDWARD (1926–   )

Former professor and chairman of thoracic and cardiovascular surgery at the University of Tennessee who earlier (1964), while working in Michael

DeBakey's department at Baylor, performed with DeBakey an early venous bypass graft of an occluded coronary artery.

GAY, WILLIAM A. (1936–   )
Cardiovascular surgeon at Cornell–New York Hospital; later the University of Utah, then Barnes Hospital in St. Louis.

GIBBON, JOHN H., JR. (1903–73)
Philadelphia surgeon who, beginning in 1935, began the development of the heart-lung machine, finally succeeding in this with a repair of an atrial septal defect in 1953. Several subsequent failures caused him to desist in further efforts, but the door had been opened for others to carry on this work.

GOFMAN, JOHN W. (1918–   )
Physicist-chemist-physician who developed a centrifuge method of separating out and identifying lipoproteins and the relationship of specific ones to the development of atherosclerosis.

GRANT, ROBERT P. (1915–66)
One of the most original thinkers and contributors to the field of electrocardiography. He later was associated with the National Heart Institute in the Grants and Training Branch (1959–61) and the National Institutes of Health (1962), finally becoming director of the National Heart Institute in 1966 shortly before his untimely death at the age of fifty-one.

GREEN, GEORGE E. (1932–   )
New York–based surgeon who introduced the technique of using magnifying lenses in the performance of coronary artery bypass grafting, especially with the internal mammary artery.

GREGG, ALAN (1890–1957)
Influential figure in medical research and education through his positions at the Rockefeller Foundation in the Divisions of Medical Education and Medical Science (1922–31), and thereafter as vice president of the foundation. His service in the fields of public health, medical education, and research spanned over forty years.

GREGG, DONALD E. (1902–83)
One of the outstanding physiologists who emerged from Carl Wiggers's laboratory at Western Reserve. Gregg became the world expert on the normal and abnormal coronary circulation, first at Western Reserve (1930–44) and

then, after obtaining a medical degree at the University of Rochester, spent the bulk of his later career as chief of the Department of Cardiorespiratory Diseases at Walter Reed Army Institute of Research (from 1950 on).

Gross, Robert E. (1905–88)

Surgeon at Children's Hospital in Boston who, in 1938, performed one of the earliest operations for correction of a congenital cardiac defect by ligating a patent ductus arteriosus (an abnormal persistence of a connection between the pulmonary artery and the aorta).

Groves, Lawrence K. (1922–   )

Cleveland Clinic surgeon who worked with Donald Effler, René Favaloro, and Mason Sones during the period when coronary bypass surgery was being developed at that institution.

Gruentzig, Andreas (1939–85)

German-born cardiologist who, stimulated by the work of Charles Dotter on arterial occlusion in the lower extremities, developed the technique of coronary angioplasty in 1979 while working in Zurich. He later moved to Emory to continue this and other investigative work before being killed in the crash of his airplane in 1985.

Halsted, William S. (1852–1922)

Founding chairman of the Department of Surgery of the Johns Hopkins University Medical School (1889–1922) who, along with William Osler (Medicine), William Welch (Pathology), and Howard Kelly (Obstetrics and Gynecology), established that institution's reputation for excellence.

Hamilton, William F. (1893–1964)

Chairman, Department of Physiology, of the Medical College of Georgia (1934–60) and prominent researcher in cardiovascular problems; especially noteworthy was his contribution to indicator-dilution theory (the Stewart-Hamilton principle), which is useful in determining cardiac output.

Harken, Dwight E. (1910–93)

Thoracic surgeon at Harvard and the Peter Bent Brigham Hospital in Boston. In addition to his work on mitral stenosis, paralleling that of Charles Bailey, he inserted the first intracardiac ball-in-cage valve and made an early contribution to the appreciation of diastolic augmentation, which he termed "counterpulsation."

HARRISON, TINSLEY R. (1900–79)

Alabama physician-cardiologist who, among other posts, developed three new departments of medicine (University of North Carolina, Bowman Gray, and the University of Alabama at Birmingham). Major contributions included his monograph, *Failure of the Circulation,* and his textbook of medicine.

HARVEY, A. McGHEE (1911–98)

Leading physician at Johns Hopkins, where he worked for over fifty years, eventually heading its Department of Medicine for twenty-seven years.

HARVEY, RÉJANE M. (1917–   )

Professor of Medicine, Columbia University College of Physicians and Surgeons, where she became director of the Pulmonary Division and collaborated frequently with Irené Ferrer and André Cournand.

HASTINGS, A. BAIRD (1895–1987)

Biochemist at Harvard with major contributions to knowledge about the regulation of blood acid-base balance, the role of calcium, and the regulation of glucose metabolism.

HECHT, HANS H. (1913–71)

Swiss-born cardiologist and member of the nucleus of outstanding internists assembled by Dr. Maxwell M. Wintrobe in building his department at the University of Utah. He left there after a number of years to become chairman, Department of Medicine, at the University of Chicago.

HERRICK, JAMES B. (1861–1954)

Distinguished Chicago physician whose investigations covered a number of medical areas. He is most remembered for his publication in 1912 of the report "Clinical Features of Sudden Obstruction of the Coronary Arteries," in which he pointed out that patients could survive from this disease, which had previously been thought to be uniformly fatal.

HUFNAGEL, CHARLES (1916–89)

Surgical protégé of Robert Gross who later joined the faculty at Georgetown University College of Medicine. He is best known for his development, in the pre–open-heart surgery era, of a ball-valve device to be placed in the aorta for relief of severe aortic regurgitation.

Huggins, Charles B. (1901–97)

American surgeon and researcher most remembered for his finding that the injection of female hormones could control cancers of the male prostate gland. This discovery introduced the concept of endocrine inhibition of tumor growth in the cancer field.

Hunter, John (1728–93)

English surgeon, anatomist, and physiologist with wide-ranging interests in many branches of natural history. At his death, in addition to a number of medical works, he left his personal museum containing over ten thousand items, which were finally donated by the government to the Royal College of Surgeons.

Jarvik, Robert K. (1946–   )

Designer of the artificial heart that was inserted into the initial patients in the Utah program of heart transplantation, beginning with Barney Clark in 1982.

Jones, T. Duckett (1899–1954)

A graduate of the medical school of the University of Virginia, Duckett later migrated to Boston and Harvard. In Boston he worked at the Massachusetts General Hospital and also the House of the Good Samaritan, where he directed the research department from 1929 to 1947. He is responsible for the Jones Criteria for the diagnosis of rheumatic fever (1944), his primary interest, thus creating some order out of the preexisting diagnostic chaos that had led to many errors.

Katz, Louis N. (1897–1973)

One of the giants of twentieth-century cardiology, Katz started out in the physiology laboratory of Carl Wiggers in Western Reserve and then moved to Chicago and the Michael Reese Hospital, where he trained a great number of top-notch future investigators as well as performed outstanding work in electrocardiography, atherosclerosis, hypertension, and hemodynamics.

Kay, Earle B. (1911–2000)

Cleveland surgeon who developed a number of closed-heart procedures between 1946 and 1956. Later, he and Frederick Cross developed a rotating–disc pump-oxygenator. Kay also contributed to the design of artificial heart valves, among his other surgical accomplishments.

KEEFER, CHESTER S. (1897–1972)

Prominent medical figure who, following training at Johns Hopkins, Billings Hospital (Chicago), and Peiping Union Medical College, came to Boston in 1930 for a ten-year stint at the Thorndike Memorial Laboratory at Boston City Hospital before moving to Boston University, where he became chief of medicine (1940–59) and later dean (1955–72).

KEITH, JOHN D. (1909–89)

Professor of pediatrics at the University of Toronto and author, with Richard Rowe and Peter Vlad, of the outstanding monograph *Heart Disease in Infancy and Childhood* (1958).

KETY, SEYMOUR S. (1916–2000)

A major figure in biological psychiatry, Kety developed the nitrous oxide method for determining cerebral blood flow with E. F. Schmidt. This technique was later applied by Richard Bing and others to study coronary blood flow and metabolism.

KEYS, ANCEL (1904–   )

Physiologist who made major contributions to our understanding of the effects of high altitude on humans as well as the biology of starvation and the influence of diet on the development of atherosclerosis.

KILLIP, THOMAS III (1927–   )

Chief of cardiology at Cornell–New York Hospital (1961–74). An authority on acute coronary care, Killip introduced a helpful clinical categorization of patients early in the course of myocardial infarction that had prognostic significance in terms of expected mortality (Killip Classes I–IV)

KIRSCHNER, MARTIN (1879–1942)

Leading German surgeon and teacher at Heidelberg who performed the first successful pulmonary embolectomy.

KORNBERG, ARTHUR (1918–   )

Although an M.D. by training, Kornberg distinguished himself in basic science and was awarded the Nobel Prize in 1959 for his work on DNA replication.

KOROTKOFF, NIKOLAI S. (1874–1920)

Russian vascular surgeon who devised the auscultatory method of measuring arterial blood pressure (1905). The sounds by which we measure systolic and diastolic pressure still bear his name.

KOUWENHOVEN, WILLIAM B. (1886–1975)
Johns Hopkins professor of electrical engineering who, with associates, began working in 1928 on cardiac arrest (ventricular fibrillation) induced by accidents in the electrical industry. This work finally led to the modern resuscitative method of "closed chest cardiac massage" with defibrillation, introduced by Kouwenhoven and Dr. James Jude in 1960.

KULLER, LEWIS H. (1934–   )
Epidemiologist-physician who has performed important population studies on sudden death, coronary heart disease, and related topics.

LANGENDORF, RICHARD (1908–87)
Czech cardiologist who preceded Alfred Pick in emigrating to Michael Reese Hospital in Chicago to work with Louis Katz during the years of Nazi domination in Europe. When he was reunited with Pick after World War II at Michael Reese Hospital, they collaborated on important studies analyzing complex cardiac arrhythmias.

LASKER, MARY (1900–1994)
Philanthropist who, in 1942, with her husband, Albert, set up the Lasker Foundation to support basic and clinical medical research.

LERICHE, RENÉ (1879–1955)
A director of the surgical clinic in Strasbourg, France, during the early part of the twentieth century. Leriche is remembered for describing the syndrome that bears his name; it involves buttock and thigh pain on exertion that results from obstruction of the terminal aorta as it divides into the iliac arteries.

LEV, MAURICE (1908–94)
Pathologist whose knowledge of congenital heart diseases was encyclopedic and who assisted many cardiologists and cardiac surgeons in understanding the anatomy and physiology of these diseases in their approaches to diagnosis and treatment.

LEVINE, SAMUEL A. (1891–1966)
Professor of medicine at Harvard and cardiologist at the Peter Bent Brigham Hospital. Author of the books *Clinical Heart Disease* (5th ed., 1958) and

Coronary Thrombosis (1929). An esteemed teacher of his specialty in Boston as well as on the national scene.

LEWIS, F. JOHN (1916–   )

Minnesota surgeon in Owen Wangensteen's department who performed the first successful open-heart surgery. It was done using hypothermia to close an atrial septal defect.

LEWIS, (SIR) THOMAS (1881–1945)

Inheriting the mantle of his older colleague James Mackensie, this Welsh-born clinician and cardiovascular physiologist was one of the earliest physicians in Great Britain to recognize the potential of the electrocardiograph. His books, *Clinical Disorders of the Heart Beat* (1912) and *Diseases of the Heart* (1933), became instant classics. From the University College Hospital in London from 1902 until his death, his outpouring of research and teaching strongly influenced subsequent generations of cardiologists in Great Britain and elsewhere.

LIKOFF, WILLIAM (1912–87)

Prominent leader in American clinical cardiology at Hahnemann Medical College in Philadelphia.

LILLEHEI, C. WALTON (1918–99)

University of Minnesota surgeon who made many important contributions to open-heart surgery, especially in the areas of congenital defects and valvular heart disease.

LINDBERGH, CHARLES A. (1902–74)

The famous aviator "adopted" Alexis Carrel as a surrogate father and, for a time in the early thirties, worked with him and Richard Bing at the Rockefeller Institute on a perfusion system to maintain the viability of isolated organs outside the body.

LONG, PERRIN H. (1899–1965)

Best known for his work on the introduction of sulfonamides in the treatment of infections. After twenty-two years at Johns Hopkins, Long became chairman of the Department of Medicine at the State University of New York–Downstate Medical Center in Brooklyn. He held this post ten years (1951–61) until illness forced his resignation.

LONGCOPE, WARFIELD T. (1877–1953)

After receiving his M.D. from Johns Hopkins in 1901, Longcope, for the major portion of his career (1922–46), was professor of medicine at his alma mater, where he exerted a major influence on its faculty and students.

LOWER, RICHARD R. (1929–   )

Early investigator in cardiac transplantation who, with Norman Shumway, developed the operative technique for this procedure.

LOWN, BERNARD (1921–   )

Born in Lithuania, Lown underwent medical training in the United States at Johns Hopkins. At the Harvard School of Public Health he and associates developed the DC defibrillator. He has also been active in international peace efforts, for which he was a corecipient of the Nobel Peace Prize in 1985.

LUDWIG, CARL (1816–95)

Circulatory physiologist and director of the Leipzig Physiological Institute, beginning in 1869, where many later leaders in the field profited from his teaching and encouragement.

LUISADA, ALDO A. (1901–87)

Italian-born cardiologist who worked primarily at the Chicago Medical School. Using graphic recording techniques, he made extensive studies of the heart sounds, murmurs, and pressure pulses in normal and diseased hearts.

MACKENZIE, (SIR) JAMES (1853–1925)

Beginning as a general practitioner in Scotland, he developed an early interest in heart disease and became, in essence, the founder of modern British cardiology through his work on graphic recordings of the pulse (1902) and his clinical observations in his textbook, *Diseases of the Heart* (1908).

MALM, JAMES R. (1925–   )

Surgeon at Columbia-Presbyterian Hospital in New York City who helped develop infant cardiac surgery at that institution.

MAROKO, PETER R. (1936–92)

Polish-born cardiologist, raised in Brazil, whose original investigative approaches for evaluating myocardial ischemia came to fruition through his association with Eugene Braunwald. He later went to Deborah Hospital in New Jersey before his untimely death.

MASTER, ARTHUR M. (1895–1973)

Cardiologist at Mount Sinai Hospital in New York City who, with Bernard Oppenheimer, introduced an early exercise test with electrocardiographic monitoring for the detection of coronary artery disease (the "Master 2-Step Test").

MATAS, RUDOLPH (1860–1938)

New Orleans surgeon who made many important contributions, including the use of spinal anesthesia, a device for assisting respiration intraoperatively, and improvement of the technique for surgery involving arterial aneurysms.

MAYO, CHARLES H. (1865–1939) AND MAYO, WILLIAM J. (1861–1939)

Sons of William W. Mayo (1819–1911) and founders of the Mayo Clinic in Rochester, Minnesota. The elder Mayo was retired when the clinic opened, and it was his sons who developed the institution at St. Mary's Hospital. The Mayo Clinic opened in 1889 and the Clinic Building in 1914.

McINTOSH, HENRY D. (1921–   )

Influential cardiologist at Duke (1956–70) and later the VA Hospital in Houston, Texas.

McNAMARA, DANIEL G. (1922–98)

Early leader in pediatric cardiology, trained by Helen Taussig, and later head of pediatric cardiology at Baylor-Texas Children's Hospital in Houston.

MELNICK, JOSEPH L. (1914–2001)

A founder of modern virology who worked at Baylor College of Medicine for over forty years.

MELROSE, DENNIS G. (1921–   )

South African–born, British-trained surgeon who stressed the need for elective cardiac arrest for proper performance of open-heart surgery, introducing the use of potassium citrate for this purpose.

MINOT, GEORGE R. (1885–1950)

Recipient with George Whipple and William P. Murphy of the Nobel Prize in medicine in 1934 for the introduction of successful liver therapy for pernicious anemia. Director of the Thorndike Memorial Laboratory at the Boston City Hospital from 1928 until his death.

MIROWSKI, MICHEL (1924–90)

Polish-born cardiologist who eventually emigrated to the United States and the Sinai Hospital in Baltimore, where he was responsible for developing the automatic implantable cardioverter-defibrillator.

MOORE, CARL V. (1908–72)

Hematologist and chairman of the Department of Medicine at Washington University at St. Louis (1955–72).

MOORE, FRANCIS D. (1913–2001)

Distinguished professor of surgery at Harvard, best known for his development of radioactive isotopic techniques to determine body water and electrolyte changes related to surgery.

MORROW, ANDREW GLENN (1922–82)

Surgeon at the National Institutes of Health who was responsible for many surgical innovations in the treatment of valvular heart disease as well as developing the surgical procedure for relief of hypertrophic obstructive cardiomyopathy (HOCM).

MURPHY, WILLIAM P. (1892–1987)

Boston internist who shared the Nobel Prize in 1934 with George Whipple and George Minot for the liver treatment of pernicious anemia.

MUSTARD, WILLIAM T. (1914–87)

Canadian surgeon who developed the operation bearing his name for the surgical treatment of transposition of the great vessels.

NADAS, ALEXANDER S. (1914–2000)

A graduate of the Budapest Medical School in Hungary who came to the United States in 1938 and eventually became the pediatric cardiologist at the Children's Hospital in Boston. His textbook, *Pediatric Cardiology,* published in 1957, served as an important guide for budding cardiologists, many of whom emerged from his tutelage over the years.

NOSÉ, YUKIHITO (1932–   )

Japanese-born surgeon whose life has been devoted to the development of artificial organs and who worked under Willem Kolff and Adrian Kantrowitz before joining the Department of Surgery at Baylor with Michael DeBakey.

NUTTING, MARY ADELAIDE (1858–1948)

With Lavinia Dock (aunt of William Dock), one of the pioneers in the development of American nursing. She coauthored with Lavinia Dock an exhaustive four-volume *History of Nursing,* which was first published in 1907.

OCHSNER, ALTON (1896–1979)

Prominent surgeon who, in 1942, founded the New Orleans clinic that bears his name. Among Ochsner's many contributions to medicine and surgery, his work linking cigarette smoking to lung cancer and other maladies was probably his most important.

OLIVER, JEAN REDMAN (1889–1976)

Professor of pathology, State University of New York–Downstate Medical Center (formerly the Long Island College of Medicine). Oliver was most noted for his work on kidney structure through meticulous micro-dissections.

OSLER, (SIR) WILLIAM (1849–1919)

Most distinguished of all American physicians, although Canadian-born and destined in later years to become Regius Professor of Medicine at Oxford. Greatly admired for his bedside teaching methods, textbook of medicine, and general philosophy, Osler was one of four clinical figures who established Johns Hopkins as a great medical institution. (The others were Welch in pathology, Halsted in surgery, and Kelly in obstetrics and gynecology.)

OUDOT, JACQUES (1913–53)

French surgeon who, in 1950, performed the first successful surgery on a patient with the Leriche syndrome (obstruction at the distal bifurcation of the aorta). He repeated this feat in four additional patients over the subsequent two years.

PAGE, IRVINE H. (1901–91)

Hypertension researcher whose investigations led to the discovery of the vasopressor substance, angiotensin. Much of his work was done at the Cleveland Clinic.

PAUL, OGLESBY (1916–   )

Harvard-trained physician, Boston-based except for a period in Chicago when he led the Western Electric Study on coronary heart disease. He is the author of a definitive biography of Paul Dudley White.

PICK, ALFRED (1907–82)

Czech-born cardiologist who joined Louis Katz's group at Michael Reese Hospital after World War II, and an important contributor to research in electrocardiography and the study of complex arrhythmias.

PICKERING, (SIR) GEORGE W. (1904–80)

Protégé of Sir Thomas Lewis and later Regius Professor of Medicine at Oxford and an authority on hypertension.

PITTMAN, JAMES A., JR. (1927–   )

Endocrinologist and nuclear medicine specialist who was dean at the University of Alabama Medical School in Birmingham for much of the time Kirklin worked there as head of surgery.

POUTASSE, EUGENE F. (1918–   )

Urologist at the Cleveland Clinic during the period Kolff and Favaloro worked there.

PROUDFIT, WILLIAM L. (1914–   )

Cardiologist at the Cleveland Clinic who worked closely with René Favaloro and Mason Sones in making clinical correlations to their work on coronary bypass surgery.

RAVDIN, ISIDORE (1894–1972)

Professor and chairman of the Department of Surgery at the University of Pennsylvania in the post–World War II years.

REGAN, TIMOTHY J. (1924–2001)

Chief of cardiology at the New Jersey Medical School (1965–93), where his laboratory and clinical observations provided important insights into the relationships among smoking, alcohol, diabetes, and heart disease.

RICHARDS, DICKINSON W. (1895–1973)

Physiologist-physician at Columbia University's College of Physicians and Surgeons in New York (1927–73). A longtime collaborator with André Cournand, with whom he shared the Nobel Prize along with Werner Forssman in 1956 for the introduction of cardiac catheterization.

ROBERTS, WILLIAM C. (1932–   )

Pathologist, currently editor of the *American Journal of Cardiology,* who has specialized in cardiovascular disease.

RODBARD, SIMON (1911–75)

Gifted physician-physiologist with unique approaches to research who began his career with Louis Katz at Michael Reese Hospital in Chicago. He later moved to the University of California and the City of Hope in Duarte, where he remained the director of cardiology until his death.

ROENTGEN, WILHELM CONRAD (1845–1923)

German physicist and discoverer of X-rays, for which he received the first Nobel Prize in physics in 1901.

ROPES, MARIAN (1903–94)

Distinguished rheumatologist at the Massachusetts General Hospital who was an authority on lupus erythematosis, and who trained many of the current leading figures in the field.

ROSS, RICHARD S. (1924–   )

Johns Hopkins cardiologist and later dean.

ROWE, RICHARD D. (1923–88)

A New Zealand native who, following his early training, came to the Hospital for Sick Children in Toronto, where John Keith was professor of pediatrics. Keith, Rowe, and Peter Vlad of the University of Iowa College of Medicine produced *Heart Disease in Infancy and Childhood* (1958), which, like the texts of Helen B. Taussig and Alexander S. Nadas, was a guiding light for those entering the field of pediatric cardiology in its infancy.

RUSHMER, ROBERT F. (1914–2001)

M.D./Ph.D. who headed the Department of Physiology at the University of Washington School of Medicine until 1985 and who introduced many bioengineering concepts to the study of the circulation.

RUSSEK, HENRY I. (1911–90)

Consultant in cardiovascular disease at the U.S. Marine Hospital in Staten Island who performed a number of clinical studies on the effectiveness of antianginal drugs.

SABIN, ALBERT B. (1907–93)

Prominent virologist with a long career at the Rockefeller Institute and the University of Cincinnati, capped by the development of an oral live attenuated virus vaccine against poliomyelitis.

SABISTON, DAVID C., JR. (1924–   )

Johns Hopkins–trained surgeon who later headed the program in cardio-vascular surgery at Duke (1964–96) and who edited two of the leading text-books in surgery (*The Biological Basis of Surgical Practice* and *Surgery of the Chest*) through many editions.

SARNOFF, STANLEY J. (1917–90)

Brilliant cardiovascular investigator in cardiac physiology at the NIH who stimulated a reexamination of cardiac function as expressed in Starling's Law of the Heart. This, in turn, led to further work by Eugene Braunwald and his colleagues on the same problem.

SAUERBRUCH, ERNST FERDINAND (1875–1951)

Outstanding German surgeon who developed a negative pressure cabinet that would permit operations on the opened chest without causing collapse of the lungs (1904). At the Charité Hospital in Berlin he dominated German surgery for years until his career was overtaken by senility he did not recog-nize, with disastrous results to his patients. Legal actions were finally under-taken to prevent his continued practice.

SCHLESINGER, MONROE J. (1892–1955)

Pathologist at Beth Israel Hospital in Boston who devised a method of postmortem injection of the coronary arteries with a radiopaque gel-like material to reveal the status of the coronary circulation; he pursued these investigations with Herrman Blumgart, Paul Zoll, and others.

SENNING ÅKE (1915–2000)

Swedish cardiovascular surgeon responsible for a number of surgical inno-vations. These included the first use of an implantable permanent pace-maker, a methodology advanced soon after by American surgeon William Chardack and the engineer Wilson Greatbach.

SHILEY, DON (1920–   )

Engineer who worked with Albert Starr and others in the development of a number of types of prosthetic heart valves.

SHUMWAY, NORMAN E. (1923–   )

Head of the cardiac transplantation team at Stanford University who, more than anyone else, pursued the problems of rejection et cetera. His work led to the establishment of cardiac transplantation as an almost routine procedure after many failures in the first blush of activity following Christiaan Barnard's first human heart transplant in Cape Town.

SMITH, FRED M. (1888–1946)

Protégé of James B. Herrick at Rush Medical School in Chicago, remembered primarily for laboratory studies involving ligation of the coronary arteries in dogs to demonstrate the associated electrocardiographic changes. This work led to the recognition of similar changes in the electrocardiograms of humans in the course of nonfatal myocardial infarctions.

SMITH, HOMER W. (1895–1962)

Professor of physiology and biophysics at New York University School of Medicine (1928–61). He was at the fore of much research done there during his tenure and as much a philosopher as an investigator of kidney function. His book *From Fish to Philosopher: The Story of Our Internal Environment* (1953) reveals the man as well as his science.

SMITHWICK, REGINALD H. (1899–1987)

Boston surgeon who, in the period before effective and conveniently taken antihypertensive drugs became available, used sympathetic denervation for the treatment of severe hypertension in over 2,500 patients between 1940 and 1955.

SMITHY, HORACE G. (1914–48)

Extraordinarily gifted young South Carolina surgeon who, with Charles Bailey, Russell Brock, and Dwight Harken, successfully introduced the operative approach for the relief of mitral stenosis and helped usher in a new era of "closed" direct surgery upon the heart before open-heart surgery became possible.

SOBEL, BURTON E. (1937–   )

Graduate of Eugene Braunwald's program at the NIH who became cardiologist-in-chief at the Barnes Hospital in St. Louis (1973–93) and, later, chief of medicine at the University of Vermont in Burlington.

SONES, F. MASON (1918–85)

Cleveland Clinic cardiologist (1950–75) who pioneered cineangiography and selective coronary arteriography in the diagnosis of coronary heart disease.

SONNENBLICK, EDMUND H. (1932–   )

One of Braunwald's team at the NIH who performed important basic studies using the papillary muscle preparation and who is now professor of medicine at the Albert Einstein College of Medicine in the Bronx, New York.

SOUTTAR, (SIR) HENRY S. (1875–1964)

British surgeon who manually dilated the stenotic mitral valve of a patient in 1925. However, the operation did not catch on because the medical community at the time resisted the idea that the problem with mitral stenosis was mechanical rather than one involving the myocardium. Souttar therefore received no further referrals for this procedure.

STARLING, ERNEST H. (1866–1927)

Physiologist at the University of London who made many contributions to this field, such as explaining the basis of fluid exchanges between tissues (the Starling Hypothesis) and developing a heart-lung preparation in dogs that enabled him and his associates to determine various factors governing the performance of the heart (Starling's Law of the Heart) and its metabolism.

STARR, ISAAC (1895–1989)

Cardiovascular physiologist at the University of Pennsylvania who promoted the use of the ballistocardiograph, an apparatus that recorded, noninvasively, the movements of the body that resulted from the beating of the heart.

STEAD, EUGENE A. (1908–   )

Legendary departmental chairman in medicine who, after graduating from Emory, trained in Boston and then returned to Atlanta to become chairman of medicine at Emory (1942–48). He then assumed the same position at Duke (1948–68). Many future departmental chairmen emerged from Stead's training programs; he also made significant research contributions.

STEINBERG, ISRAEL (1902–83)

Radiologist at Cornell–New York Hospital who made many contributions to the field of cardiac diagnosis.

SZENT-GYÖRGY, ALBERT (1893–1986)

Colorful Hungarian-born biochemist who is most noted for the discovery of vitamin C as the antiscurvy factor as well as his work on the muscle components necessary for contraction. He received the Nobel Prize in 1937 for the vitamin C work.

TAUSSIG, HELEN B. (1898–1986)

Johns Hopkins pediatrician-cardiologist who, through her clinic for children with congenital and other heart diseases, laid the foundations of modern pediatric cardiology. With surgeon Alfred Blalock she was responsible for the introduction of the "blue baby" operation (Blalock-Taussig procedure) for certain cyanotic congenital cardiac defects. She also trained many of the leading pediatric cardiologists of the twentieth century.

THOMAS, VIVIEN (1910–85)

Gifted African-American laboratory worker who became an invaluable assistant—some would say collaborator—to Alfred Blalock in his cardio-vascular surgical research.

VARCO, RICHARD L. (1912–)

Talented staff surgeon at the University of Minnesota whose support of and cooperation with Walton Lillehei was important in carrying forth the work to develop an open-heart surgical program at that institution.

VATNER, STEPHEN F. (1940–)

Laboratory investigator whose work on animal models of myocardial ischemia has provided important information applicable to clinically observed human coronary heart disease. Currently he is professor of medicine at the New Jersey Medical School in Newark, New Jersey.

VINEBERG, ARTHUR M. (1903–88)

Canadian cardiac surgeon who, in the precoronary bypass era, devised the Vineberg procedure, in which an internal mammary artery, implanted in the muscle of the heart or omentum, could be sutured to the heart to provide revascularization to ischemic heart muscle in patients with coronary artery disease.

VISSCHER, MAURICE B. (1901–83)

Leading American physiologist at the University of Minnesota who was one of the last fellows of Ernest Starling in London. He also spent time with A. J. Carlson at the University of Chicago before returning to Minnesota, where he became chairman of the physiology department and intimately involved in the cardiac surgical program being developed there under Owen Wangensteen and C. Walton Lillehei.

WANGENSTEEN, OWEN H. (1898–1981)

Chief of surgery at the University of Minnesota for almost forty years (1930–67), where he built one of the nation's outstanding departments.

Although primarily known for his own work on gastrointestinal problems, he presided during a period of innovation and rapid development in the field of cardiac surgery, spurred on by C. Walton Lillehei, Richard A. DeWall, and others who worked under him in the department.

WARREN, JAMES V. (1915–90)

Harvard-trained physician who, following his initial postgraduate years at the Peter Bent Brigham Hospital under Soma Weiss, joined Eugene Stead at Emory, where important early studies in cardiac dynamics were performed. Warren went on to have a distinguished career at Emory and then Ohio State, where he served as chairman of medicine for eighteen years (1961–79).

WEINSTEIN, LOUIS (1909–2000)

Considered by most of his contemporaries to be the most gifted intuitive infectious disease expert of his time, this Boston physician was also a superior investigator and mentor to innumerable acolytes who have since populated the field.

WEISS, SOMA (1899–1942)

Hungarian-born physician who emigrated to the United States in his youth, eventually joining the Harvard medical faculty in 1925. A brilliant career led to his appointment as Hersey Professor of Medicine there until his untimely death at forty-three.

WENCKEBACH, KAREL F. (1864–1941)

Dutch cardiologist whose major pioneering work in electrocardiography was done during his tenure as professor at Groningen and Vienna.

WHIPPLE, ALLEN O. (1881–1963)

First full-time chairman of surgery at Columbia's College of Physicians and Surgeons (1921–46). Best remembered for his development of radical surgery for cancer of the pancreas, the Whipple procedure (pancreatoduodenectomy plus partial stomach removal.)

WHITE, PAUL DUDLEY (1886–1973)

One of the world's best-known and most beloved cardiologists, White was based at Harvard's Massachusetts General Hospital for virtually his entire professional life. His activities as author of an important monograph on heart disease, as a founder of the American Heart Association, and as an investigator of, among other subjects, the epidemiology of coronary heart disease, made him well known to the medical world. His public recognition derived from his treatment of President Dwight Eisenhower during the latter's myocardial infarction in 1955.

WIGGERS, CARL J. (1883–1963)

As chairman of physiology at Western Reserve, to which he came in 1918 and where he worked until 1953, Wiggers became the leading circulatory physiologist of our time, training many others in this discipline. Of these, thirty-seven went on to become departmental chairmen or research directors at other medical centers.

WILLIAMS, ROBERT H. (1909–80)

Hopkins-, Harvard-, and Vanderbilt-trained endocrinologist whose textbook on the subject (1950) became the leader in the field. He served as professor and chairman, Department of Medicine at the University of Washington in Seattle until his death.

WILSON, FRANK N. (1890–1952)

Early researcher in various aspects of electrocardiography who applied and extended much of the earlier work of Einthoven.

WINTROBE, MAXWELL M. (1901–86)

Canadian-born chairman of medicine at the University of Utah (1943–67) and one of the world's leading hematologists, whose text on the subject became the primary resource for all those in hematology and internal medicine during this time.

WOOD, EARL H. (1912–   )

M.D.-physiologist under Maurice Visscher at the University of Minnesota who later spent the bulk of his career at the Mayo Clinic and became an important member of John Kirklin's group in starting the open-heart program there. Through his work on oximeters, strain gauges, and indicator-dilution techniques, Wood made groundbreaking contributions to the development of clinical cardiac catheterization.

WOOD, PAUL H. (1907–62)

Brilliant cardiologist at Postgraduate Medical School at Hammersmith Hospital, London, who was responsible for numerous important clinical studies, and whose textbook, *Diseases of the Heart and Circulation* (1950), is a classic of its kind. A great researcher, clinician, and teacher, he was also known for his frequent vitriol.

NOTES

---

1. The injectable mercurials were the first effective diuretics introduced for congestive heart failure and other fluid-retaining disorders. The article reporting this finding was P. Saxl and R. Helig, Über die diuretische Wirking von novasural—und angeren Quecksilberinjektionen, *Wien Clin Wchnschr* 1920; 33:943–945. For a direct personal account of how this breakthrough came about, see A. Vogl, The discovery of the organic mercurial diuretics, *Am Heart J* 1950; 39:881–883. For a broader view on the same subject, see A. B. Weisse, Mercury Finally Makes It, in *Medical Odysseys: The Different and Sometimes Unexpected Pathways to Twentieth-Century Medical Discoveries* (New Brunswick, N.J.: Rutgers University Press, 1991), 4–15.

2. Ballistocardiography involves the optical recording of the impulses imparted to the patient's body by the ejection of blood from the heart, with the patient placed on a specially designed table for such recordings. Although he did not discover the technique, ISAAC STARR (1895–1989) of the University of Pennsylvania pioneered it during the first decades of the century. In the late forties, when the then-current instrument was selling for $3,200 on the market, Dock devised an equally good one at a cost of $20 to construct. In 1953 he coauthored a monograph on its uses: W. Dock, H. Mandelbaum, and R. A. Mandelbaum, *Ballistocardiography: The Application of the Direct Ballistocardiograph to Clinical Medicine* (St. Louis: C. V. Mosby, 1953). Although at one time there was considerable interest in the technique, it is rarely, if ever, used by clinicians today.

3. W. Dock, Mode of production of the first heart sound, *Arch Int Med* 1933; 51:737–746.

4. W. Dock, Korotkoff's sounds, *N Engl J Med* 1980; 302:1264–1266.

5. W. Dock, Use and abuse of bed rest, *NY State J Med* 1944; 44:724–730.

6. *Time*, April 24, 1944, 44, 46.

7. W. Dock, Apical localization of phthisis, *Am Rev Tuberc* 1946; 53:297–305.

8. W. Dock, The predilection of atherosclerosis for the coronary arteries, *JAMA* 1946; 131:875–878. In this study Dock examined sections of the coro-

nary arteries of infants who had died, and he found that the intima of the coronaries, already known to be thicker than in other arteries of the same size in the body, were thicker in males than in females and therefore might account for the earlier predilection for coronary heart disease in men compared to women.

9. GEORGE R. MINOT and WILLIAM P. MURPHY demonstrated the effectiveness of liver feeding in the treatment of pernicious anemia and for this work received a Nobel Prize in medicine along with pathologist George Whipple in 1934.

CHAPTER 2 · ANDRÉ COURNAND

1. For an excellent history of cardiac catheterization from 1844 to the present, see A. Cournand, Cardiac catheterization. Development of the technique, its contributions to experimental medicine, and its initial applications in man, *Acta Med Scand* 1975; suppl 579:1–32. For a broader account of early cardiac physiology, see The Heart, in Circulation of the Blood: Men and Ideas, ed. A. P. Fishman and D. W. Richards (New York: Oxford University Press, 1964), 1–351.

2. A. J. Benatt, Cardiac catheterization: A historical note, *Lancet* 1949; 1:746.

3. See Cournand, Cardiac catheterization, 24.

4. A.V.S. Lambert, F. B. Berry, A. Cournand, and D. W. Richards, Pulmonary and circulatory function before and after thoracoplasty, *J Thorac Surg* 1938; 7:302–325.

5. A. Cournand and H. A. Ranges, Catheterization of the right auricle in man, *Proc Soc Exp Biol & Med* 1941; 46:462–466. This article reported the findings in four patients. It was followed by a paper in 1942 dealing with thirteen patients (many of whom, as in the initial study, had cancer), which tried unsuccessfully to correlate catheterization outputs with the ballistocardiogram (A. Cournand et al., Comparison of the normal ballistocardiogram and a direct Fick method for measuring cardiac output in man, *J Clin Invest* 1942; 21:287–294). A later paper established normal values as determined in thirty-three cardiovascular normals: A. Cournand et al., Measurement of cardiac output in man using the technique of catheterization of the right auricle or ventricle, *J Clin Invest* 1945; 24:106–116.

CHAPTER 3 · MARY ALLEN ENGLE

1. M. E. Abbott, *Atlas of Congenital Heart Disease* (New York: American Heart Association, 1936).

2. R. E. Gross and J. P. Hubbard, Surgical ligation of a patent ductus arteriosus. Report of a first successful case, *JAMA* 1939; 112:729–731.

3. C. Crafoord and G. Nylin, Congenital coarctation of the aorta and its surgical treatment, *J Thorac Surg* 1945; 14:347–361.

4. A. Blalock and H. B. Taussig, The surgical treatment of malformations of the heart in which there is pulmonary stenosis or pulmonary atresia, *JAMA* 1945; 128:189–202.

5. S. E. Levy and A. Blalock, Experimental observations of the effects of connecting by suture the left main pulmonary artery to the systemic circulation, *J Thorac Surg* 1939; 8:525–530.

6. C. Ferencz, Reflections on her eighty-eight years in historical milestones. Helen Brooke Taussig: 1898–1986 (ed. D. G. McNamara), *J Am Coll Cardiol* 1987; 10:662–671. (This was one of a number of posthumous tributes to Dr. Taussig by fellows who trained under her, including Dr. Engle.)

7. H. B. Taussig, *Congenital Malformations of the Heart* (New York: Commonwealth Fund, 1947). A revised edition was published by Harvard University Press in 1960.

8. M. A. Engle, Ventricular septal defects in infancy, *Pediatrics* 1954; 14:16–27.

9. M. A. Engle, T.P.B. Payne, C. Bruins, and H. B. Taussig, Ebstein's Anomaly of the tricuspid valve. Report of three cases and analysis of clinical syndrome, *Circulation* 1950; 1:1246–1260.

CHAPTER 4 · RICHARD J. BING

1. R. J. Bing, ed., *Cardiology: The Evolution of the Science and the Art,* 2d ed. (New Brunswick, N.J.: Rutgers University Press, 1999).

2. Lindbergh's sister-in-law suffered from rheumatic heart disease (mitral stenosis), and Lindbergh became interested in the possibility of using a mechanical pump to circulate the blood so that surgery could be performed directly upon the diseased valve. This led to his meeting with ALEXIS CARREL at the Rockefeller Institute and their joint effort to develop such a pump. This subject is covered well in A. Scott Berg's biography of Lindbergh (New York: Berkley Books, 1998). See also R. J. Bing, Lindbergh and the biological sciences (A personal reminiscence), *Texas Heart Inst J* 1987; 14:68–74.

3. For Bing's recollections of Carrel, see R. J. Bing, Carrel. A personal reminiscence, *JAMA* 1983; 250:3297–3298. See also G. M. Lawrie,The scientific contributions of Alexis Carrel, *Clin Cardiol* 1987; 10:428–430.

4. Bing's publications on congenital heart disease include the first reported hemodynamic studies of some twenty different congenital heart defects. See D. G. McNamara, Contributions of Richard Bing to the field of congenital heart disease, *J Appl Cardiol* 1989; 4:351–356.

5. H. B. Taussig and R. J. Bing, Complete transposition of the aorta and a levo-position of the pulmonary artery, *Am Heart J* 1949; 37:551–559.

6. W. P. Longmire, Jr., *Alfred Blalock: His Life and Times* (n.p., 1991).

7. M. C. Sosman and L. Dexter, Venous catheterization of the heart, *Radiology* 1947; 48:441–462.

8. C. L. Evans and M. Matsuoka, The effect of various mechanical conditions on the gaseous metabolism and efficiency of the mammalian heart, *J Physiol* 1914; 49: 379–405.

9. S. S. Kety and C. F. Schmidt, The determination of cerebral blood flow in man by the use of nitrous oxide in low concentrations, *Am J Physiol* 1945; 143:53–66.

10. R. J. Bing, L. D. Vandam, F. Gregoire, J. C. Handelsman, W. T. Goodale, and J. E. Eckenhoff, Catheterization of the coronary sinus and the middle cardiac vein in man, *Proc Soc Exper Biol & Med* 1947; 66:239–240; and R. J. Bing, M. M. Hammond, J. C. Handelsman, S. R. Powers, F. C. Spencer, J. E. Eckenhoff, W. T. Goodale, J. H. Hafkenschiel, and S. S. Kety, The measurement of coronary blood flow, oxygen consumption, and efficiency of the left ventricle in man, *Am Heart J* 1949; 38:1–24.

11. R. J. Bing, Metabolism of the Heart, in *Harvey Lecture Series* (New York: Academic Press, 1954–55), 27–70.

CHAPTER 5 · CHARLES P. BAILEY

1. E. C. Cutler and S. A. Levine, Cardiotomy and valvotomy for mitral stenosis. Experimental observations and clinical notes concerning an operated case with recovery, *Boston Med & Surg J* 1923; 188:1023–1027.

2. H. S. Souttar, The surgical treatment of mitral stenosis, *Br Med J* 1925; 2:603–606.

3. Rheumatic fever, when it affects the heart, causes a pancarditis; that is, the heart muscle, valves, and pericardium are all involved. As the disease progresses over the years, the mechanical effects of valve dysfunction become paramount, emphasizing the need for valve surgery as it is practiced today. However, in the early part of the twentieth century, the two leading British cardiologists, SIR JAMES MACKENZIE and THOMAS LEWIS, whose influence was very great, both emphasized the myocardial effects of the disease rather than the valvular component in causing disability, heart failure, and death, thus discouraging any surgical approach to the problem. For an excellent discussion of this topic, see A. Hollman, *Sir Thomas Lewis* (Berlin: Springer-Verlag, 1977), 172–174.

4. Ludwig Rehn (1849–1930) opened the door to direct surgery upon the heart with his case report: Penetrating cardiac wounds and cardiac suture, *Arch Klin Chir* 1897; 55:315–329. This report stimulated other attempts, many of which, including his own, were summarized by Luther Hill (1862–1946) in: A report of a case of successful suturing of the heart and table of thirty-seven other cases of suturing by different operators with various terminations and conclusions drawn, *Med Rec* 1902; 62:846–848. Both articles are reproduced in *Classics of Cardiology*, vol 3, ed. J. A. Callahan, T. E. Keys, and J. D. Key (Malabar, Fla.: Krieger, 1983). Neither of these articles, however, had the immediate impact on the practice of surgery that DWIGHT E. HARKEN's report probably had when he successfully removed shell frag-

ments from the hearts of wounded soldiers in World War II: D. E. Harken, Foreign bodies in and in relation to the thoracic blood vessels and heart, *Surg Gyn Obst* 1946; 83: 117–125.

5. For years, THEODOR BILLROTH was probably criticized unjustly for including this dictum as part of his published teaching regarding cardiac surgery. Rudolph Nissen, a German surgeon who assisted the great ERNST SAUER-BRUCH in the preparation of the second volume (1925) of his book on thoracic surgery, was assigned by his chief to trace the source of this statement. Nissen tracked down a surviving assistant of Billroth's, a Dr. von Eiselberg, who recalled Billroth making this remark in passing but never publishing it (R. Nissen, Billroth and cardiac surgery [letter] *Lancet* 1963; 2:250–251). Searches by others to find this opinion in Billroth's papers and monographs have similarly failed to document this opposition to cardiac surgery as part of his official position on the subject.

6. C. P. Bailey, The surgical treatment of mitral stenosis (mitral commissurotomy), *Dis Chest* 1949; 15:377–397.

7. That this continues to be a problem has been documented in the Institute of Medicine report indicating that between 44,000 and 98,000 hospital deaths per year in the United States are due to errors: L. T. Kohn, J. M. Corrigan, and M. S. Donaldson, eds., *To Err Is Human: Building a Better and Safer Health Care System* (Washington D.C.: National Academy Press, 2000).

CHAPTER 6 • JOHN W. KIRKLIN

1. Although there had been earlier investigations involving the perfusion of isolated organs, the first acknowledged serious effort to provide clinically effective cardiopulmonary bypass (perfusion of the whole body by mechanical means to exclude the heart and lungs) was carried out by DR. JOHN H. GIBBON, JR., of Jefferson Medical College, whose efforts spanned a period of almost twenty years (1934–53) until his first success (J. H. Gibbon, Jr., Application of a mechanical heart and lung apparatus to cardiac surgery, *Minnesota Med* 1954; 37:171–180; and The development of the heart-lung apparatus, *Am J Surg* 1978; 135:608–619). After subsequent failures, Gibbon discontinued his efforts in the field, and the challenge to continue this work was taken up by the University of Minnesota and the Mayo Clinic.

2. The remarkable and long-lasting results of these forty-five operations were summarized years later by C. WALTON LILLEHEI: C. W. Lillehei, R. L. Varco, M. Cohen, H. E. Warden, C. Patton, and J. H. Moller, The first open-heart repairs of ventricular septal defect, atrioventricular communis, and Tetralogy of Fallot using extracorporeal circulation by cross-circulation. A thirty-year follow-up, *Ann Thorac Surg* 1986; 41:4–21.

3. R. A. DeWall, H. E. Warden, R. C. Read, V. L. Gott, N. R. Ziegler, R. L. Varco, and C. W. Lillehei, A simple, expendable, artificial oxygenator for open heart surgery, *Surg Clin NA* 1956; 36:1025–1034.

4. J. W. Kirklin, J. W. DuShane, R. T. Patrick, D. E. Donald, P. S. Hetzel, P. S. Harshbarger, and E. H. Wood, Intracardiac surgery with the aid of a mechanical pump-oxygenator system (Gibbon type): Report of eight cases, *Proc Staff Meet Mayo Clin* 1955; 30:201–206.

5. J. W. Kirklin and B. G. Barratt-Boyes, *Cardiac Surgery*, 2d ed. (New York: Churchill Livingstone, 1993).

6. Letter, Richard A. DeWall to A.B.W., April 11, 2000.

7. Notably, in his biography, *One Life*, CHRISTIAAN BARNARD, who, as a fellow at the University of Minnesota, visited other institutions, writes: "Kirklin never held back. Thanks to his knowledge, we changed catheters, suction systems, and he taught me how to close a ventricular septal defect without causing heart block" (204).

8. Kirklin et al., Intracardiac surgery with the aid of a mechanical pump-oxygenator system (Gibbon type): Report of eight cases.

9. British surgeons A. T. Andreason and F. Watson found that, in dogs, when the complete venous return to the right side of the heart was eliminated, with the exception of the flow from the azygos vein, viability could be maintained for a considerable time without any evidence of harm (Experimental cardiovascular surgery [the azygos factor], *Brit J Surg* 1952; 39:548–551). Lillehei's group confirmed this finding in the laboratory and then translated it into much lower flows with cardiopulmonary bypass in humans than had previously been thought safe. This modification avoided the flooding of the operative field that often occurred at higher flow rates on the heart-lung machine and was thought to be a great advantage by the University of Minnesota group. Obviously, Kirklin was skeptical about it and utilized higher flow rates. Today the question is moot. With the modern membrane oxygenators utilized universally, flows are started in the low normal range and then lowered with the induction of hypothermia and the associated reduction in body metabolism. Adjustments are then made during surgery according to individual variations in response.

10. Without detracting from Dr. Lillehei's accomplishments, it is interesting to note that, whereas he introduced electrical pacemaking for patients who developed complete heart block as a result of accidental destruction of the conduction pathway between atria and ventricles (bundle of His) in the repair of ventricular septal defects, Kirklin went to a knowledgeable pathologist, MAURICE LEV, to learn the exact anatomical position of this conduction bundle in patients so that he could avoid creating this problem in the first place during surgery.

11. Dr. Kirklin understates his contributions to many aspects of associated problems that arose as side effects of total cardiopulmonary bypass, as evidenced by the many publications from his group that address these problems and which are included in his bibliography.

12. Dr. DeWall: "Never, in the forty-eight years that I knew Walt, did I ever hear him discuss his income or even express an interest in his income. I know he

was very casual about his billing of patients." Dr. Lillehei performed many surgeries gratis. His healthy economic state later in life derived primarily from good stock investments made with his military income during World War II and, in part, from his position as a clinical director of the company making the St. Jude heart valves. This and other aspects of Dr. Lillehei's career and personality are well covered in a recent biography: G. Wayne Miller, *King of Hearts: The True Story of the Maverick Who Pioneered Open Heart Surgery* (New York: Times Books, 2000).

13. Perhaps, more precisely "difficult to *understand*" was what the flamboyant Lillehei represented to the straight-as-an-arrow Kirklin. DeWall: "I never found Walt difficult, even when I first met him and had nothing to offer. In my experience his office was always open to anyone who wanted to see him and talk, preferably about medicine and research." For further insights by several contemporaries about Lillehei, the man and surgeon, see C. Walton Lillehei surgical symposium, *J Thorac Cardiovasc Surg* 1989; 98:805–851.

14. This, no doubt, is true and, as suggested by DeWall, may have been related to his barely surviving a lymphosarcoma after extensive surgery as a young man. With the threat of recurrence hanging over Lillehei, DeWall writes, "I believe he was determined to live to the maximum degree both in his work and play regardless of the consequences." Also see Miller, *King of Hearts* for further details.

CHAPTER 7 · ARTHUR C. GUYTON

1. J. H. Comroe, Jr., and R. D. Dripps, Ben Franklin and open heart surgery, *Circ Res* 1974; 35:661–669.

2. The current edition: A. C. Guyton and J. E. Hall, *Textbook of Medical Physiology*, 10th ed. (Philadelphia: W. B. Saunders, 2000).

3. Warm Springs, Georgia, was the location of a hospital and poliomyelitis rehabilitation center started by another polio victim, Franklin D. Roosevelt, who purchased the property in 1926 after personally experiencing the soothing and revitalizing effects of the waters there. With the later introduction of effective polio vaccines and the marked decrease in the incidence of polio, the facility gradually became outmoded and was permanently closed in 1979.

4. Although other physiological forebears may have held their positions longer than Dr. Guyton, ERNEST H. STARLING was not one of them. He became professor of physiology at the University College, London, in 1899 and died in 1927 after having accepted another professorship, and falling far short of Guyton's tenure record.

5. Guyton's paper that appeared in this notable symposium was: Determination of cardiac output by equating venous return curves with cardiac response curves, *Physiol Rev* 1955; 35:123–129. Many consider his theory on venous return and cardiac performance his most important conceptual contribution.

6. C. Brinson and J. Quinn, *Arthur C. Guyton: His Life, His Family, His Achievements* (Jackson, Miss.: Oakdale Press, 1974).

7. G. Pickering, *Creative Malady* (New York: Oxford University Press, 1974).

CHAPTER 8 · ALBERT STARR

1. For a detailed account of the Starr-Edwards collaboration, see A. M. Matthews, The development of the Starr-Edwards heart valve, *Texas Heart Inst J* 1998; 25:282–293.

2. It should be noted that, at about the same time Starr was working on a caged-ball prosthesis in the mitral position, Dwight E. Harken was attempting to correct aortic regurgitation with a similarly designed valve (D. E. Harken, H. S. Soroff, W. J. Taylor, A. A. Lefemine, S. K. Gupta, and S. Lunzer, Partial and complete prostheses in aortic insufficiency, *J Thorac Cardiovasc Surg* 1960; 40:744–762). However, among the five patients in whom this procedure was attempted, there was only one survivor.

3. These results were published in the following paper: A. Starr and M. L. Edwards, Mitral replacement. Clinical experience with a ball-valve prosthesis, *Ann Surg* 1961; 154:726–740. The two deaths among the eight patients included the patient with the air embolis and one who died eleven days postoperatively from renal failure and a cerebrovascular accident.

4. A. Starr, The thoracic surgical industrial complex, *Ann Thorac Surg* 1986; 42:124–133.

5. An evaluation of the Starr-Edwards valve, after three decades of implantations, showed that it compared favorably to more recently introduced valve prostheses with a variety of designs. J. S. Swanson and A. Starr, The ball valve experience over three decades, *Ann Thorac Surg* 1989; 48:551–552.

CHAPTER 9 · PAUL M. ZOLL

1. For reviews, see P. M. Zoll, Historical development of cardiac pacemakers, *Progr Cardiovasc Dis* 1972; 14:421–429. See also W. B. Fye, Ventricular fibrillation and defibrillation: Historical perspectives with emphasis on the contributions of John MacWilliam, Carl Wiggers, and William Kouwenhoven, *Circulation* 1985; 71:858–865; and B. Lüderitz, *History of the Disorders of Cardiac Rhythm* (Armonk, N.Y.: Futura, 1995).

2. P. M. Zoll, Resuscitation of the heart in ventricular standstill by external electric stimulation, *N Engl J Med* 1952; 247:768–771.

3. J. L. Prevost and F. Battelli, Quelques effets des décharges électriques sur le coeur des mammifères, *J Physiol et de Path Gén* 1900; 2:40–52.

4. C. S. Beck, W. H. Pritchard, and H. S. Feil, Ventricular fibrillation of long duration abolished by electric shock, *JAMA* 1947; 135:985–986.

5. P. M. Zoll, A. J. Linenthal, W. Gibson, M. H. Paul, and L. R. Norman, Termination of ventricular fibrillation in man by externally applied electric countershock, *N Engl J Med* 1956; 254:727–732.

6. W. B. Kouwenhoven, J. R. Jude, and G. G. Knickerbocker, Closed-chest cardiac massage, *JAMA* 1960; 173:1064–1067.

7. D. E. Harken, Foreign bodies in and in relation to the thoracic blood vessels and heart, *Surg Gyn Obst* 1956; 83:117–125.

8. Beginning in 1940, at Beth Israel Hospital in Boston, Blumgart, using the postmortem injection technique developed by his colleague in pathology, Monroe J. Schlesinger, began a decade-long study of the coronary circulation in patients who had had manifestations of coronary disease during life. Among the still-valid findings in this series of reports was that collateral vessels develop following coronary artery occlusion.

9. A. S. Hyman, Resuscitation of the stopped heart by intracardiac therapy, *Arch Int Med* 1932; 50:283–305.

10. Beck, Pritchard, and Feil, Ventricular fibrillation of long duration abolished by electric shock.

11. Zoll, Resuscitation of the heart in ventricular standstill by external electric stimulation.

12. P. M. Zoll, A. J. Linenthal, W. Gibson, M. H. Paul, and L. R. Norman, Intravenous drug therapy in Stokes-Adams Disease, *Circulation* 1958; 17:325–339.

13. P. M. Zoll, H. A. Frank, L.R.N. Zarsky, A. J. Linenthal, and A. H. Belgard, Long-term electric stimulation of the heart for Stokes-Adams Disease, *Ann Surg* 1961; 154:330–346.

14. W. M. Chardack, A. A. Gage, and W. Greatbatch, A transistorized, self-contained, implantable pacemaker for the long-term correction of complete heart block, *Surgery* 1960; 48:643–654. (Although Chardack is frequently given credit for this innovation, Åke Senning actually mentions prior use in Sweden of an implantable pacemaker in his discussion of a presentation at a surgical meeting. See *J Thorac Cardiovasc Surg* 1959; 38:639. Senning's patient finally died at the age of eighty-six in 2001, outlasting twenty-six pacemakers as well as Senning, who died in 2000.)

15. S. Furman and J. B. Schwedel, An intracardiac pacemaker for Stokes-Adams seizures, *N Engl J Med*; 1959; 261:943–948.

16. P. M. Zoll, A. J. Linenthal, L. R. Norman, M. H. Paul, and W. Gibson, Treatment of unexpected cardiac arrest by external electric stimulation of the heart, *N Engl J Med* 1956; 254:541–546.

17. Kouwenhoven mentions this in his recounting of the development of the Hopkins version of the defibrillator: The development of the defibrillator, *Ann Int Med* 1969; 71:454.

18. B. Lown, R. Amarasingham, and J. Neuman, New method for terminating cardiac arrhythmias. Use of a synchronized capacitor discharge, *JAMA* 1962; 182:548–595. The controversy between Lown and Zoll regarding DC- or AC-powered devices did not involve patients in ventricular fibrillation but rather other patients with less serious arrhythmias who, Lown warned, could have their arrhythmias worsened by use of AC current. He based this

opinion on unpublished observations in dogs included in the aforementioned paper. Lown reported that in dogs initially in normal sinus rhythm, "ventricular fibrillation occurred in every 5 [AC] shocks." Zoll's position is reflected in his remarks contained in this conversation. However, the views of Lown ultimately prevailed, and the DC defibrillator is now the standard one employed.

19. H. W. Day, An intensive coronary care area, *Dis Chest* 1963; 44:423–427. Day was, no doubt, aware of an earlier article by Desmond Julian (Treatment of cardiac arrest in acute myocardial infarction, *Lancet* 1961;2:840–844), the first to advocate the use of a specialized coronary care unit for these patients. Shortly after the establishment of Day's unit, several other successful programs were initiated in the United States and elsewhere, leading to the general acceptance of this concept to salvage patients with cardiac arrest in acute myocardial infarction (H. W. Day, History of coronary care units, *Am J Cardiol* 1972; 30:405–407).

CHAPTER 10 · MICHAEL E. DEBAKEY

1. M. DeBakey, A simple continuous-flow blood transfusion instrument, *New Orleans Med & Surg J* 1934; 87:386–389.

2. Few discoveries or inventions are without precursors. It has been pointed out that the roller pump did not originate with DeBakey but with Porter and Bradley in 1885 (D. A. Cooley, Development of the roller pump for use in the cardiopulmonary bypass circuit, *Texas Heart Inst J* 1987; 14:113–118). However, DeBakey clearly acknowledges here the previous work on pumps that he found during his library search, and it was DeBakey, not Porter and Bradley, who suggested the applicability of the roller pump to John H. Gibbon, Jr., at a time when he was bogged down in making his heart-lung machine operable.

3. In a way, along with ALTON OCHSNER, RUDOLPH MATAS may have helped map out DeBakey's future professional course, given his own early report on the treatment of aneurysms (R. Matas, Traumatic aneurysm of the left brachial artery, *Medical News* Oct. 27, 1888; 53:462–466). RENÉ LERICHE, with whom DeBakey spent time in Strasbourg, was also interested in arterial disease and no doubt added to DeBakey's interest in such problems.

4. M. E. DeBakey, The National Library of Medicine. Evolution of a premier information center, *JAMA* 1991; 266:1252–1258.

5. For an excellent historical summary of these developments, with many major ones occurring during the fifties and sixties, see M. E. DeBakey, The development of vascular surgery, *Am J Surg* 1979; 139:697–738.

6. M. E. DeBakey, Successful carotid endarterectomy for cerebrovascular insufficiency. Nineteen-year follow-up, *JAMA* 1975; 233:1083–1085.

7. H. E. Garrett, E. W. Dennis, and M. E. DeBakey, Aortocoronary bypass with saphenous vein graft. Seven-year follow-up, *JAMA* 1973; 223:792–794.

8. D. C. Sabiston, Jr., The coronary circulation, *Johns Hopkins Med J* 1974; 134:314–329.

9. DeBakey's earlier experience with left ventricular bypass in patients unable to be weaned off the heart-lung machine appears in the following report: M. E. DeBakey, Left ventricular bypass pump for cardiac assistance, *Am J Cardiol* 1971; 27:3–11. His more recent development of a modern, compact device for even long-term support of the failing heart appears as: M. E. DeBakey, Development of a ventricular assist device, *Artificial Organs* 1997; 21:1149–1153.

10. The great schism that developed between DeBakey and his former protégé and collaborator, Denton Cooley, as a result of this controversy received a great deal of publicity at the time and remains fresh in the minds of those active in medicine and surgery during that period. One recounting of these events, including the professional surgical climate at Baylor during the sixties, appears in the journalist Thomas Thompson's book *Hearts* (New York: McCall, 1971), 211–217. Another appears in surgeon Stephen Westaby's book *Landmarks in Cardiac Surgery* (Oxford: Isis Medical Media, 1988), 282–285.

   There are two extreme views about Cooley regarding this episode: one holds that his action represented a daring, innovative, and humanitarian effort to save a dying patient's life and advance the status of heart surgery; the other view is that this was a reckless, illegal, and foolish attempt at self-aggrandizement. The truth, I suspect, lies somewhere in between.

11. M. E. DeBakey, Development of a ventricular assist device, *Artificial Organs* 1997; 21:1150.

12. The great German surgeon Ferdinand Sauerbruch (1875–1951) showed signs of what we would now call Alzheimer's disease late in life, but he insisted on continuing to perform surgery, with disastrous results. The story of his tragic deterioration is recounted by Jurgen Thorwald in his book *The Dismissal*.

CHAPTER 11 · RENÉ G. FAVALORO

1. J. B. Herrick, Clinical features of sudden obstruction of the coronary arteries, *JAMA* 1912; 59:2015–2020.

2. For a brief historical review of the surgical approaches to coronary heart disease, see Dr. Favaloro's book *Surgical Treatment of Coronary Arteriosclerosis* (Baltimore: Williams and Wilkins, 1970). Additional material on this subject is included at the end of his autobiography: *The Challenging Dream of Heart Surgery* (Boston: Little, Brown, 1994).

3. F. M. Sones and E. K. Shirey, Cine coronary arteriography, *Mod Concepts Cardiovasc Dis* 1962; 31:735–738.

4. A. Carrel, On the experimental surgery of the thoracic aorta and the heart, *Ann Surg* 1910; 52:83–95.

5. The first person who performed saphenous vein coronary bypass surgery in a patient was DAVID SABISTON at Johns Hopkins in 1962 (D. C. Sabiston, Jr., The coronary circulation, *Johns Hopkins Med J* 1974; 134:314–329). DeBakey's group did the same surgery in 1964 (H. E. Garrett, E. W. Dennis, and M. E. DeBakey, Aortocoronary bypass with saphenous vein graft. Seven-year follow-up, *JAMA* 1973; 223:792–794). The frequent problem of saphenous vein bypass occlusion after several months led to the use of the internal mammary arteries for this purpose, usually in conjunction with saphenous grafts. In this procedure, an internal mammary artery is detached from its normal course, running down the inner aspect of the sternum, and inserted beyond the obstruction in a diseased coronary artery. The internal mammaries have been shown to remain patent for many years. Experimental work on these mammaries was begun by Canadian surgeon Gordon Murray in the fifties. The first clinical application was performed by Robert Goetz in 1960 at the Bronx Municipal Hospital, although the case was not reported in the literature. Russian surgeon Vasily I. Kollessev published his results in multiple patients in 1966. However, it was GEORGE E. GREEN at New York University who became the major proponent and popularizer of this technique.

6. Dr. Favaloro's personal and professional history up to the time of his departure from the Cleveland Clinic in 1971 is covered in his autobiography, *The Challenging Dream of Heart Surgery.*

7. W. L. Proudfit, and E. K. Shirey, Selective cine coronary arteriography. Correlation with clinical findings in 1,000 patients, *Circulation* 1966; 33:901–910.

8. Sones and Shirey, Cine coronary arteriography.

9. See note 5.

10. R. G. Favaloro, Critical analysis of coronary bypass graft surgery: A 30-year journey, *J Am Coll Cardiol* 1998; 31 (suppl B): 1B–63B. (Contains 1,066 references.)

CHAPTER 12 · ADRIAN KANTROWITZ

1. A. Kantrowitz, A method of holding galea hemostats in craniotomies, *J Neurosurg* 1944; 1:392.

2. The surgery is described in: A. Kantrowitz and A. Kantrowitz, Experimental artificial left heart to permit surgical exposure of the mitral valve in cats, *Proc Soc Exp Biol & Med* 1950; 74:193–198. The filming of the mitral valve was reported in: A. Kantrowitz, E. S. Hurwitt, and A. Herskovitz, A cinematographic study of the function of the mitral valve in situ, *Surg Forum* 1952; 2:204–206.

3. A. Kantrowitz and A. Kantrowitz, Experimental augmentation of coronary flow by retardation of the arterial pressure pulse, *Surgery* 1953; 34:678–687.

4. Both these cases are described in: A. Kantrowitz, T. Akutsu, A. Chaptal, J. Krakauer, A. R. Kantrowitz, and R. T. Jones, A clinical experience with an implanted mechanical auxiliary ventricle, *JAMA* 1966; 197:97–101.

5. S. D. Moulopoulos, S. Topaz, and W. J. Kolff, Diastolic balloon pumping (with carbon dioxide) in the aorta—a mechanical assistance for the failing circulation, *Am Heart J* 1962; 63:669–675. "Counterpulsation," the term for this technique commonly employed later on, came from a study in dogs by Dwight Harken's group, using an external "mechanical ventricle": R. H. Clauss et al., Assisted circulation I. The arterial counterpulsator, *J Thorac Cardiovasc Surg* 1961; 41:447–458.

6. A. Kantrowitz, S. Tjønneland, P. S. Freed, S. J. Phillips, A. N. Butner, and J. L. Sherman, Initial clinical experience with intraaortic balloon pumping in cardiogenic shock, *JAMA* 1968; 203:113–118.

7. S. Scheidt, G. Wilner, H. Mueller, D. Summers, M. Lesch, G. Wolff, J. Krakauer, M. Rubenfire, P. Fleming, G. Noon, N. Oldham, T. Killip, and A. Kantrowitz, Intra-aortic balloon counterpulsation in cardiogenic shock. Report of a cooperative clinical trial, *N Engl J Med* 1973; 288:979–984.

8. A. Kantrowitz, Electronic physiologic aids, *Proc 3d IBM Med Symp* 1961, 549.

9. The events and controversies surrounding this period are reviewed by Dr. Kantrowitz in: A. Kantrowitz, America's first human heart transplantation. The concept, the planning, and the furor, *ASAIO J* 1998; 44:244–252.

10. In 1943 Isaac Starr at the University of Pennsylvania performed experiments in which over 75 percent of the right ventricle in dogs was cauterized, with no significant change in central venous or systemic pressures (I. Starr, W. A. Jeffers, and R. H. Meade, The absence of conspicuous increments in venous pressure after severe damage to the right ventricle of the dog, with a discussion of the relation between clinical congestive heart failure and heart disease, *Am Heart J* 1943; 26:291–301.

CHAPTER 13 • WILLEM J. KOLFF

1. For Dr. Kolff's reminiscences about his early years in Holland and the development of the artificial kidney, see A. B. Weisse, *Conversations in Medicine* (New York: New York University Press, 1984).

2. Published in November of 1998 was a very informative Festschrift in honor of Dr. Kolff, containing a number of tributes and reviews of his work by former associates and trainees: *Artificial Organs* 1998; 22:917–1001.

3. As Dr. Kolff points out, one difficulty involved the initially slow response of the surgeons in taking up open-heart surgery. However, his main problem in Cleveland concerned the differences in emphasis and outlook between him and Irvine Page about the future role of the artificial kidney, which Kolff championed and about which Page was not enthusiastic. (See Weisse, *Conversations in Medicine.*)

4. S. D. Moulopoulos, S. Topaz, and W. J. Kolff, Diastolic balloon pumping (with carbon dioxide) in the aorta—a mechanical assistance to the failing circulation, *Am Heart J* 1962; 63:669–675.

5. T. Akutsu and W. J. Kolff, Permanent substitute for valves and hearts, *Trans Am Soc Artif Intern Organs* 1958; 4:230–232.

6. W. C. DeVries, J. L. Anderson, L. D. Joyce, F. L. Anderson, E. H. Hammond, R. K. Jarvik, and W. J. Kolff, Clinical use of the total artificial heart, *N Engl J Med* 1984; 310:273–278.

7. W. J. Kolff, D. B. Effler, L. K. Groves, G. Peereboom, P. Moraca, S. Aoyama, and F. M. Sones, Disposable membrane oxygenator (heart-lung machine) and its use in experimental surgery and elective cardiac arrest in open-heart surgery, *Cleveland Clin Quart* 1956; 23:69–114.

8. Four cases, including Barney Clarke, are reported in: W. C. DeVries, The permanent artificial heart. Four cases, *JAMA* 1988; 259:849–859.

9. J. G. Copeland, Current status and future directions for a total artificial heart with a past, *Artificial Organs* 1998; 22:998–1001.

CHAPTER 14 · JEREMIAH STAMLER

1. This dismal period in America's political life is reflected in law professor Arthur Kinoy's book *Rights on Trial: The Odyssey of a People's Lawyer* (Cambridge, Mass: Harvard University Press, 1983). For his contribution to the successful defense of Stamler, see pp. 297–301.

2. This was a long-term prospective study in over three thousand men.

3. A. Keys, ed., Coronary heart disease in seven countries, *Circulation* 1970; 41 (suppl 4) 1–199. This five-year study of 12,770 men between the ages of forty and fifty-nine was conducted in Greece, the Netherlands, Yugoslavia, Italy, Japan, the United States, and Finland to determine the prevalence and incidence of coronary heart disease, with an emphasis on the varying diets observed. Prevalence (ECG evidence) was related to blood pressure and serum cholesterol. Highest rates were found in the United States, eastern Finland, and the Netherlands, and they appeared to be related to the high amounts of saturated fats in the diet and consequent high average levels of serum cholesterol.

4. A. Blakeslee and J. Stamler, *Your Heart Has Nine Lives* (Englewood Cliffs, N.J.: Prentice-Hall, 1963).

5. A. B. Weisse, P. D. Abiuso, and I. S. Thind, Acute myocardial infarction in Newark, NJ. A study of racial incidence, *Arch Int Med* 1977; 137:1402–1405.

6. In 1974, two San Francisco cardiologists, MEYER FRIEDMAN and Ray Rosenman, published *Type A Behavior and Your Heart,* in which they proposed that those with a Type A personality (aggressive, impatient, time-constrained) were much more likely to develop coronary heart disease that those at the other behavior extreme, the Type B personalities (relaxed, imperturbable, and easygoing). As he was developing this concept in the fifties and sixties, Friedman was, for a time, the attending physician to the author, who served as an intern at Mount Zion Hospital in 1958–59. Friedman, who appeared to the staff as a thoughtful, avuncular, pipe-smoking type, presented himself as a Type B until he had his own myocardial infarction, after which he reclassified himself as Type A. Nevertheless, he still lived to the age of ninety!

7. The initial findings of the Multiple Risk Factor Intervention Trial (MRFIT) did not demonstrate clear differences in the development of coronary heart disease between those with specific interventions and those who received ordinary medical care. It is believed that this result may have been related to the fact that many of those receiving ordinary care had also received adequate treatment for their hypertension, made changes in their diet, and stopped smoking. Therefore the differences between the two groups in major risk factors was much lower than expected, so that the trial was weak in statistical power for its primary end point, coronary mortality. This inference is supported by data from recent MRFIT analyses showing significant lower cardiac and cardiovascular rates for combined end points, such as are used in more recent trials (e.g., coronary death plus nonfatal myocardial infarction plus unstable angina, etc.). Moreover, as Dr. Stamler points out, other useful knowledge has been obtained as a result of initiating this trial.

8. J. Stamler, R. Stamler, J. D. Neaton, D. Wentwork, M. L. Daviglus, D. Garside, A. R. Dyer, K. Liu, and P. Greenland, Low risk-factor profile and long-term cardiovascular and noncardiovascular mortality and life expectancy, *JAMA* 1999; 282:2012–2018.

CHAPTER 15 • EUGENE BRAUNWALD

1. Dr. Braunwald's first nine years in Vienna, and his family's harrowing escape from the Nazis, are covered in: W. C. Roberts and E. Braunwald, A conversation with the editor, *Am J Cardiol* 1998; 82:93–108.

2. E. Braunwald, H. L. Moscovitz, S. S. Amram, R. B. Lasser, S. O. Sapin, A. Himmelstein, M. M. Ravitch, and A. J. Gordon, The hemodynamics of the left side of the heart as studied by simultaneous left atrial, left ventricular, and aortic pressures; particular reference to mitral stenosis, *Circulation* 1955; 12:69–81.

3. S. W. Patterson, H. Piper, and E. H. Starling, The regulation of the heart beat, *J Physiol* 1914; 48:465–513; and C. L. Evans and Y. Matsuoka, The effect of various mechanical conditions on the gaseous metabolism and efficiency of the mammalian heart, *J Physiol* 1915; 49:378–405.

4. S. J. Sarnoff and E. Berglund, Ventricular function I. Starling's law of the heart studied by means of simultaneous right and left ventricular function curves in the dog, *Circulation* 1954; 9:706–718.

5. A summary of previous work in this area plus his own appears in: E. Braunwald, Thirteenth Annual Bowditch Lecture. The determinants of myocardial oxygen consumption, *Physiologist* 1969; 12:65–93.

6. Evans and Matsuoka, The effect of various mechanical conditions on the gaseous metabolism and efficiency of the mammalian heart.

7. Gregg's monograph on the coronary circulation has become a classic (D. E. Gregg, *The Coronary Circulation in Health and Disease* [Philadelphia: Lea and Febiger, 1950]).

8. See chapter 6, "John W. Kirklin," and the reference cited in note 2 of that chapter.

9. S. A. Levine, *Clinical Heart Disease,* 5th ed. (Philadelphia: W. B. Saunders, 1958), 111–112.

10. A. G. Morrow and E. Braunwald, Functional aortic stenosis: A malformation characterized by resistance to left ventricular outflow without anatomic obstruction, *Circulation* 1959; 20:181–189.

11. E. Braunwald, C. T. Lambrew, S. D. Rockoff, J. R. Ross, Jr., G. E. Pierce, and A. G. Morrow, Idiopathic hypertrophic subaortic stenosis (analysis of 64 patients), *Circulation* 1964; 30 (suppl 4): 1–213.

12. A. B. Weisse, P. D. Abiuso, and I. S. Thind, Acute myocardial infarction in Newark, NJ. A study of racial incidence, *Arch Int Med* 1977; 137:1402–1405. It was once mistakenly believed that acute myocardial infarction was rare in blacks. When investigated in Newark, it was found that this disease is at least as common among blacks as among whites, and that many of the former were dying out-of-hospital before even reaching an emergency room. The situation in Newark was undoubtedly mirrored in Washington, D.C., and in other medically underserved black communities.

13. Based on their own early research in the field, Braunwald and Maroko authored an important editorial at a critical time to stimulate research in the protection of jeopardized but still viable heart muscle in acute myocardial infarction: E. Braunwald and P. R. Maroko, The reduction of infarct size—an idea whose time has come. *Circulation* 1974; 50:206–209.

CHAPTER 16 · J. WILLIS HURST

1. P. D. White, *Heart Disease* (New York: Macmillan, 1931). (The fourth and last edition of this work appeared in 1951.)

2. For a personal appreciation of Dr. White, see J. W. Hurst, Paul Dudley White. To know him better, *Am J Cardiol* 1985; 56:169–178.

3. E. S. Brannon, H. S. Weens, and J. V. Warren, Atrial septal defect: Study of hemodynamics by the technique of right heart catheterization, *Am J Med Sci* 1945; 210:480–491.

4. J. W. Hurst and J.C. Cain, *LBJ: To Know Him Better* (Austin: Lyndon Baines Johnson School of Public Health, 1995).

5. For a model of how a departmental history should be written, see J. W. Hurst, *The Quest for Excellence: The History of the Department of Medicine at Emory University School of Medicine (1834–1986)* (Atlanta: Scholars Press, 1997).

6. For a good assessment of Gruentzig, see J. W. Hurst, Tribute: Andreas Roland Gruentzig (1939–1985): A private perspective, *Circulation* 1986; 73:606–610.

7. J. W. Hurst and R. B. Logue, eds., *The Heart* (New York: McGraw-Hill, 1966).

8. R. P. Grant, *Clinical Electrocardiograpy: The Spatial Vector Approach* (New York: McGraw-Hill, 1957).

9. Dr. Hurst has published many articles and several books on electrocardiography. Included among the latter are: J. W. Hurst and G. C. Woodson, Jr., *An Atlas of Spatial Vector Electrocardiography* (New York: Blakiston, 1952); J. W. Hurst and R. J. Myerburg, *Introduction to Electrocardiography,* 2d ed. (New York: McGraw-Hill, 1973); and J. W. Hurst, *Ventricular Electrocardiography* (New York: Gower Medical Publishing, 1991).

CHAPTER 17 · THE TWENTY-FIRST CENTURY

1. M. C. Morice, RAVEL results: Sirolimus-coated stent may usher in "a new era," *Heartwire News,* Sept. 4, 2001.

2. M. F. Newman, J. L. Kirchner, B. Phillips-Bute, V. Gover, H. Grocott, R. H. Jones, D. B. Mark, J. G. Reves, and J. A. Blumenthal, Longitudinal assessment of neurocognitive function after coronary-artery bypass surgery, *N Engl J Med* 2001; 344: 395-402.

3. E. A. Rose, A. C. Gelijns, A. J. Moscowitz, D. F. Hertzan, L. W. Stevenson, W. Dembitsky, J. W. Long, D. D. Ascheim, A. R. Tierney, R. G. Levitan, J. T. Watson, and P. Meier, Long-term use of a left ventricular assist device for end-stage heart failure, *N Engl J Med* 2001; 345: 1435-1443.

4. S. B. Freedman and J. M. Isner, Therapeutic angiogenesis for coronary artery disease, *Ann Int Med* 2002; 136:54-71.

5. A. P. Beltrami, K. Urbanek, J. Kajstura, S. Yan, N. Finato, R. Bussani, B. Nadal-Ginard, F. Silvestri, A. Leri, C. A. Beltrami, and P. Anversa, Evidence that human cardiac myocytes divide after myocardial infarction, *N Engl J Med* 2001; 344:1750-1757.

6. F. Quaini, K. Urbanek, A. P. Beltrami, N. Finato, C. A. Beltrami, B. Nadal-Ginard, J. Kajstura, A. Leri, and P. Anversa, Chimerism of the transplanted heart, *N Engl J Med* 2002; 346: 5-15.

7. M. S. Gottleib, The future of an epidemic, *New York Times,* June 5, 2001.

SELECTED BIBLIOGRAPHY

Acierno, L. J. *The History of Cardiology.* New York: Parthenon Publishing, 1994.

> Probably the most comprehensive current history in English. Although it falters a bit on medical therapy and the latter part of the twentieth century, the rest of the long history of cardiology is masterfully done in fine style, with over 4,200 references.

Bing, R. J. *Cardiology: The Evolution of the Science and the Art.* 2d ed. New Brunswick, N.J.: Rutgers University Press, 1999.

> Another solid history, infused with Bing's wisdom and wit.

Classics in Cardiology. Vols. 1 and 2, ed. F. A. Willius and T. E. Keys. Vols. 3 and 4, ed. J. A. Callahan, D. C. McGoon, and J. D. Key. Malabar, Fla.: Robert E. Krieger, 1983–89.

> A four-volume series, which contains reprints of classic articles about cardiology, with English translations provided when necessary.

Comroe, J. H. *Retrospectroscope: Insights into Medical Discovery.* Menlo Park, Calif.: Von Gehr Press, 1977.

> An entertaining and eye-opening collection of essays on how, why, and where research is done.

Fishman, A. P., and D. W. Richards, eds. *Circulation of the Blood: Men and Ideas.* New York: Oxford University Press, 1964.

> A classic collection of historical essays on many aspects of the circulation.

Fye, W. B. *American Cardiology: The History of a Specialty and Its College.* Baltimore: Johns Hopkins University Press, 1996.

> A comprehensive and well-documented account of the individuals, programs, and institutions that led to the preeminence of twentieth-century American cardiology.

Lüderitz, B. *History of the Disorders of Cardiac Rhythm.* Armonk, N.Y.: Futura Publishing, 1995.

A short but beautifully illustrated and well-written account.

Opportunities for Medical Research in the Twenty-first Century. JAMA 2001; 285(5).

A special issue devoted to this subject.

Silverman, M. E., P. R. Fleming, et al., eds. *British Cardiology in the Twentieth Century.* London: Springer-Verlag, 2000.

The view from Great Britain.

Westaby, S. *Landmarks in Cardiac Surgery.* Oxford: Isis Medical Media, 1997.

A handsome but exasperating book in search of an editor. Despite the many typographical errors and misspellings, it is valuable for its presentation of a surgeon's viewpoint, many excellent photographs, and the inclusion of details on a number of important surgeons that may not be found elsewhere.

Name Index

Pages in boldface refer to interviews or entries in the Biographical Notes.

Subject Index

acquired immunodeficiency syndrome (AIDS), 199

AICD, *see* automatic implantable cardioverter-defibrillator

AMI, *see* myocardial infarction, acute

angioplasty, coronary, *see* percutaneous transluminal coronary angioplasty (PTCA)

aortic aneurysms, surgery for, 188–192

aortic dissection, *see* aortic aneurysms

aortic valve surgery, 148; for aortic regurgitation, 139; for aortic stenosis, 148–149

artificial kidney, 251, 258, 260, 270, 397n1

atherosclerosis: distribution of, 201; experimental, 275, 278, 281–283, 286

automatic implantable cardioverter-defibrillator (AICD), 157

azygos vein factor, 98–99, 390n9

ballistocardiography, 15, 385n2

Batista operation, 199, 238

Baylor College of Medicine, 178, 197

Bellevue Hospital (New York), 5, 30, 33–37, 61–63, 302, 305–306

Beth Israel Hospital (Boston) 155, 158–171, 318, 322–323

Blalock-Taussig procedure, 41

blue baby operation, *see* Blalock-Taussig procedure

bubble oxygenator, 94

bundle of His, 99, 154

CABG (coronary artery bypass graft), *see* coronary artery surgery

cardiac arrest, resuscitation for, 156, 393n6

cardiac care units, 169, 172, 394n19

cardiac catheterization, 28–30, 32–36, 65–67, 303–304, 386nn1, 5

cardiac output: by Fick principle, 34; regulation of, 125–126, 391n5

cardiac surgery, *see* surgery, cardiac

cardiac transplantation, 221–222, 238–239

cardiomyoplasty, 151

cardiopulmonary bypass, *see* heart-lung machine; surgery, cardiac

cardioversion, 156, 393–394n18. *See also* ventricular fibrillation

Carlsberg Institute, 59–60

Case Western Reserve School of Medicine, 229

Chicago People's Gas Study, 291

cholesterol: as coronary risk factor (*see* coronary heart disease); experimental studies involving, 277, 281–283

Cleveland Clinic, 208–211, 214–216, 250–254, 261–262

coarctation of the aorta, 40*fig.*; surgery for, 41

Columbia-Presbyterian Medical Center (New York), 31, 61, 63, 135–136

congenital heart disease, 39, 54–55; surgery for (*see* Blalock-Taussig procedure; cross-circulation surgery; *specific entities*)

Cornell Medical School, *see* New York Hospital–Cornell

About the Author

Dr. Allen B. Weisse has been on the New Jersey medical scene since 1963, when he joined the faculty of Seton Hall College of Medicine (now called the New Jersey Medical School). He has remained in New Jersey with that institution for over thirty years, actively engaged in teaching, patient care, medical research, and community service.

He is the author of *Medicine: State of the Art* (Dial, 1984), the award-winning *Conversations in Medicine* (NYU Press, 1984), *Medical Odysseys: The Different and Sometimes Unexpected Pathways to Twentieth-Century Medical Discoveries* (Rutgers University Press, 1991), and *The Staff and the Serpent: Pertinent and Impertinent Observations on the World of Medicine* (Southern Illinois University Press, 1998). He has been a frequent contributor to *Hospital Practice* and *Perspectives in Biology and Medicine*.

Recent past-president of the Medical History Society of New Jersey and a member of the American Association for the History of Medicine and the American Osler Society, he lectures frequently throughout the United States on a variety of subjects related to medical history and ethics as well as cardiovascular disease. In 1997, in order to devote himself more fully to his writing and historical interests, he resigned his full-time position as professor of medicine at the New Jersey Medical School, although he remains on the faculty as a clinical professor, stimulating new generations of students and house officers to explore the past and move knowledgeably into the future of American medicine.